Science
and Football
II

Other Titles Available From E & FN Spon

Intermittent High Intensity Exercise
Edited by D. MacLeod

Foods, Nutrition and Sports Performance
Edited by C. Williams and J.T. Devlin

Biomechanics and Medicine in Swimming
Edited by D. MacLaren, T. Reilly
and A. Lees

Science and Football
Edited by T. Reilly, K. Davids, W.J. Murphy
and A. Lees

Physiology of Sports
Edited by T. Reilly, N. Secher, P. Snell
and C. Williams

Kinanthropometry IV
Edited by W. Duquet and J.A.P. Day

Sport and Physical Activity
Edited by T. Williams and L. Almond

Effective Writing
Improving scientific, technical and business communication
Second edition
C. Turk and J. Kirkman

Science and Football II

Edited by

T. Reilly
J. Clarys
and
A. Stibbe

Proceedings of the
Second World Congress of
Science and Football
Eindhoven, Netherlands
22nd–25th May 1991

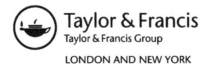

Taylor & Francis
Taylor & Francis Group

LONDON AND NEW YORK

First Published by Taylor & Francis in 1993

Reprinted 2001
by Taylor & Francis
2 Park Square, Milton Park,
Abingdon, Oxon, OX14 4RN

711 Third Avenue,
New York,
NY 10017

Taylor & Francis is an imprint of the Taylor & Francis Group

First issued in paperback 2011

A Catalogue record for this book is available from the British Library

Library of Congress Cataloging-in-Publication Data available

ISBN13: 978-0-419-17850-7 (hbk)
ISBN13: 978-0-415-51193-3 (pbk)

Second World Congress of Science and Football
Eindhoven, 22–25 May 1991

Contents

xiii

Preface

The Second World Congress of Science and Football was held at Eindhoven, May 22–25, 1991, at the magnificent Veldhoven Congress site.
This event followed the inaugural Congress at Liverpool in 1987 set up
under the initiative of the World Commission of Sports Biomechanics. In
both instances the Congress was supported by the governing bodies of
the various football codes – American, Australian Rules and Gaelic
football, Rugby League and Union and Association football (soccer).

The Second Congress was organized under the auspices of the Medical
Staff of PSV Eindhoven – and the Departments of Surgery at the
University Hospital Maastricht, St Lucas Hospital Amsterdam, the
Department of Orthopaedic Surgery of the Academic Medical Centre
Amsterdam and St Anna's Hospital Geldrop.

The organizers of this Congress were fortunate to have generous
sponsorship from Philips, Eindhoven. Delegates had the opportunity to
experience the training facilities of its club, P.S.V. Eindhoven, where the
demonstration game of Gaelic football and the delegates' own soccer
match were held. The club also hosted the workshop on isokinetic
training and the sumptuous banquet at its fabled stadium. The en-
thusiastic involvement of the club's management (Bobby Robson),
medical (C. van den Hoogenband) and support staff in the formal
programme of the Congress contributed much to its enjoyment.

The philosophy underpinning this Congress is to bring together, every
four years, those scientists whose research is directly related to football
and practitioners of football interested in obtaining current information
about its scientific aspects. In this way an attempt is made to bridge the
gap between research and practice so that scientific knowledge about
football can be communicated and applied. The Congress themes are
related to all the football codes and the common threads among these are
teased out in the formal presentations, workshops and seminars of the
Congress programme.

Patrons of the Congress included the International Council of Sport
Science and Physical Education, the International Society of Biomechanics
and the World Commission of Sports Biomechanics. A particularly strong
'football medicine' component of this Congress was due to the supportive
involvement of the European Association of Football Team Physicians.

Whilst the primary focus of this section of the Congress was on soccer, the work-shops and practical demonstrations concerned with treatment, rehabilitation and prevention were relevant to all the football codes.

Overall the Congress programme included 164 oral presentations, 90 posters, 9 instructional courses and various workshops. The chairperson of the Scientific Committee, Professor Jan Clarys, planned the scheduling of the programme with an attention to detail that was admirable. The awesome task of regulating this programme on-site was adroitly executed by Otto Stibbe. The Organizing Committee under the guidance of Professor Co Greep deserves credit for its work whilst the Organizing Secretariat provided the administrative drive to the well-oiled organization machine.

This record of events of the Congress might not have been documented without the backing of a consortium of academic institutions. These included the University Hospital Maastricht, the Academic Medical Centre at the University of Amsterdam, Vrije Universiteit Brussels and the Liverpool Polytechnic (now Liverpool John Moores University). In particular we thank Professor Rene Marti and Professor Co Greep whose financial support is gratefully acknowledged.

Delegates from all over the world attended the Congress, ranging from Albania to Zambia. For four days football was the focus of every conversation. It will be once again when the Congress convenes for the third time in 1995.

Thomas Reilly, May 1992
Chair, Steering Group on Football of the
World Commission of Sport Biomechanics
(a service group of the International
Council for Sport Science and Physical
Education and the International Society
of Biomechanics)

Introduction

The football games are intrinsically attractive to millions of people worldwide. Watching or playing provide untold enjoyment to those attending or participating in play. Events such as the World Cup excite human emotions and curiosities in a manner that almost defies reason. Approaching and analysing football phenomena in an objective manner pose no mean challenge to both professionals in the football business and to sports science researchers. The proceedings of Science and Football II, the Second World Congress of Science and Football held at Eindhoven in the Netherlands, provide a record of selected research reports related to the football games.

The Proceedings give an indication of current work utilizing scientific approaches towards furthering understanding of factors impinging on football. Included in this volume is less than one-third of the contributions to the Congress programme. The onus on contributors to provide camera ready copy of manuscripts to the editors may have deterred some from preparing their reports. Others failed to satisfy the quality control standard of the peer review process to which all submissions were subjected. The 84 papers selected for publication provide a good balance of topics and are representative of the content of the Congress programme.

The book is divided into eleven Parts, each containing a group of related papers. This is three less than in the Proceedings of the First World Congress on Science and Football. As far as possible we tried to retain the titles of Parts contained in the previous volume but have combined topics in some instances e.g. management and coaching, biomechanics of skills and equipment. Inevitably there are papers that could rest easily in one of two Parts and we trust the location allotted to these papers is not incongruous. There is a more substantial 'football medicine' part in this volume compared to its predecessor and there is a new section devoted to youth in football.

A number of people deserve thanks for enabling us to realize this publication. We are grateful to the contributors for their painstaking preparations of manuscripts in conformity with the publisher's guidelines. The input of referees of the papers was much appreciated. We thank Anne, May, Mary, Sue, Sue and Val (at Liverpool Polytechnic) for re-typing some manuscripts. The wizardry of Adam Coldwells in executing corrections to the computer discs provided by some authors helped to speed up the preparation of the book.

Finally, we acknowledge the support of the consortium of institutions - University Hospital Maastricht, Academic Medical Centre of the University of Amsterdam, the Free University of Brussels and Liverpool Polytechnic (now Liverpool John Moores University) – who made the production of this book possible.

T. Reilly
J. Clarys
A. Stibbe

PART ONE

Science and Football: Opening Address

SCIENCE AND FOOTBALL : AN INTRODUCTION

T. REILLY
Centre for Sport and Exercise Sciences, The Liverpool Polytechnic,
Liverpool, England.

1 Introduction

This overview of science and football provides an opportunity of
articulating the philosophy of the Congress of Science and Football,
and of forging a link between the First World Congress at Liverpool
in 1987 and the present event. It presents also a personal perspective of achievements so far in research applied to football in its
various codes. The Congress is geared towards representatives of all
the football codes - American, Australian Rules, Gaelic, Rugby League
and Union, and soccer. Indeed the inaugural Congress at Liverpool
in 1987 was the occasion when formal representatives from all the
football codes came together for the very first time.

The audience at such a meeting is inevitably varied in background.
The sprinkling of academics and practitioners includes scientists,
statisticians, teachers, medical, paramedical and engineering
expertise on the one hand and managers, coaches, trainers, players,
game officials and supporters on the other. A major objective is to
effect a bridge between theorists and practitioners so that there is
dialogue and debate between them.

This formula for cross-fertilisation is endorsed by the International Council for Sport, Science and Physical Education and also
the World Commission of Sports Biomechanics. Their programme of
scientific conferences allied to specific sports started with
swimming and its inaugural meeting in Brussels in 1970. Meetings are
held every four years, the sixth symposium for biomechanics and
medicine in swimming having been held at Liverpool in 1990. The most
recent addition to the calendar was the First World Scientific
Conference of Golf, held prior to the 1990 British Open at St.
Andrews. In the normal schedule of events the Third World Congress
of Science and Football will take place in 1995.

Football, in one or other of its forms, is unique in its universal
appeal. It can give national identity an expression for both
developing countries, such as Cameroun in its 1990 World Cup
performances, and space-age nations. It reflects also common themes
and origins among the football games, rugby as legend has it having
sprung from a foul play in soccer and then developing into separate
codes and Australian Rules evolving from the version of Gaelic
football imported by Irish immigrants. Many skills and tactics are
common to two or more of the football codes and there are many
instances of top players switching to alternative football codes
without undue difficulty.

3

Before proceeding to a scientific description of football, I wish to underline the important role that football has in contemporary culture. I can do so by referring to observations at a qualifying match for the 1970 World Cup for soccer between Nigeria and Cameroun. The game was held in Douala in ambient temperatures exceeding 30°C. At this time the Biafran War was still unresolved whilst civil disturbances were being crushed in the countries neighbouring on Cameroun. Yet life according to the conventions of competitive soccer went on; these have a logic which sometimes supercedes analysis.

2 Behaviour Analysis

The first hallmark of science is rigorous observation. This provides data which allow description of events in progress and ultimately some inferences that afford insight into the events being observed. This process is illustrated by some of our early observations on professional soccer on Merseyside.

Soccer practitioners are mainly concerned with performance. A scientific approach towards analysing the game can employ an ergonomics perspective as a broad thrust. This can operate on a number of fronts by studying:-

   i) work-rate during matches;
  ii) severity of training;
 iii) fitness of players;
  iv) psychological stress;
   v) physical stress and injuries;
  vi) daily energy expenditure

In this paper consideration is restricted to the performance aspects and the physiological investigations. The detailed findings have been reported elsewhere (Reilly, 1979; Reilly, 1986; Reilly, 1990).

In one of the first applications of motion analysis to professional soccer, the premise was that work-rate could be expressed in gross terms as total distance covered in a game, since this determines the energy expenditure. Obtaining work-rate profiles required careful observations of specific activities of individual players throughout a complete game. Co-operation with the club groundsman was necessary to devise a grid of the pitch in 1 m bands and visual cues both on the pitch and alongside the sideline were used. The method of coding the type and intensity of behaviour onto a tape-recorder from a vantage point overlooking the half-way line was cross-checked using film analysis and stride characteristics of players. The work-rate profiles indicated the nature of game demands, implicated fitness requirements for play and generated the reference data for devising training programmes.

The main categories of activity were classed as jogging, cruising, sprinting, walking and moving backwards. On average there is a change in intensity every 6 s, a burst of effort every 30 s and an all-out sprint every 90 s. The overall distance covered, including that by the goalkeeper, is about 9 km, most of the activity being sub-maximal and aerobic. The distance covered in possession of the ball is about 2% of the total. So, put another way, if you merely

activity
classes

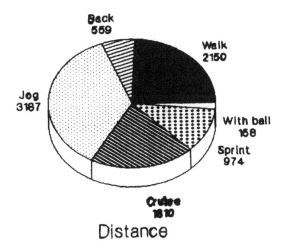

Fig.1. Distance covered (m) for classes of activity in soccer.

watch the ball you miss 98% of the activity! This is evident on inspection of pie diagrams of the breakdown (Figure 1). Of course superimposed on this profile are the frequent accelerations, decelerations, angled runs, moving backwards and game-related actions such as jumping and tackling that add to the demands of match-play.

Average values may disguise differences between playing positions. In soccer, for example, the greatest distance is covered by midfield players, the least among outfield players by the centre-backs. The positional role may be reflected also in discrete activities e.g. the greater call on midfielders and strikers to sprint. Overall the game is essentially aerobic, as evidenced by the cruising and jogging profiles of players, the highest work-rate being associated with the highest $\dot{V}O_2$max. The specificity of demands on the defenders who spend a lot of time back-pedalling is noted. Similar profiles of other games can be built up so that appropriate training programmes can be formulated. Gaelic football, for example, is played on a pitch 40% longer than soccer or rugby but has 15 a-side. The profile of activity is very similar to soccer when one player is followed. Game-related activity accounts for 1.3% of the total work and in the main players are exercising submaximally with occasional sprints mostly "off the ball" (Figure 2).

Indeed when we look at the work-level in distance covered per minute, Australian Rules and soccer are the most demanding, Rugby Union and American Football the least (Figure 3). This is reflected in the values at top level of $\dot{V}O_2$max which show the games players

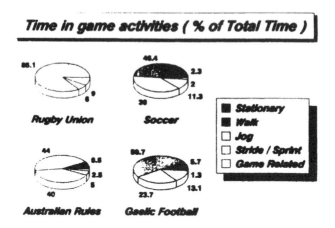

Fig. 2. Relative time spent in various categories of activity in four football codes.

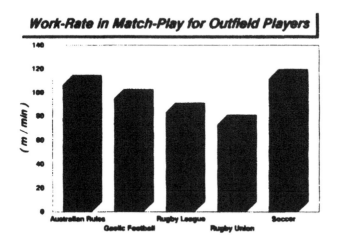

Fig. 3. Work-rate in match-play for the various football codes.

6

that are highest in $\dot{V}O_2$max. It is offset by the strength and muscle
power needed for American football and Rugby League in particular
(Figure 4).

The distance covered in various activities underlines this. Much
of the striding and sprinting in Rugby Union, for example, is to
support the player on the ball.

Time in activity categories related to total time shows that
except for game-related activities the profiles for soccer,
Australian Rules, Gaelic football and Rugby Union are comparable -
mostly low-level aerobic exercise. The high game-related activity in
Rugby is dictated by the time spent in scrummaging, an activity that
is the subject of biomechanical and medical considerations.

Of course there are extreme anaerobic demands on all games,
whether these are the jumping and timing skills of Australian Rules
players or the sprints of the Rugby and American football games.
These show that the activities in the game cannnot be directly extra-
polated from isolated running. An example is seen in dribbling,
which it is possible to simulate in laboratory conditions. The
protocol required a player to dribble on the treadmill, with the ball
being returned to him via a rebound box at a rate compatible with
what is done in the game (Reilly and Ball, 1984).

The data showed that there is a linear increment in both oxygen
consumption and blood lactate at each speed of dribbling. One of the
implications is of course that it might be best for players to train
with the ball. One of the contributing factors to the added energy
cost is the change in stride rate, the best dribblers using the
change in stride rate to deceive opponents.

Additional physiological costs are also evident when players move
backwards or sideways. This is reflected both in oxygen consumption
and perception of effort (Reilly and Bowen, 1984). It suggests also
that these features need to be built into the training programme.

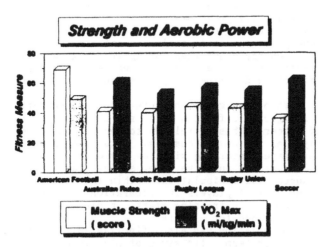

Fig. 4. Typical values of muscle strength (arbitrary scores based
          on strength data reported in the literature) and $\dot{V}O_2$max of
          players at high levels of competition in the various
          football codes.

3 Training

It was possible to look at the training programme of First Division
players using long-range radio telemetry (Reilly and Thomas, 1979).
During training the elements may be classified into warm-up,
calisthenics, fitness (weight-training or running), skills, drills,
games; the programme started with warm-up and flexibility work, and
fitness work. Most emphasis was placed on games either short-sided
or full-sided simulations of match-play. The latter has allowed us
to compare work-rate and heart rates during real play and calculate
energy expenditure levels.

The heart rate data indicate that players work hardest during
their games. When figures include goalkeepers, the average heart
rate is 157 beats/min : otherwise the values are about 160 beats/min.
It was estimated that on average outfield players operate at 75-80%
$\dot{V}O_2$max, which is comparable with high standard marathon running. The
calculation is achieved by obtaining HR-$\dot{V}O_2$max regression lines in
the laboratory and both HR and work-rate in friendly matches.

It is common practice for coaches to use performance tests during
training to monitor fitness. The argument is that they are more
user-friendly than laboratory tests such as $\dot{V}O_2$max. Such tests tend
to have poor reliability with professional players. This gets worse
the longer the duration of the test. Players want to show
improvement when it is important and so underperform on the first
test.

4 Habitual Activity

The training of footballers is varied sensibly from day to day,
showing a cycle of energy expenditure during the week. The mid-week
peak is followed by a lowering in preparation for mid-week
competition. This preparation is enhanced if the training is
supplemented by a dietary programme.

Reilly and Thomas (1979) examined how professional players do
expend their energy once outside their occupational context. They
spend very little energy other than during training and playing.
Most of their activity is sedentary or lying resting and so it
appears justifiable to describe the professional footballer as "homo
recumbans".

The highest rate of energy expenditure is during competition and
this leads to fatigue as reflected in a drop in work-rate in the
second half of soccer. This is related to reduced energy stores in
the form of glycogen in the leg muscles. Data from Saltin (1973)
have shown that players starting with low glycogen level in their
muscles cover less ground and have fewer sprints late in the game.

One of our successful manipulations within the English League has
been to alter the diet of players in preparation for competition.
Thus, once the tapering in training starts, a diet high in carbohydrate (CHO) is provided for players.

This kind of manipulation was also effective in the World Cup as
evidenced by the Irish team. Its style of play is extremely
demanding in terms of work-rate, since opponents are not allowed to
build up moves from the defence. The players faded towards the end
of their game against the Netherlands in 1988 in the European Nations
finals, but this was not so in Italy in 1990 when players had a
suitable diet rich in CHO and adequate time to restore glycogen
stores between matches.

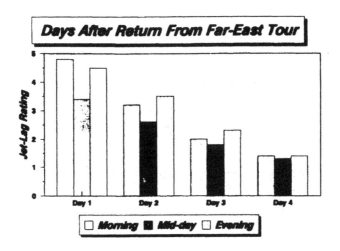

Fig. 5. Mean jet-lag ratings (scale 0 to 10) of soccer players for 4
days after returning to England from Japan. Values were
zero on Day 5.

One of the other successes in applying science to football has
been with teams travelling abroad – e.g. Rugby League international
teams and Rugby Union clubs going to New Zealand and to North
America. With such trips players' performances are affected by
jet-lag. The most notable examples were the English soccer clubs
competing in Japan and coming home to play important matches within 5
days.   In one experimental case players of an English League First
Division team came off the plane at Manchester on Sunday morning and
went straight to the training ground to use exercise to help re-tune
their biological clocks. The reduction in jet-lag rating showed they
were practically clear within 4 days of returning home (Figure 5).
This compares to control conditions with the same phase shift where
jet-lag is experienced at some time of day for about 10 days. After
the trip the team may not have won but at least they weren't jet-
lagged.

5 Notation Analysis

Teams are judged on their ability to score – a goal, a try or touch-
down or whatever. Consequently much has been written about how goals
are scored. This has led to a different type of analysis of play,
largely for tactical purposes. A computer overlay is used for the
computerised notation analysis system of Hughes (1988), modelled on
the playing pitch. The 128 cells are programmed so that with each
move the position on the field, the player involved, and the action

9

and its outcome are all recorded. This allows patterns of play to be discerned and this type of analysis is a powerful tool for the coach. A task for the future is to align this technqiue with work-rate analysis so that a more complete analysis of play is obtained.

Notation analysis is also useful in identifying precursors of injury such as errors. This starts a chain of events leading to an accident, sometimes causing injury. An example was the mistimed tackle of Tottenham's Paul Gascoigne in the 1991 F.A. Cup Final, which placed one of the world's most expensive players on the sidelines for the next year. Sports medicine personnel will also be keen to exploit modern technology for monitoring fitness of players recovering from injury, or of using fitness data as a basis for intervention training.

6 Overview

Only a sample of topics that come under the umbrella of Science and Football has been touched upon in this presentation. Biomechanics and sports medicine personnel will wish to know more about the equipment, particularly boots and surfaces, which might cause injury as well as about behaviour within the game. Psychologists, coaches and managers will want to understand more about stress and how to relieve it. The sociologists and administrators will wish to remind us that we are dealing with group dynamics and crowd behaviour, often unpredictable. The teachers and coaches, of whatever code, will seek to find out and discuss the best methods of nurturing footballing talent. There is a thirst for knowledge reflected in various ways. There are further Conferences of Football following this present one:-

i) The FIFA Congress in Brugge in October, 1991;

ii) the Rugby World Cup Conference on the Biology of Intermittent Activity preceding the Rugby World Cup semi-finals in Edinburgh in October, 1991.

iii) The Third World Congress of Science and Football in 1995.

There is now good reference material on Science and Football - e.g. the Proceedings of the First World Congress (Reilly et al., 1988). Coaching magazines, such as that of the Gaelic Athletics Association, have more scientific articles in their content. The European Society of Team Physicians in Football has its own publication (called Science and Football) and the First Diploma in Science and Football, which is a one-year course at Liverpool Polytechnic, started in September 1991.

Despite this emphasis on science, it must be recognised that football is an art represented by the craft of Cruyff, the guile of Maradona, the genius of David Campese, Ellery Hanley and artists in the other football codes. At top level there are few compromises, as shown by the man-handling of the games' top players. There is plenty to question and debate. Practitioners can seek help from the scientists without loss of security. The researchers thus consulted must come up with good solid answers, or else they let down their disciplines.

7 References

Hughes, M. (1988) Computerised notation analysis in field games. Ergonomics, 31, 1585-1592.

Reilly, T. (1979) What Research Tells the Coach about Soccer, AAHPERD, Washington.

Reilly, T. (1986) Fundamental studies in soccer, in Sportspiel-furschung : Diagnose Prognose (eds H. Kasler and R. Andresen), Verlag Ingrid Czwalina, Hamburg, pp. 114-120.

Reilly, T. (1990) Football, in Physiology of Sports (eds T. Reilly, N. Secher, P. Snell and C. Williams), E. and F.N. Spon, London, pp.371-425.

Reilly, T. and Ball, D. (1984) The net psychological cost of dribbling a soccer ball. Res. Quart. Exerc. Sport, 55, 267-271.

Reilly, T. and Bowen, T. (1984) Exertional costs of changes in directional modes of running. Percept. Motor Skills, 58, 49-50.

Reilly, T. and Thomas, V. (1979) Estimated daily energy expenditures of professional association footballers. Ergonomics, 22, 541-548.

Reilly, T. Lees, A. Davids, K. and Murphy, W.J. (eds) (1988) Science and Football. E. and F.N. Spon, London.

Saltin, B. (1973) Metabolic fundamentals in exercise. Med. Sci. Sports, 5, 137-146.

PART TWO

Physical Fitness
Profiles of Footballers

ANAEROBIC PERFORMANCE AND BODY COMPOSITION OF INTERNATIONAL
RUGBY UNION PLAYERS

W. BELL, D. COBNER, S-M COOPER and S.J. PHILLIPS
CARDIFF INSTITUTE OF HIGHER EDUCATION, CARDIFF, WALES, UK

1 Introduction

The game of rugby union football demands a wide variety of playing skills; as a result
there tends to be a fairly high degree of player specialisation. This diversity of
performance has two immediate consequences. The first concerns the structural
characteristics of players, the second the functional demands of the playing positions
themselves. For optimal performance, therefore, it is necessary to identify and
respond to both these factors.

Morphological characteristics have been shown to be associated with playing
position; for example, in size and shape (Bell,1973a), skinfold distribution and body
proportions (Bell,1973b), and body composition (Bell,1979; 1980). Aerobic fitness
has been investigated by Williams et al. (1973), Bell (1980), Maud (1983) and
Maud and Shultz et al. (1988), and anaerobic performance by Cheetham et al.
(1988), Rigg and Reilly (1988) and Ueno et al. (1988).

The relationship between physical fitness and body composition is of considerable
importance in rugby football. Even supposing the desired amount and intensity of
training are being carried out, optimal physical fitness will be obtained only when the
fat and fat-free components of body composition are appropriate to meet the
structural, physiological and performance needs of the individual. In this sense body
composition sets the base line for the attainment of optimal fitness. In a game so
variable in its physiological demands differing admixtures of aerobic and anaerobic
fitness are required by the various positions. The attainment of optimal fitness,
therefore will depend upon the correctness with which decisions are made regarding
these requirements.

The main purpose of the present investigation was to identify the status of anaerobic
performance and body composition in international rugby players and to establish the
relationship between the various expressions of anaerobic performance and the
components of body composition

2 Methods

Players were regular members of a national squad. They were listed originally
according to playing position. For forwards (n=11) these were props (2), hookers
(2), locks (3), No 8's (2), and flankers (2). In the backs (n=5) there was one
player in each position at scrum-half, outside-half, centre, wing and full-back.

Ideally it is desirable to analyse the characteristics of players according to playing
position; this was prohibited in the present series by the relatively small numbers of

players in each position. Players were therefore assembled in groups according to the similarity of their physiological requirements. On these grounds props and locks were combined to establish one group (n=5); hookers, flankers and No 8's a second (n=6); and backs a third (n=5). The mean age of the total sample was 24.2 years.

Stature was measured to the nearest 0.1 cm using a fixed Harpenden stadiometer (Weiner and Lourie, 1981). Body mass was recorded on a beam balance to the closest 0.1 kg. Body density was determined by hydrostatic weighing with simultaneous measurement of underwater weighing. Total body fat (TBF) was calculated from body density using the equation of Siri (1956); fat-free mass (FFM) was determined by the subtraction of TBF from total body mass.

Anaerobic performance was assessed with a friction belt cycle ergometer (Monark 864) using a basket weight loading system interfaced to a microcomputer. The seat, handlebars and toe clips were adjusted to suit the needs of the subject. Each individual was allowed a 5 min submaximal warm-up followed by a 5 s sprint using the actual test load. After a brief recovery period the subject maintained a pedal frequency of 60 rev/min before the full braking force was applied. Subjects then pedalled maximally in a seated position for a continuous period of 30 s (BASS, 1988).

3 Results

To identify significant differences between playing positions a one-way analysis of variance (ANOVA) was carried out on all variables. Where a difference was found post hoc analyses were employed using the Scheffe test.

The descriptive statistics for height and body mass together with body density and the absolute and relative amounts of TBF and FFM are given in Table 1. No significant differences were evident in height between the playing units (P>0.05). In body mass there were significant differences between the three playing units (P<0.05). Props and locks were heaviest (103 kg) followed by hookers and the back row (101 kg), then backs (85 kg). Post-hoc analyses confirmed the differences between backs and each of the two forward units as being significant. Of the components of body composition only absolute amounts of FFM were significant (P<0.05). Once again the differences occurred between the backs and each of the forward playing units. Relative amounts of body fat were greater in props and locks (16%) with similar amounts being present in hookers and the back row (12%), and backs (13%), but these differences were not significant (P>0.05).

Results for anaerobic performance (Table 2) showed no significant differences between the playing units in any of the variables measured (P>0.05). Table 3 contrasts the zero-order coefficients of correlation for the forward playing units between anaerobic performance, FFM and body mass (P>0.05). In props and locks, and hookers and back row players, coefficients were positive, and consistently larger between FFM and anaerobic performance than they were between body mass and anaerobic performance.

First-order partial coefficients of correlation between anaerobic performance and FFM (with body mass held constant), were substantially larger for hookers and back row players (0.58 to 0.73) than they were for props and locks (0.21 to 0.56). Coefficients between anaerobic performance and body mass (with FFM held constant) were negative; values were greater for hookers and back row players (-0.47 to -0.70) than for props and locks (-0.06 to -0.32). None of the coefficients was significant (P>0.05).

Table 1. Mean values ± SD for height, body mass, and components of body composition for international rugby players * = P<0.05, NS = P>0.05

		Props Locks (n=5)	Hookers Back row (n=6)	Backs (n=5)	
Height	(cm)	190.7 ± 11.4	184.8 ± 7.9	178.1 ± 6.3	NS
Body Mass	(kg)	102.5 ± 2.6	100.9 ± 12.8	84.98 ± 7.0	*
Density	(g/ml)	1.063 ± 0.008	1.071 ± 0.01	1.069 ± 0.01	NS
FFM	(kg)	86.6 ± 5.3	88.1 ± 8.4	74.0 ± 9.0	*
TBF	(kg)	15.9 ± 3.5	12.8 ± 5.7	11.0 ± 3.1	NS
FFM	(%)	84.5 ± 3.6	87.7 ± 4.6	86.9 ± 4.4	NS
TBF	(%)	15.5 ± 3.6	12.3 ± 4.6	13.1 ± 4.4	NS

Table 2. Mean values ± SD for anaerobic performance of international rugby players NS = P>0.05

		Props Locks (n=5)	Hookers Back row (n=6)	Backs (n=5)	
Total Work	(kJ)	29.4 ± 5.3	34.1 ± 8.1	29.9 ± 3.6	NS
Peak Power	(W)	1342 ± 261	1388 ± 315	1336 ± 134	NS
PPO/Mass	(W/kg)	9.7 ± 1.6	11.3 ± 1.9	12.1 ± 1.9	NS
PPO/FFM	(W/kg)	11.4 ± 1.8	12.8 ± 2.2	14.1 ± 2.7	NS
Mean Power	(W)	991.7 ± 179	1144 ± 279	1013 ± 131	NS
Fatigue Index	(W/s)	-28.4 ± 10.0	-21.9 ± 8.4	-28.31 ± 4.9	NS

Table 3. Zero-order coefficients of correlation between anaerobic performance and body mass and FFM according to playing unit (P>0.05)

		FFM		Body Mass	
		Props Locks (n=5)	Hookers Back row (n=6)	Props Locks (n=5)	Hookers Back row (n=6)
Total work	(kJ)	0.55	0.75	0.43	0.65
Peak power	(W)	0.56	0.60	0.31	0.50
PPO/Mass	(W/kg)	0.48	0.23	0.32	0.15
PPO/FFM	(W/kg)	0.26	0.49	0.18	0.38
Mean Power	(W)	0.57	0.75	0.44	0.65

4 Discussion

There were no significant differences in height between the three playing units (Table 1). The reason for this was the manner in which positions were aggregated. When positional samples are small, the customary practice is to combine positions to increase sample size. The weakness in doing this without first testing for homogeneity is that it may well conceal differences between positions which may otherwise be apparent. When analysed by position, differences in height between forward positions are known to be significant (Bell,1980).

Body mass is often a decisive factor in the constitution of players and contributes greatly to functional performance, more so in forwards than backs. The significantly larger mass of the two forward playing units compared to backs is not, therefore, surprising. Although mass is of considerable importance in rugby forwards, it is not mass per se that is of primary concern, but rather the proportion of TBF to FFM.

As a group, props and locks were heavier than hookers and back row players; in contrast, the FFM in hookers and back row players (88 kg), was greater, marginally, than it was in props and locks (87 kg). The corollary of this was that the fat mass of props and locks was greater (16 kg) than that of hookers and back row players (13 kg). In relative terms these values were equivalent to 16% TBF in props and locks, and 12% TBF in hookers and back row players. In part, these compositional differences may well reflect positional requirements; for example, props and locks provide the cornerstone at set pieces such as scrummages and line-outs, while hookers, flankers and No 8's require a greater capacity for power and mobility in open play. At the same time these differences may well indicate more than optimal amounts of TBF. Levels of body composition in the present group of international players, however, are more favourable for performance than those of college-based players (Bell, 1980).

In making comparisons between players of large body mass the use of relative fat may be misleading. For example, a prop 178 cm tall, weighing 120 kg and with 10% body fat, will carry 12 kg of fat. A centre of the same height and percent body fat, but weighing only 80 kg, will carry only 8 kg of fat. The prop is actually carrying 50% more fat than the centre even though he is of the same height and relative fat. Consideration should be given to frame size and physique when making individual comparisons and decisions.

Since the FFM responds to training in a more productive way than TBF, in principle, it is advantageous to increase the FFM at the expense of TBF, at least to an amount which is commensurate with structural, physiological and functional requirements. Because fat, muscle and bone are largely independent (Tanner,1964), there seems no good reason why players in any position should not attain optimal ratios of body composition.

There were no significant differences ($P>0.05$) between the three playing units in any of the expressions of anaerobic performance (Table 2). However, hookers and back row players, despite their smaller body mass, produced a greater amount of total work (34 kJ), peak power output (1388 W), and mean power output (1144 W), than either props and locks, or backs. Rigg and Reilly (1988) also found higher amounts of power output in back row players compared to other playing units.

When peak power output was expressed in relation to body mass, backs had the largest values (12.1 W/kg) and props and locks the smallest (9.7 W/kg). This finding has also been identified in treadmill sprinting : 10.1 W/kg for backs and 9.0 W/kg for forwards (Cheetham et al., 1988). Exactly the same relationship holds true for FFM (14.1 W/kg for backs and 11.4 W/kg for props and locks).

Present values of anaerobic performance are greater than those found for rugby players by other studies (Cheetham et al.,1988; Holmyard et al.,1988; Rigg and

18

Reilly,1988; Ueno et al.,1988). The only exception is the high relative value of peak power output in Japanese players (Ueno et al.,1988). Although the absolute values of peak power output are less in Japanese players, because of their smaller body mass, the relative values of peak power output are actually higher (13.0 to 13.7 W/kg compared to 9.7 to 12.1 W/kg). That is, they have a larger power to body mass ratio. Absolute and relative aspects of anaerobic performance both make their contribution to the game at set pieces and open play, respectively.

Deterioration of anaerobic performance as measured by work decrement was least in hookers and back row players (-22 W/s) and greatest in props and locks, and backs (-28 W/s). Cheetham et al. (1988) found those forwards with a high peak power output experienced the greatest amount of fatigue, and had the largest increases in blood lactate concentration.

Coefficients of correlation were greater between FFM and anaerobic performance than between body mass and anaerobic performance (Table 3). This was true in both props and locks (0.26-0.57 versus 0.18-0.44), and hookers and back row players (0.23-0.75 versus 0.15-0.65), and supports the view that FFM contributes more to the production of anaerobic performance than body mass. The association was also stronger in hookers and back row players than it was for props and locks; this is demonstrated by the greater absolute amounts of anaerobic performance in hookers and back row players compared to props and locks. In forwards TBF correlates either negatively or weakly with anaerobic performance; that is, the greater the amount of TBF the poorer the anaerobic performance.

When body mass is held constant the correlations between FFM and anaerobic performance generally diminish, indicating that body mass does in fact make some contribution to anaerobic performance. The coefficients for props and locks are actually lower (0.21-0.56) than those of hookers and back row players (0.58-0.73) which suggests that props and locks would benefit from an increase in FFM. It is important that the increase in FFM occurs at the expense of TBF so that body mass is not reduced.

Coefficients of correlation between body mass and anaerobic performance, with FFM held constant, are all negative; that is, as body mass increases anaerobic performance decreases. Thus any increase in body mass attributed solely to TBF will be disadvantageous and reduce anaerobic performance.

We have expressed the view earlier that for functional purposes relative amounts of TBF and FFM are more important than body mass itself. The logic of this is that the greater the FFM the greater the potential for strength, speed, power, aerobic and anaerobic fitness; all are necessary prerequisites for optimal physical fitness in rugby players.

We conclude that all players should identify the optimal status of body composition bearing in mind their playing positions. Absolute levels of anaerobic performance were greatest in hookers and back row players and lowest in props and locks. When standardised in relation to body size backs had the highest anaerobic performance. The correlations between anaerobic performance and FFM were greater than those between anaerobic performance and body mass. When body mass was held constant the correlations between FFM and anaerobic performance diminished; with FFM held constant the correlations between body mass and anaerobic performance were negative. It is clear that anaerobic performance will be improved by increasing FFM at the expense of TBF.

5 References

Bell, W. (1973a) Anthropometry of the young adult college rugby player in Wales. Brit. J. Sports Med., 7, 298-299.

Bell, W. (1973b) Distribution of skinfolds and differences in body proportions in young adult rugby players. J. Sports Med. Phys. Fit., 13, 69-73.

Bell, W. (1979) Body composition of rugby union football players. Brit. J. Sports Med., 13, 19-23.

Bell, W. (1980) Body composition and maximal aerobic power of rugby union forwards. J. Sports Med. Phys. Fit., 20, 447-451.

British Association Sports Sciences (1988) Position statement on the assessment of the elite athlete. B.A.S.S., Leeds.

Cheetham, M. E., Hazeldine, R. J., Robinson, A. and Williams, C. (1988). Power output of rugby forwards during maximal treadmill running, in Science and Footba (eds T. Reilly, A. Lees, K. Davids and W.J. Murphy), E & F N Spon, London, pp. 206-210.

Holmyard, D.J., Cheetham, M.E., Lakomy H.K.A. and Williams, C. (1988) Effect of recovery duration on performance during multiple treadmill sprints, in Science and Football (eds T. Reilly, A. Lees, K. Davids and W.J.Murphy), E & F N Spon, London, pp.134-142.

Maud, P.J. (1983) Physiological and anthropometric parameters that describe a rugby team. Brit. J. Sports Med., 17, 16-23.

Maud, P.J. and Shultz, B.B. (1984) The US national rugby team; a physiological and anthropometric assessment. Physician Sportsmed.,12, 86-89.

Rigg, P. and Reilly, T. (1988). A fitness profile and anthropometric analysis of first and second class rugby union players, in Science and Football (eds T. Reilly, A. Lees, K. Davids and W.J. Murphy), E & F N Spon, London, pp.194-200.

Siri, W.E. (1956). Body composition from fluid spaces and density. Berkeley, California: Donner Lab Med Physics, University California Report 3349.

Tanner, J.M. (1964) The Physique of the Olympic Athlete. Allen & Unwin, London.

Ueno, Y., Watai, E. and Ishii, K. (1988). Aerobic and anaerobic power of rugby football players, in Science and Football (eds T. Reilly, A.Lees, K.Davids and W.J. Murphy), E. & F N Spon, London, pp. 201-205.

Weiner, J.S. and Lourie, J.A. (1981) Practical Human Biology. Academic Press, London.

Williams, C., Reid, R.M. and Coutts, R. (1973). Observations on the aerobic power of University rugby players and professional soccer players. Brit. J. Sports Med., 7, 390-391.

SEASONAL VARIATIONS IN THE ANTHROPOMETRIC AND PHYSIOLOGICAL CHARACTERISTICS OF INTERNATIONAL RUGBY UNION PLAYERS

D. J. HOLMYARD AND R.J. HAZELDINE

Department of Physical Education, Sports Science and Recreation Management
Loughborough University, Loughborough, Leics., LE11 3TU, England.

1 Introduction

The seasonal nature of Rugby Union imposes varied physiological stresses on the player. During the playing season, there are demanding playing and training commitments and soft tissue injuries frequently occur as a result of the high impact collisions common to the game. However, during the off-season, activity and fitness training are largely self-regulated. In The British Isles, the game has become increasingly competitive over the last few seasons with the advent of new league structures. This has placed greater performance demands upon players. International players are expected to perform at a consistently high level for approximately 30 weeks of the 35 week season, including two months of peak performance during the Five Nations Championship. In years when there is a World Cup or a major tour, performance and fitness levels need to be maintained for even longer periods.

Experience from other sports would suggest that such sustained 'peaking' would ultimately be counter-productive to performance, in terms of lost training and accumulated fatigue. At best, players can only aim to maintain high levels of fitness demonstrated in the early season. The limited time for fitness preparation during the playing season, combined with the limited recovery time available between successive matches could lead to a decline in fitness levels as the season progresses. However, no studies have monitored the fitness levels of Rugby Union players throughout a season.

Changes in physiological characteristics of soccer players throughout a season have been described by Brewer (1990) and the effects of training on soccer players have been investigated by Bangsbo and Mizuno (1988) and Islegen and Akgun (1988). Of the literature specific to rugby, most studies have reported the physiological and anthropometric characteristics of players (Williams et al., 1973; Bell, 1979, 1980; Maud, 1983; Maud & Shultz, 1984; Cheetham et al., 1988; Ueno et al., 1988 ; Rigg and Reilly, 1988). In studies which have compared between playing positions, differences have been observed between the forwards (ball winners) and backs (ball carriers). Interpositional differences have been demonstrated to be more pronounced at higher playing levels. These differences include height, body mass, percent body fat, speed and maximal power output (Maud & Shultz, 1984; Rigg and Reilly, 1988). The subjects used in these studies have not been truly elite international players and whether or not these findings hold true for this group remains to be demonstrated.

It was the purpose of this study to assess the seasonal variations in physiological and anthropometric characteristics of elite Rugby Union players and secondly to examine any differences in these characteristics between backs and forwards, at this level.

2 Methods

In this study 18 subjects from the English national Rugby Union squad were measured on selected anthropometric and physiological characteristics on five occasions, at 2-3 month intervals, over a 12-month period. During this period the players were following a training programme designed (i) to lead to a long term increase in general fitness and (ii) to achieve peak levels of fitness in January for the major international matches. The tests were conducted in a field environment at national squad training weekends which took place during the playing seasons (September-April) 1989-90 and 1990-91 and the off-season (May-August) between them. The players were assessed in January 1990 (mid-season), April 1990 (end of season), June 1990 (early off-season), September 1990 (pre-season) and January 1991 (mid-season). The subjects were sub-divided into positional categories: 9 forwards (2 props, 2 hookers, 2 locks, 3 back row) and 9 backs (2 scrum halves, 2 fly halves, 1 centre, 3 wings, 1 full back).

The parameters assessed on each player were height, body mass, estimated body fat percent, predicted maximum oxygen uptake, speed and anaerobic capacity. Body fat percent was estimated using skinfold measurements (Durnin & Womersley, 1974). Maximum oxygen uptake was predicted from the players' performance on the 'Multistage Fitness Test' using the method validated by Ramsbottom et al. (1988). Speed was assessed from the time taken to cover a 30 m distance. Players sprinted from a standing start one metre behind an electronic beam. Timing began once the first beam was broken and stopped when the player crossed the beam of the finish line. A 20 m high intensity shuttle run test (HISRT) was used to predict maximal accumulated oxygen deficit (MAOD), which was used as an index of anaerobic capacity (Medbo et al., 1988; Ramsbottom et al., 1990)These tests formed part of a larger battery of fitness tests, which took place at the beginning of squad sessions. The tests discussed are the ones for which a complete set of data was collected, with the exception of the HISRT, which was conducted on 4 of the 5 occasions.

A one-way analysis of variance was used to examine changes in the means of the data for the whole group of players (n=18) over the five testing sessions. A students t-test was used to assess differences in the means of forwards and backs at any one session.

3 Results

The physical characteristics of the subjects in January 1991 are shown in Table 1. The age, height and body mass of the subjects are within the ranges previously reported for first class rugby union club players (Maud and Schultz, 1984; Rigg and Reilly, 1988). The forwards were older, taller ($p < 0.05$) and heavier ($p < 0.01$) than the backs.

Table 1. Physical characteristics (Means ± SD)

	Age (Yrs.)	Height (m)	Body Mass (kg)	
Fowards	29.2 ± 2.3	1.84 ± 0.11	100.3 ± 10.4	
Backs	26.9 ± 1.5	1.75 ± 0.02	83.0 ± 5.2	
				* p<0.05
	*	*	* *	* * p<0.01

There was a significant fall in percent body fat for the whole group during the period of assessment ($p < 0.001$), (see Figure 1). The sub-group of forwards had a higher percent body fat than the backs ($p < 0.01$ - $p < 0.05$) on all occasions except at the June test session (e.g. 13.3 ± 1.9 and 11.4 ± 1.5 % for forwards and backs respectively in January 1991). The mean body fat percentages reported in this study are somewhat greater than those previously reported by the same method. The largest falls in percent body fat occurred during the off season (April-September) and the first half of the playing season (September-January). Body fat remained at the same level during the

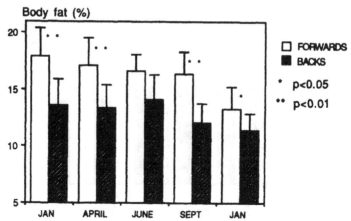

Fig.1. Body composition Jan. 1990 - Jan. 1991. (Means ± SD)

second half of the season (January-April).There was a significant increase in predicted maximum oxygen uptake for the whole group during the period of assessment (p< 0.001), (see Figure 2). The backs exhibited a significantly higher predicted maximum oxygen uptake than the forwards in January 1990 (mid-season) and April (end of season). However, in June, September and January 1991, the aerobic power of the backs and forwards were not significantly different. The lowest values for both forwards and backs were in April. The aerobic power values are somewhat higher than those that have previously been predicted (Bell, 1980; Maud and Schultz, 1884), or directly measured (Ueno et al., 1988) for Rugby Union players. This was particularly so towards the end of the assessment period (e.g. 58.0±3.9 and 59.6±2.3 ml/kg/min. for the forwards and backs respectively in January 1991). There was a steady increase in aerobic power throughout the off-season, no further improvement during the first half of the season and a fall in aerobic power during the second half of the season.

There was a significant improvement in sprint performance for the whole group during

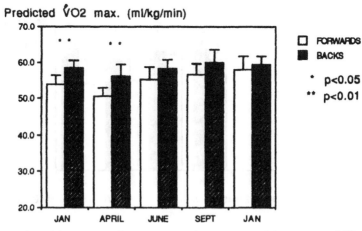

Fig.2. Aerobic power Jan. 1990 - Jan. 1991. (Means ± SD)

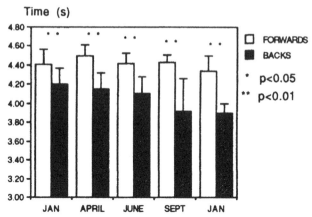

Fig.3. 30m Sprint times Jan. 1990-Jan. 1991 (Means ± SD)

the period of assessment (see Figure 3). The fastest mean time was recorded in January 1991(4.34 ± 0.16 and 3.90 ± 0.10s for the sub-groups of forwards and backs respectively). At all times of testing the sub-group of backs were significantly faster than the forwards (p< 0.01). The greatest improvement in sprint performance occurred during the off-season for the backs, but during the first half of the playing season for the forwards. These differences may have been a result of personal preferences in off-season training.

There were no significant changes overall, in the mean MAOD of the whole group throughout the study (see Figure 4). The predicted mean MAOD of the forwards and backs was not significantly different, except in January 1990 when the backs had a significantly higher value than the forwards (p< 0.05). The anaerobic capacity of the backs showed a marked improvement during the first half of the season. This was not the case with the forwards.

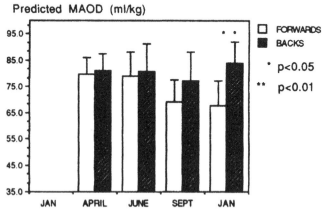

Fig.4. Anaerobic capacity Jan. 1990 - Jan. 1991. (Means ± SD)

4 Conclusions

The results demonstrate that the elite international rugby union players in this study experienced significant improvements in body composition, aerobic power and speed, but no significant changes in anaerobic power during the 12 months of assessment. This finding lends support to the effectiveness of the training programme in eliciting long term improvements in fitness. During the off-season there were decreases in percent body fat and increases in aerobic power. However, apart from a decrease in percent body fat during the first half of the playing season there were no further improvements in these characteristics during the playing season, and actually a small decline in aerobic power was noted. It is unclear whether this decline is due to a reduction in fitness per se, or is a result of accumulated match fatigue. Improvements in speed were demonstrated during the first half of the season whilst anaerobic capacity remained somewhat constant throughout the assessment period. It would appear from this evidence that improvements in particular aspects of fitness are specific to the time of the season. The major improvements in body composition and aerobic power occurred during the off-season. During the playing season these aspects of fitness remained relatively constant, while there was an improvement in speed. There was a relative lack of variation in anaerobic capacity throughout the assessment period. The sensitivity to training, of the anaerobic capacity test used in this study, has not been fully established. This result is therefore not conclusive evidence of a lack of seasonal variation in this fitness variable.

Significant interpositional differences were found in the anthropometric and physiological characteristics of elite international players. The most pronounced of these differences between backs and forwards were in body mass, body fat and speed. Predicted aerobic power and anaerobic capacity did not distinguish well between backs and forwards.

5 References

Bangsbo, J. and Mizuno, M. (1988) Morphological and metabolic alterations in soccer players with detraining and their relation to performance, in **Science and Football** (eds T. Reilly, A. Lees, K. Davids and W.J. Murphy), London, E. & F.N. Spon, pp 114-124.

Bell, W. (1979) Body composition of rugby union football players. **Brit. J. Sports Med.**, 13, 19-23.

Bell, W. (1980). Body composition and maximal aerobic power of rugby union forwards. **J. Sports Med. Phys. Fit.**, 20, 447-451.

Brewer, J. (1990) Changes in selected physiological characteristics of an English first division soccer squad during a league season. **J. Sports Sci.**, 8, 76-77.

Cheetham, M.E., Hazeldine, R.J., Robinson, A. and Williams, C. (1988) Power output of rugby forwards during maximal treadmill sprinting, in **Science and Football** (eds T. Reilly, A. Lees, K. Davids and W.J. Murphy). London, E. & F.N. Spon, pp 206-210.

Durnin, and Womersley, J. (1974) Body fat assessment from total-body density and its estimation from skinfold thickness measurements on 481 men and women aged 16 to 72 years. **Brit. J. Nutr.**, 32, 169-179.

Islegen, C. and Akgun (1988) Effects of 6 weeks pre-seasonal training on physical fitness among soccer players, in **Science and Football** (eds T. Reilly, A. Lees, K. Davids and W.J. Murphy). London, E. & F.N. Spon, pp 125-129.

Maud, P.J. (1983) Physiological and anthropometric parameters that describe a rugby team. **Brit. J. Sports Med.**, 17, 16-23.

Maud, P.J. and Shultz, B.B. (1984) The US National rugby team: A physiological and anthropometric assessment. **Phys. Sportsmed.**, 12(9), 86-99.

Medbo, J.I. Mohn, A.C., Tabata, I., Bahr, R., Vaage, O. and Sejersted, O. (1988) Anaerobic capacity determined by maximal accumulated oxygen deficit. **J. Appl. Physiol.**, 64, 50-60.

Ramsbottom, R., Hazeldine, R., Nevill, A. and Williams, C. (1990) Shuttle run performance and maximal accumulated oxygen deficit. **J. Sports Sci.**, 8, 292.

Rigg. P and Reilly, T. (1988) A fitness profile and anthropometric analysis of first and second class rugby union players, in **Science and Football** (eds T. Reilly, A. Lees, K. Davids and W.J. Murphy). London, E. & F.N. Spon, pp 194-200.

Ueno, Y., Watai, E. and Ishii. K. (1988) Aerobic and anaerobic power of rugby football players, in **Science and Football** (eds T. Reilly, A. Lees, K. Davids and W.J. Murphy). London, E. & F.N. Spon, pp 201-205.

Williams, C., Reid, R. and Coutts, R. (1973) Observations on the aerobic power of university rugby players and professional soccer players. **Brit. J. Sports Med.**, 7, 390-391.

ANTHROPOMETRIC AND FITNESS PROFILES OF ELITE FEMALE RUGBY UNION PLAYERS

WENDY J. KIRBY and T. REILLY
Centre for Sport and Exercise Sciences, Liverpool Polytechnic, Liverpool, L3 3AF, England.

1 Introduction

The increase in women's participation in competitive games is reflected in the growing popularity of Women's Rugby Union football. The acceptance of the sport culminated in the holding of the first World Cup in Wales during April 1991. Up to now there has been little attention given to the game by researchers.

Men's Rugby Union teams have been examined by various research groups (see Reilly, 1990) in terms of anthropometric, muscular fitness and physiological fitness profiles. The data have been used for descriptive profiling and for examination of differences both between positional groups and levels of participation (Rigg and Reilly, 1988). Body size and fitness profiles tend to be specific to positional categories: this specificity is more strongly governed by positional role in first class compared to second class levels of play. The extent to which this influence of positional role on fitness profiles manifests itself in the women's game has not been established.

The aims of this study were to:- (i) provide a comprehensive profile of anthropometric and physiological measures in first class Women's Rugby Union players; (ii) examine differences in such profiles between playing positions.

2 Methods

Thirty-nine females (20 forwards, aged 24.6±3.1 years; 19 backs aged 23.4±2.8 years) participated in the study. They had played the game of Rugby Union for an average of over four full years and had attained regional squad standard or above. They were drawn from Wasps R.U.F.C., Richmond R.U.F.C., Liverpool Polytechnic 1st XV and the North of England Representative Squad. Five were full internationals. The sample comprised 12 backs (full and three-quarters), 7 half-backs, 9 front row, 3 second row and 8 back row forwards.

Anthropometric measures included height, body mass and percent body fat estimated from skinfold thicknesses (Durnin and Womersley, 1974). Somatotype was determined according to Heath and Carter (1967). Grip strength was measured with a dynamometer and back strength with a 'back and leg' dynamometer (Takei Kiki Kogyo, Tokyo). The standing broad jump and vertical jump were used as indices of 'explosive' leg muscle performance (Clarke, 1967). Aerobic power

($\dot{V}O_2$max) was predicted from performance on a progressive 20 m shuttle run test (Ramsbottom et al., 1988).

Results were analysed using normal descriptive statistics. A series of ANOVA tests was used to examine differences between positional groups and to isolate features of selected playing positions. A P value of 0.05 was taken to indicate significance.

3 Results and Discussion

The forwards as a group were heavier but not significantly taller than the backs. This was reflected in the higher ponderal index (height divided by cubed root of body mass) among the backs. The difference is due possibly to fat free mass since the two groups were similar in estimated percent body fat. This contrasts with findings of lower adipose tissue (17.5%) in backs than in forwards (22.6%) in U.S.A. women collegiate players (Sedlock et al., 1988), a factor which might lead to selection of positional roles at the collegiate level.

The proposition of a positional differentiation according to lean body mass is supported by the somatotype measures, the forwards having greater mesomorphy and lower ectomorphy than the backs. These differences reflect the differing requirements of forward play from back play, the greater body mass and muscularity being advantageous in set plays of scrummages, rucks and mauls. The differences in body mass may at least in part be accounted for by skeletal factors, since the forwards had the greater limb girths and bone diameters (P<0.05).

Table 1. Comparison of forwards (n=20) and backs (n=19)

	Forwards	Backs
Height (cm)	168.5±7.9	165.5±3.9
Body Mass (kg)	68.9±6.6	60.8±5.7 **
Ponderal Index	12.5±0.4	12.8±0.4 *
% Body Fat	21.2±1.7	20.2±2.1
Somatotype:		
Endomorphy	3.0±0.5	2.8±0.5
Mesomorphy	4.8±0.7	3.9±0.9 **
Ectomorphy	2.5±1.0	3.1±0.8 *
Strength:		
Grip (N)	370.8±41.2	360.1±41.2
Back (N)	1020.2±1000.0	947.6±147.1
Power:		
Broad Jump (cm)	187.7±14.3	190.8±14.1
Vertical Jump (cm)	35.4±3.3	36.9±2.7
Predicted $\dot{V}O_2$max (ml/kg/min)	43.8±4.8	47.3±4.0

*Indicates P<0.05 ; **Indicates P<0.01

The somatotype of the Rugby Union players differed from that of the hockey players studied by Reilly and Bretherton (1986). Both forwards and backs had higher mesomorphy values than the female hockey groups. They were also lower in endomorphy, an observation reinforced by the lower values for estimated percent body fat. Ectomorphy values were higher than for the hockey players, but this applied only to the Rugby Union backs.

The greater muscularity in the forwards was not reflected in the static strength tests (grip and back) which did not differ significantly between the groups. A similar result was found for the jump tests. The grip strength and jump performances of the women Rugby Union players were similar to those observed in elite and county standard female hockey players (Reilly and Bretherton, 1986). The hockey players were closer in anthropometric profile to the backs than to the forwards, except that they were more endomorphic (3.2) and less ectomorphic (2.5).

Further univariate analysis of the data showed that the consideration of the forwards as a group disguised specific positional characteristics. Second row players tended to be tall and heavy, along with players in the No.8 position. These features would be an advantage in winning the ball in line-outs. Players at No.8 also scored highly in the muscular strength tests. Front row players were shortest and lightest of the forwards whilst prop forwards were heavy relative to stature. Props had significantly higher back strength values than the remaining forwards except for No.8 players, which would reflect the scrummaging requirements of this role.

The performance on the shuttle run test was better for the backs than for the forwards. For each group the observed values were higher than those noted by Sedlock et al. (1988) for American collegiate players. The average value of estimated $\dot{V}O_2$ max for the backs was close to the 47.9 ml/kg/min observed by Colquhoun and Chad (1986) for Australian national female soccer players. The highest estimated aerobic power was found in full-backs ($\bar{x}$ = 51.0 ml/kg/min), followed by fly-halves (48.5 ml/kg/min): props had the poorest values (39.4 ml/kg/min on average), a factor which would impair their mobility in extended periods of open play.

In general the results corroborate trends noted previously in male Rugby Union players (Reilly, 1990). They highlight the need to consider positional requirements when interpreting fitness test data in female players.

4 References

Clarke, H.H. (1967) Application of Measurement to Health and Physical Education. Prentice-Hall, New York.

Colquhoun, D. and Chad, K.L. (1986) Physiological characteristics of Australian female soccer players after a competitive season. Austr. J. Sci. Med. Sport, 18 (No.3), 9-12.

Durnin, J.V.G.A. and Womersley, J. (1974) Body fat assessed from total body density and its estimation from skinfold thickness: measurements on 481 men and women aged 16 to 72 years. Brit. J. Nutr., 32, 77-97.

Heath, B.H. and Carter, J.E.L. (1967) A modified somatotype method. Amer. J. Phys. Anthrop., 27, 57-74.

Ramsbottom, R., Brewer, J. and Williams, C. (1988) A progressive shuttle run test to estimate maximal oxygen uptake. Brit. J. Sports Med., 22, 141-144.

Reilly, T. (1990) Football, in Physiology of Sports (eds T.Reilly, N.Secher, P.Snell and C.Williams). E. and F.N. Spon, London, pp. 371–425.

Reilly, T. and Bretherton, S. (1986) Multivariate analysis of fitness of female field hockey players, in Perspectives in Kinanthropometry (ed J.A.P.Day). Human Kinetics, Champaign, III, pp. 135–142.

Rigg, P. and Reilly, T. (1988) A fitness profile and anthropometric analysis of first and second class Rugby Union players, in Science and Football (eds T.Reilly, A.Lees, K.Davids and V.J.Murphy). E. and F.N. Spon, London, pp. 194–200.

Sedlock, D.A., Fitzgerald, P.I. and Knowlton, R.G. (1988) Body composition and performance of collegiate women rugby players. Res. Quart. Exerc. Sport, 59, 78–82.

MEASUREMENT OF SPRINTING SPEED OF PROFESSIONAL AND AMATEUR SOCCER PLAYERS

E. KOLLATH, Deutsche Sporthochschule, Köln, Germany
K. QUADE, Bundesinstitut für Sportwissenschaft, Köln

1 Introduction

Practical experience shows that in soccer speed plays an important role. An accelerated pace of the game calls for rapid execution of typical movements by every member in a team. In many instances, successful implementation of certain technical or tactical manoeuvres by different team members is tied up with the degree of velocity deployed.

A look at the pertinent literature reveals that sprints from standing have been most frequently tested. According to Föhrenbach et al. (1986) the distance best suited for assessment of maximal running velocity is 30 m.
The aims of this study were to determine:
  a) The differences that exist between amateur and professional players in 5, 10, and 20 and 30 m sprint times.
  b) The differences that exist between defensive and offensive players.
  c) How faster players gain their advantage in individual sections of the overall distance.

2 Methods

The experimental measurements were carried out on 20 National League professionals, all members of the first team of FC Köln and 19 top class amateur players. The participants performed two 30 m sprints in a roofed running facility, with a recovery of 3 minutes. Five photoelectric cells and reflectors were used. The cells were positioned at 0, 5, 10, 20 and 30 meters. The immediate data available for intermediate times were further treated by computer to yield individual intermediate mean velocities.

In order to minimize the risk of faulty reactions, the photoelectric cells were placed at shoulder to head high. Nevertheless for the split times an error in measurement of ± 0.02 s must be taken into consideration. The corresponding errors for the mean velocities are ± 0.1 m/s in a 5 m interval and ± 0.15 m/s in 10 m intervals.

3 Results and Discussion

3.1 Differences between professional and amateur players

Table 1. Intermediate time and final results of professional and amateur soccer players in 30 m sprints.

	Time (s) after			
	5 m	10 m	20 m	30 m
Profess. (n = 20) x + SD	1,03 ± 0,08	1,79 ± 0,09	3,03 ± 0,11	4,19 ± 0,14
Amateurs (n = 19) x + SD	1,07 + 0,07	1,88 + 0,10	3,15 + 0,12	4,33 + 0,16
Sign. (P)	>0.05	<0.05	<0.05	<0.05

Table 1 shows that the professionals reached all interval marks earlier on average than their amateur rivals. There were significant differences (P < 0.05) in the 10 m, 20 m, and 30 m times. The difference between the groups constantly increased. The professional group started with a 0.04 s lead at the 5 m mark and ended with a 0.14 s advantage. This may explain the persistently increasing lead of the professionals over the amateurs.

Owing to the faster running speed, the professionals were on average 19 cm ahead of the amateurs after 5 m and 121 cm ahead by 30 m (Fig. 1). It follows from the corresponding percentages that the amateurs are about half way behind the professionals already by the first 10 m of the overall distance. This result suggests that in order to perform well in the 30 m sprint, the quick dash at the beginning must be given special attention.

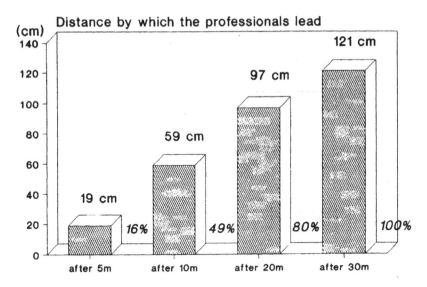

Fig. 1. Lead of professional soccer players over amateurs in 30m sprints (mean values).

3.2 Differences between offensive and defensive players

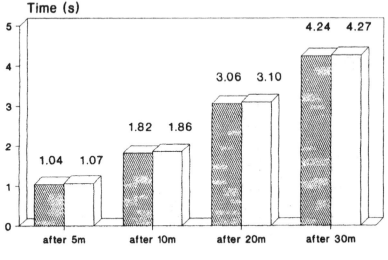

Fig. 2. Split time and final results (mean values) of offensive and defensive players (professionals and amateurs jointly).

Figure 2 illustrates that the differences between the observed mean values of offensive and defensive players are

≤ 0.04 s. In terms of statistical relevance, there are no significant differences (P > 0.05). Defensive players were as fast as offensive players in both sections of the total 30 m. This implied that in top-class professional and amateur soccer the speed requirement of offensive and defensive players is similar. This should be paralleled in training.

3.3 Individual differences in the sections of the 30 m run. The ways in which less efficient sprinters in our population were falling behind their competitors may now be considered.

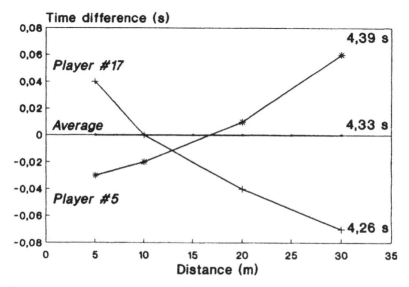

Fig. 3. Development of time lag (amateur no. 5) and advantage (amateur no. 17) with respect to the group's average.

Compared with the group average result of 4.33 s, the 30 m time achieved by amateur no. 17 (4.26 s) was not the result of faster initial acceleration. He examplifies a relatively poor acceleration capacity at the beginning of the sprint. Only after a running distance of 10 m will he show better split time results than the group average and in the end he drew away with a 0.07 s lead.

   The running time of amateur no. 5 was exactly in the opposite direction. Until about half way of the total distance, he did better than the average, but then accumulated a time lag of 0.06 s (corresponding to 42 cm). Comparisons with other players revealed that identical 30 m times often resulted from different split times.

Another example illustrates the way the sprint
performance of the fastest and the slowest runner among the
professionals differed in our investigation. For this
purpose, the mean velocities of these two participants were
compared in the four running sections (Fig. 4).

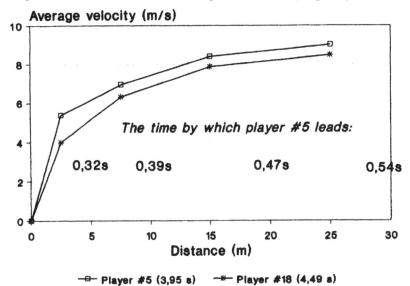

Fig. 4. Average velocity of the fastest and slowest player.

Professional no. 5 performed better over the total distance
than professional no. 18. The most interesting fact,
however, is that professional no. 18 had built up a major
share of his backlog already by the first 5 m, by the end
of which he was 0.32 s behind. At the 30 m mark, the
difference amounted to 0.54 s.

4 Conclusions

The results show that experimental analysis of the sprint
capacity of football players may contribute a good deal to
viewing this important element of physical fitness in a
more objective light. The comparatively simple equipment -
a couple of photoelectric cells - allows the coach to
assess the running speed of his team in detail.
   The findings of our survey leave no doubt about the fact
that even simple kinematic parameters, such as split times
and mean velocities obtained in certain sections of the
total running distance, are indicative of individual strong
points and weak points in sprinting performance. Once the
coach has been given this kind of information, he may take

the initiative to train acceleration capacities of his team members in a fast start, or try to enhance maximal speed.

In this context it is necessary to mention a method of measurement not well known or much used so far for determination of running speed, the ultra-sound method. It is based on the "Acoustic Doppler Effect" and allows the measurement of running velocity as a function of time.

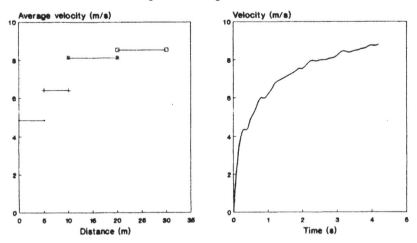

Fig. 5. Speed measurement by two different methods.

In the case of the photoelectric cells, the velocity data are restricted to mean values achieved at certain intervals (Fig. 5, left side). The ultra-sound method in contrast yields a continuous velocity curve (Fig. 5, right side). The decision on which method should be chosen depends on the objective pursued. Wherever the main interest lies in knowing certain split times or the final time in sprints, photoelectric cells will suffice. Where additional information on momentary running velocity is required, the ultra-sound method is to be preferred.

5 References

Föhrenbach, R., Hollmann, W., Mader, A., Thiele, W. (1986) Testverfahren und metabolisch orientierte Intensitätssteuerung im Sprinttraining mit submaximaler Belastungsstruktur. Leistungssport, 5, 15-24.

Geese, R. (1990) Konditionsdiagnose im Fußball. Leistungssport, 4, 23-28.

PHYSIOLOGICAL PROFILE OF TOP CROATION SOCCER PLAYERS

B.R. MATKOVIC, S. JANKOVIC AND S. HEIMER
Faculty of Physical Education, University of Zagreb, Croatia.

1 Introduction

Soccer is probably the popular game world-wide but there is still
limited scientific information available concerning the physiological
characteristics of professional soccer players (Raven et al., 1976;
Thomas and Reilly, 1979; Bale, 1986; Reilly et al., 1988). Due to
the fact that the game lasts one hour and a half, sometimes even
longer than the official timing, it requires a good aerobic capacity.
Soccer also comprises activities like sprints, and jumps in attack
and defence. These short lasting activities are performed over the
entire game, so both aerobic and anaerobic capacity are required from
athletes. Our research aimed to establish the functional capability
of the professional soccer players in Croatia with an emphasis on
their aerobic capability.

2 Methods

Measurements were performed on 44 soccer players (age 20–33), all
competing in the first National league. Maximal aerobic power and
other cardiorespiratory measures (oxygen pulse, ventilatory
equivalent) were directly measured on a treadmill during a continuous
test. For this experimental work the ergopneumo-test electronic
equipment of Erich Jaeger (West Germany) was utilized.
 The following measures of respiratory function were performed at
rest: forced vital capacity (FVC), forced expiratory volume in the
first second (FEV_1), Tiffeneau's index (TIFF). Further, the heart
volume was measured using a modification of the method of Rohrer and
Musshoff (Medved, 1987).

3 Results and discussion

The results for the functional capacity of soccer players are shown
in Table 1. Basic results of respiratory function for athletes at
rest are far above population average values of similar age and
height (Heimer et al., 1985). Several researchers (Vaccaro et al.,
1975) believe that sport training develops hypertrophy of the
respiratory muscles. That may cause the higher values of lung
function. As both parameters are highly dependent on the respiratory

muscles' capability, whether hard training had developed this kind of hypertrophy or the athletes had started training with a better respiratory predisposition can be answered only after conducting longitudinal research.

Our results for maximal heart rate are similar to published data for soccer players and other athletes (Ekblom, 1986). The same values are under the average for non-athletes (Medved et al., 1987a). These results are in line with most of the published data. This could be indicative of the adaptation of the cardiovascular system to increased work loads.

The heart volume of a soccer player compared to a non-athlete is higher on average, compared to a volleyball or handball player it is equal, but compared to basketball players, swimmers or rowers it is significantly lower (Medved et al., 1987b). The average value of the heart volume working quotient is very good (42.4) and significantly below standard figures established by Reindel et al. (1967). These comparisons indicate a good economical and functional state of the cardiovascular and cardiopulmonary system of the soccer players investigated.

Absolute and relative maximal oxygen intake are higher than average values for non-athletes of the same age group in our country. However, it appears that our subjects have lower aerobic power compared to top players in Western Europe (Ekblom, 1986). This could be caused by the play itself. Coaches in Croatia prefer and enforce ball skills rather than physical fitness.

The average values of oxygen pulse (23.6) and its ventilation equivalent (30.3) lead us to conclude that the cardiopulmonary system of a soccer player is economical and effective.

The athletes were subdivided according to their playing position and the results of all the tests were submitted to analysis of variance (ANOVA). The goalkeepers, who are generally the least active, were tallest and heaviest and they had the highest forced vital capacity and aerobic power. When the aerobic power was expressed relative to body weight, the midfield players had the highest values. The defenders and the forwards had almost the same level of aerobic power, both in absolute and relative terms. The midfield players are probably the most active over long periods in the game.

4 Conclusion

The playing of soccer appears to require a high degree of cardio-respiratory fitness. The aerobic power of Croatian soccer players is significantly higher than the normal sedentary standards in Croatia. The high level of cardiorespiratory fitness is also shown through the values of oxygen pulse, ventilatory equivalent and heart volume working quotient. The midfield players have the highest values of $\dot{V}O_2$max expressed relative to body weight due to their intensive activity over long periods in the game. The least active, the goalkeepers, are heaviest and least fit aerobically.

Table 1.   Functional characteristics of soccer players

	Mean	SD
Age (years)	26.4	3.5
Body mass (kg)	77.5	7.1
Body height (cm)	179.1	5.9
Heart volume (ml)	888.1	134.9
Rel. heart volume (ml/kg)	12.1	1.1
Heart quotient	42.4	5.4
FVC (1)	6.0	0.7
FEV_1 (1/s)	4.9	0.6
TIFF (%)	81.7	6.2
$\dot{V}O_2$max (1/min)	4.12	0.64
$\dot{V}O_2$ (ml/kg/min)	52.07	10.71
HRmax (beats/min)	178	13
O_2 pulse (ml/bt)	23.63	3.60
$\dot{V}Eq$	30.28	5.33

5 References

Bale, P. (1986) A review of physique and performance qualities
    characteristic of games players in specific positions on the field
    of play. J. Sports Med. Phys. Fit., 26, 109-122.
Ekbolm, B. (1986) Applied physiology of soccer. Sports Med., 3,
    50-60.
Heimer, S., Matkovic, B., Medved, R., Medved, V. and Zuskin, E.
    (1985) Praktikum kinezioloske fiziologije, FFK, Zagreb.
Medved, R. (1987) Sportska Medicina. Jumena, Zagreb.
Medved, R., Matkovic, B.R., Misigoj-Durakovic, M., Pavicic, L.
    (1987a) Neki fiziolosko-funkcionalni pokazatelji djece i omladine
    muskog spola, uzrasta od 8-18. godina. Sportskomedicinski glasnik,
    3-4, 5-9.
Medved, R., Misigoj-Durakovic, M., Osvald, N. and Frankic D. (1987b)
    Srcano-volumni radni kvocijent u sportasa i spsortasica.
    Sportskomedicinski glasnik, 3-4, 19-24.
Raven, P.B., Gettman, L.R., Pollock,M.L. and Cooper, K.H. (1976) A
    physiological evaluation of profesional soccer players. Brit. J.
    Sports Med., 10, 209-216.
Reilly, T., Lees, A., Davids, K. and Murphy, W.J. (1988) Science and
    Football. E. and F.N. Spon, London.
Reindell, H., Konig, K., Roskamm, H. (1967) Funktionsdiagnostik des
    gesunden und kranken Herzens. Georg Thieme, Stuttgart.
Thomas, V., and Reilly, T. (1979) Fitness assessment of English
    league soccer players through the competitive season. Brit. J.
    Sports Med., 13, 103-109.
Vaccaro, P., Clarke, D.H. and Wrenn, J.P. (1975) Physiological
    profiles of elite women basketball players. J. Sports Med. Phys.
    Fit., 9, 45-54.

PHYSICAL PROFILE OF A FIRST DIVISION PORTUGUESE PROFESSIONAL SOCCER TEAM

Nelson Puga, Jose Ramos, Joaquim Agostinho, Isabel Lomba, Ovidio
Costa and Falcao de Freitas
Centro de Medicina Desportivo do Norte, Porto, Portugal

1 Introduction

One of the most important questions that most people involved in
football would like to have answered, is concerned with the
evaluation of the physical fitness of the players and their team. In
the laboratory the aerobic power ($\dot{V}O_2$max), ventilatory and blood
lactic acid responses to exercise, can be measured as determinants of
physical performance. The purpose of this work was to evaluate
maximal oxygen uptake, blood lactate and body composition in male
elite soccer players.

2 Methods

The sample consisted of 21 male professional soccer players from the
Portuguese First Division. They were broken down into 2 goalkeepers
(GK), 3 central defenders (CD), 2 lateral defenders (LD), 8
mid-fielders (MF) and 6 forwards (F).

As Table 1 shows, the tallest players were the goalkeepers and
central defenders respectively and the lowest heights were among the
forwards. The goalkeepers were the heaviest and the lateral
defenders the lightest of the group. The oldest were the central
defenders and the youngest of this team were the forwards.

A treadmill test was conducted using a continuous protocol. The
initial speed was 4 km/h with 2km/h increments every 3 min until
exhaustion and a constant slope of 2%. The $\dot{V}O_2$ was measured with a
Jaeger EOS Sprint equipment, and the mean ventilatory parameters were
obtained every 30 s. Blood samples were taken from the ear lobe, at
rest, 2, 3, 5 and 10 min after the exercise and lactate was
determined using an enzymatic method.

Table 1. Mean anthropometric characteristics of the players

	Goal-keepers (N=2)	Central Defenders (N=3)	Lateral Defenders (N=2)	Mid-Fielders (N=8)	Forwards (N=6)
Age (yrs)	28	29.3	26.5	28.4	25.8
Height (cm)	186	185.3	175	176.8	174.6
Body Mass	84.4	75.9	67.5	74	71.1
Body fat(%)	10.0	10.1	10.0	11.4	11.5

3 Results

For $\dot{V}O_2$ corrected for body weight (ml/kg/min) the higher values were found among lateral defenders (62.1 ml/kg/min), midfield players (61.9 ml/kg/min) and forwards (60.6 ml/kg/min). Lowest values were among the goalkeepers (52.7 ml/kg/min) and central defenders (54.8 ml/kg min), Fig. 1.

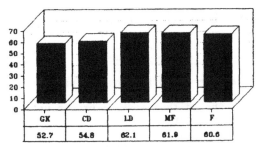

Fig. 1. The $\dot{V}O_2$max (ml/kg/min) according to playing position.

Peak lactates were highest in midfield players (MF) and forwards (F). Lateral defenders (LD) showed lowest lactacid capacity (Fig.2).

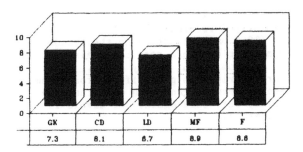

Fig. 2. Peak blood lactate (mmol/l) according to playing positions.

The maximal heart rate (HR) was lowest (184 beats/min) among the oldest sector, the central defenders (Fig. 3).
The fattest group was the forwards (11.5%). The groups with the lowest body fat percentage were goalkeepers (GK) and lateral defenders (LD).

4 Discussion and Conclusions

The physiological significance of the relationship between performance and aerobic power in soccer players remains controversial. Previous studies have demonstrated that aerobic power was not necessarily a performance limiting factor (Faina et al.

41

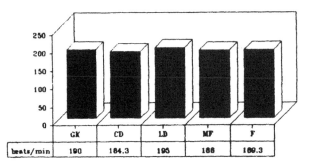

	GK	CD	LD	MF	F
beats/min	190	184.3	195	166	169.3

Fig. 3. Maximal heart rates for the different positions.

1988), while other studies showed that maximal oxygen uptake could be related to the distance covered during the game (Reilly, 1986). The present data show mean $\dot{V}O_2$max values similar to those found in the literature (Reilly et al., 1988). Considering the distribution of values in different positions on the field, our data were also similar to the literature (Reilly et al., 1988). The data suggest that different positions reflect different energy requirements. They support modern training concepts in soccer, which attempt to specialize the different activities of the performers.

Peak lactates are probably difficult to correlate with anaerobic level and performance in football. Our mean lactate values (8.2 mmol/l) were significantly lower than those 15 players from the German National Team (12.3 mmol/l) tested on the treadmill (Nowacki et al., 1988). The meaning of these results remain unclear. In the available literature (Ekblom, 1986; Reilly et al., 1988) the maximal lactate values measured during the game differ from 12 mmol/l to 5.87 mmol/l. The differences between groups in our study are very small (range 6.7 - 8.8 mmol/l) but, once again, our sample is too small to supply reliable information.

5 References

Ekblom, B. (1986) Applied physiology of soccer. Sports Med., 3, 50-60.

Faina, M., Gallozzi, C., Lupo, S., Colli, R., Sassi, R. and Marini, C. (1988) Definition of physiological profile of the soccer player, in Science and Football (eds T. Reilly, A. Lees, K. Davids, and W.J. Murphy), E and F.N. Spon, London, pp.158-163.

Nowacki, P.E., Cai, D.Y., Buhl, C. and Krummelbein, U. (1988) Biological performance of German soccer players (professionals and juniors) tested by special ergometric and treadmill methods, in Science and Football. (eds T. Reilly, A. Lees, K. Davids and W.J. Murphy) E. and F.N. Spon, London, pp.145-157.

Reilly, T. (1986) Fundamental studies on soccer. Sportswissenschaft und Sportspraxis, 57, 114-120.

Reilly, T., Lees, A., Davids, K. and Murphy, V.J. (1988) Science and Football. E. and F.N. Spon, London.

MAXIMAL AEROBIC POWER AND VENTILATORY THRESHOLD OF A TOP LEVEL SOCCER TEAM

J.H.P. VANFRAECHEM and M. TOMAS
Research Unit in Cardiorespiratory Physiology, Laboratoire de l'Effort,
I.S.E.P.K., Université Libre de Bruxelles, Brussels, Belgium

1 Introduction

The aim of this study is to establish the level of the cardiorespiratory parameters of a professional soccer team, in order to
point out practical implications concerning the training process.

2 Material and Methods

Subjects were 18 professional players of the Anderlecht RSCA soccer
team, their mean (+ SD) characteristics were : Age (Yr) : 24.7 ± 4.1,
Body Mass (kg) : 76.7 ± 6.4, Height (cm) : 181 ± 3.9, Body shape (m^2) :
1.96 ± 0.09.
  Data were collected during graded bicycle exercise with a 30 W/min
increement until volitional fatigue. All tests were administrated on
the same electronically braked ergometer (Ergoline). Respiratory values
were measured by means of the open-circuit method (Morgan pneumotacho-
graph) and the cardiac values with the Kubicek non-invasive electrical
impedance technique (IFM 400) (Kubicek et al., 1970). Respiratory
values were computed on-line and cardiac values were recorded every
2 min until exhaustion. Ventilatory threshold was assessed by means
of the Wasserman ventilatory method (1984).

3 Results

Maximal respiratory values (N = 18) were as follows : Watts : 308 ± 36,
VE (1/min) : 122 ± 27, $\dot{V}O_2$ (ml/min) : 4300 ± 521, $\dot{V}O_2$ (ml/kg/min) :
56.5 ± 7, RER : 1.07 ± 0.06, $\dot{V}E/\dot{V}O_2$: 28 ± 4, Oxygen pulse (ml/beat) :
26.3 ± 2.5.
  Maximal respiratory values were somewhat low in July, before the
beginning of the season, but ventilation efficiency is clearly assessed
through the value of the respiratory equivalent ($\dot{V}E/\dot{V}O_2 = 28$).
  The O_2pulse reached a high value of 26.3 ml/beat due to the rela-
tively low maximal HR inherent to bradycardia.
  Maximal cardiac values (N = 18) were as follows : HR (beats/min) :
166 ± 10, BPS (mmHg) : 211 ± 19, ventricular ejection time (VET) (ms) :
164 ± 23, PEP (ms) : 60 ± 11, SV (ml/beat) : 121 ± 33, cardiac output
(Q) (1/min) : 19.5 ± 5.7, EF (%) 58.3 ± 6, EDV (ml) : 209 ± 54.7.
  According to different authors, describing an inverse correlation
between HR and VET (Weissler et al., 1963 ; Vanfraechem, 1979), VET in
our study was not greatly reduced at maximal HR. Indeed, a 164 ms
ejection time at exhaustion corresponds to the LVET value recorded

below the ventilatory threshold (Tvent) in sedentary people.

Such a high value for LVET induces a great left ventricular stroke output (Weissler et al., 1969) which is required to compensate the HR bradycardia and maintain the cardiac output (Q) level.

Stroke output depends of EDV which is closely related to the venous return. So, a marked increase of EDV at maximal exercise emphasizes an optimal EF and SV.

Mean values at ventilatory threshold (Tvent) were (N = 18) : Watts 238, SV : 101 $\pm$ 30, HR : 146 $\pm$ 9, Q : 14.8 $\pm$ 4.8, $\dot{V}O_2$: 3.88 $\pm$ 0.48 (51 $\pm$ 6.4 ml/kg/min).

At ventilatory threshold, mean O_2 consumption reached 51 ml/kg:min and HR 146 b/min. This represents about 80 % of the values recorded during maximal exercise.

Power output corresponds to 77 % of the maximal power (308 W) sustained previously.

Moreover, statistically, the range of variation (CV %) is very low for the respiratory parameters but high for Q, due to the prevalent role played by the SV distribution.

4 Discussion

It is established that soccer is not a typical aerobic sport. It involves anaerobic alactic power for maximal efforts of 1 to 10 s duration, the anaerobic capacity for strenuous exercises during 20 to 45 s (ATP-PC + anaerobic glycolysis) and the lactic acid tolerance for heavy exercise lasting 1 to 8 min (anaerobic glycolysis).

Above 10 minutes and at submaximal exercise, the aerobic pathway becomes predominant (Skinner and Morgan, 1984 ; Costill, 1970 ; Gollnick and Hermansen, 1973).

The anaerobic performance training is generally based upon interval training in running and strength, 3 to 5 days per week, for 5 to 8 weeks, at maximal or near maximal intensity. The effect of training on classified anaerobic pathways depends on the duration of the training bouts versus rest, the number of repetitions, the ratio of work to rest and work intensity. It leads for anaerobic power to an ATP increase (Thorstensson et al., 1975), for anaerobic capacity to a glycolysis improvement resulting in a greater power output (Roberts et al., 1982) and for lactate tolerance to a lengthening of the performance time and a decrease of LA after standard workloads of similar duration (Houston and Thomson, 1977).

Concerning the importance of the aerobic system, which is the aim of this paper, aerobic training has been shown to cause a doubling of mitochondrial density (Holloszy et al., 1984) in muscle, resulting in a greater aerobic capacity of the muscle and for each cell, a lower demand of ATP at submaximal work.

The ATP/ADP ratio imbalance is reduced, and fat oxidation is increased, allowing carbohydrate conservation. As carbohydrate is the main fuel for anaerobic glycolysis, it is obvious that its saving, enhances the anaerobic capacity. Moreover the duration of the match is an important factor and necessitates great muscular aerobic capacity. It is thought that a value of 65 ml/kg/min $\dot{V}O_2$ max is required for top level play. According to Conley and Krahenbuhl (1980) it is clear that this $\dot{V}O_3$ max, allows a 13 % lower energy expenditure ($\dot{V}O_3$) at running speeds, from 12 to 21 km/h. To reach such values of $\dot{V}O_2$ max, a high SV is needed. In our study as a result of bradycardia, the deviation of PEP (shortening) and LVET (lengthening), decreases the PEP/LVET ratio. The linear regression between the 2 parameters is : EF % = 81.21-62.7 PEP/LVET (r = -0.96 ; P < 0.001).

The correlation between this ratio and EF is high. Both measures reflect the left ventricular contractile performance (Garrard, 1970).

A high EF corresponds to a short ratio and produces a good SV. In addition to a good EDV, linked to the venous return, the prevalent determinants of the O_2 transport system are present, to permit the maximal O_2 consumption enhancement.

In accordance with our results, to attain 65 ml/kg/min $\dot{V}O_2$ max, a 13 % increase is required. How could we realise that ?

At Tvent, HR reaches 146 beats/min at 80 % $\dot{V}O_2$ max. According to several authors (Nagle et al., 1970 ; Costill, 1970). Our data indicate that subjects are still in the aerobic pathway, below the lactate threshold.

Training at 146 beats/min represents 80 % of Karvonen's (1957) maximal HR reserve. The threshold exercise intensity necessary to produce a cardiovascular training effect, has been reported to be 60 %. So applied to field training, these basic concepts are valuable processes in developing the aerobic performance.

In conclusion, we think that top level soccer players have to reach the following maximal values : Power : > 300 W, $\dot{V}E$: > 120 l/min, $\dot{V}O_2$: > 65 ml/min/kg, anaerobic alactic power $\geqslant$ 900 W, HR : $\leqslant$ 180 beats/min, SV > 120 ml/beat, Q > 25 l/min, EF > 60 %, O_2pulse : > 25 ml/beat, $\dot{V}O_2$ at Tvent = 50 ml/min/kg, HR at Tvent = 150 beats/min.

5 References

Conley, D.L. and Krahenbuhl, G.S. (1980) Running economy and distance running performance of highly trained athletes. Med. Sci. Sports, 12, 357-360.

Costill, D.L. (1970) Metabolic responses during distance running. J. Appl. Physiol., 28, 251-255.

Gollnick and Hermansen, L. (1973) Biochemical adaptation to exercise : Anaerobic metabolism. Ex. Sport Sci. Rev., 1, 1-43.

Holloszy, J.O. and Coyle, E.F. (1984) Adaptation of skeletal muscles to endurance exercise and their metabolic consequences. J. Appl. Physiol., 56, 831-838.

Houston, M. and Thomson, J. (1977) The response of endurance adapted to adults to intensive anaerobic training. Europ. J. Appl. Physiol., 36, 207-213.

Karvonen, M.K., Kentala, M. and Mustaba, O. (1957) The effect of training heart rate. Ann. Med. Expl. Biol. Fenn., 35, 307-315.

Kubicek, W.G., Patterson, R.P., Witsae, D.A. (1970) Impedance cardiography as non-invasive method of non working cardiac function and other parameters of the cardiovascular system. Ann. N.Y. Acad. Sc., 170, 724-732.

Nagle, F.J., Robinhold, D., Howley, E., Daniels, J.T., Balesta, G. and Staedefalke, K. (1970) Lactic acid accumulation during running at submaximal aerobic demands. Med. Sci. Sports, 2, 182-186.

Roberts, A., Belleter, R. and Howald, H. (1982) Anaerobic muscle enzyme changes after interval training. Int. J. Sport Med., 3, 18-21.

Skinner, J.S., Morgan, D.W. (1984) Aspects of anaerobic performance in limits of human performance. American Academy of Physical Education Papers, 18, 31-44.

Thorstensson, A., Sjodin, B. and Karlsson, J. (1975) Enzyme activity and muscle strength after sprint training in man, Acta Physiol. Scand., 94, 313-318.

Vanfraechem, J.H.P. (1979) Stroke volume and systolic time interval adjustments during bicycle exercise. J. Appl. Physiol., 46, 588-592

Wasserman, K. (1984) The anaerobic threshold measurement to evaluate exercise performance. American Rev. Resp. Diseases, 129,suppl., 35-40.

Weissler, A.M., Harris, L.C. and White, D.G. (1963) Left ventricular ejection time index in man. J. Appl. Physiol., 18, 919-923.

Weissler, A.M., Hones, W.S. and Schoenfeld, C.D. (1969) Bedside technics for the evaluation of ventricular function in man. The Amer. J. Cardiol., 23, 577-583.

PHYSICAL FITNESS OF SOCCER PLAYERS AFFECTED BY A MAXIMAL INTERMITTENT EXERCISE "MIE."

H.NAGAHAMA, *, M.ISOKAWA**, S.SUZUKI*** AND J.O'HASHI****

*   DEPT. OF PHYSICAL EDUCATION, ASIA UNIV., TOKYO, JAPAN.
**   DEPT. OF PHYSICAL EDUCATION, TOKYO MET. UNIV., TOKYO,
     JAPAN.
*** DEPT. OF SPORTS SCIENCES, SEIKEI UNIV., TOKYO, JAPAN.
**** DEPT. OF SPORTS SCIENCES, DAITO BUNKA UNIV., SAITAMA,
     JAPAN.

1 Introduction

Soccer players cover about 10 km and need to sprint
repeatedly within irregular intervals during a 90 minute
game. They must also display some specialized skills of
soccer (Ekblom, 1986; Kirkendall, 1985; Reilly, 1986).
Considering energy delivery systems, both aerobic and
anaerobic capacities make up a soccer player's physical
fitness. Until now, studies have been made of the players'
actions by using match analysis techniques. Short duration
maximal efforts (the type of exercise used in the ATP-CP
system) appear approximately every 5 s and after 30 to 60 s
of aerobic recovery, then once again, maximal exercise is
performed (Nagahama et al., unpublished data). This pattern
of exercise is intermittent, and requires both aerobic and
anaerobic capacities (Saltin et al., 1976). There have
been, thus far, few reports made in the scientific field of
this type of study, especially involving soccer.
    Therefore, the present study has two purposes: i)to study
the maximal intermittent exercise "MIE," which is similar to
the activity found in a soccer match, with special reference
to the potentials of the three energy delivery systems;
ii)to estimate the physical fitness of soccer players with
this exercise.

2 Methods and Materials

2.1 Relationship between "MIE" and the three energy delivery systems
Thirty four volunteer soccer players who played in the First
Division of the Japanese Soccer League participated in this
study. Exercise bouts of 5 s maximal effort pedalling

repeated 20 times, were used to measure the "MIE" by using an electromagnetically braked cycle ergometer. The work load was set at 7.5% of body weight. Between each bout a 30 s active recovery period with no load was given. Blood lactate concentration was determined from a 75 ul fingertip blood sample taken after 5 min at the end of exercise by using an enzymatic method. The sum of the peak power in each bout was estimated as performance of "MIE."

On a separate day, maximal anaerobic power, 40 s power, and maximal O_2 uptake of each subject were measured for indexes of ATP-CP power, lactic power, and aerobic power, respectively.

Maximal anaerobic power (Nakamura et al., 1985) was used after the subjects performed approximately 10 s maximal pedalling on the electromagnetically braked cycle ergometer at three different loads, with 2 min rest between work.

A 40 s power test was used to assess the 'lactic' capacity. The subjects performed a 40 s maximal effort pedalling with the work load set at 7.5% of body weight. The mechanical mean power was measured during the last 10 s.

Finally, maximal O_2 uptake was measured by using the customary incremental exercise with the treadmill ergometer.

2.2 Comparison of the different levels using "MIE"

In addition to the previous subjects who were labelled the "Elite" group, 123 volunteer soccer players belonging to the Japan University Soccer League were also included. These subjects were divided into the following two sub-groups. The "Univ. 1" group players belonged to the upper league, and the "Univ. 2" group players belonged to the lower league.

The subjects of these two university groups were tested in the same way as the "Elite" group had been. Table 1 shows the characteristics of the three groups.

2.3 Statistical analyses

Differences between means were tested using an unpaired t test. Significance was set at the 0.05 level of confidence. All data are reported as mean ± SD. The Pearson correlation procedure was used to calculate the four capacities.

Table 1. Physical characteristics of the subjects.

Groups	n	Age(yrs)	Height(cm)	Body Mass(kg)
Elite	34	23.3±5.2	175.1±5.2	70.5±5.4
Univ.1(Upper)	17	19.7±1.0[*]	170.6±6.6[*]	65.2±6.8[**]
Univ.2(Lower)	106	19.9±1.1[***]	170.9±4.5[***]	62.8±4.7[***]

(*:p<0.05, **:p<0.01, ***:p<0.001, different from Elite group)

3 Results

Table 2 shows the results of the performance during the ATP-CP test, Lactic test, Aerobic test, and "MIE" test of the "Elite" group. Table 3 shows the correlation matrix for the four capacities. For the absolute value, these three energy delivery capacities were positively correlated with the performance of "MIE" (r=0.604 ~ 0.789, p<0.01). Next, at the normalized body weight, only the ATP-CP capacity was correlated with "MIE" (r=0.501, p<0.05). Finally, normalized to lean body mass, ATP-CP (r=0.539, p<0.01) and Lactic capacities (r=0.447, p<0.05) were correlated with the "MIE."

Table 2. Results of the performance of the ATP-CP power, Lactic power, Maximal O_2 uptake, and "MIE."

	ATP-CP (Anaerobic)	Lactic (Anaerobic)	Oxygen (Aerobic)	MIE
Abs.	1107.8±115.8 (watt)	475.3±47.4 (watt)	3.9±0.3 (1/min)	17023±2094 (watt)
/BW	15.9± 1.1 (watt/kg)	6.8± 0.5 (watt/kg)	55.8±4.0 (ml/kg/min)	241±19.2 (watt/kg)
/LBM	18.0± 1.2 (watt/kg)	7.8± 0.6 (watt/kg)	63.3±4.8 (ml/kg/min)	270±24.0 (watt/kg)

Figure 1 shows the performance of the "MIE" in the three groups. The performance of the "Elite" group was significantly higher than the other two groups. The performance of the "Univ. 1" group tended to be higher than that of the "Univ. 2" group but did not show the statistical significance at the normalized body weight (p>0.10).

Figure 2 shows 20 consecutive examples of mechanical peak power output in the three groups. The "Elite" group had a significantly higher power output in comparison to the other two groups from an early stage until the end of the exercise. "Univ. 1" had a significantly higher power output in comparison to the "Univ. 2" group, with the exception of the initial stage.

4 Discussion

Soccer players have to travel approximately 10 km during a game (Ekblom, 1986; Kirkendall, 1985; Reilly, 1986), and also need to sprint repeatedly. In other words, they must do both short duration maximal exercise and moderate endurance exercise. The present study has indicated that both aerobic and anaerobic energy delivery systems are necessary for "MIE," which is similar activity to that found

Table 3. The relationship between three energy delivery
capacities and the "MIE."

Absolute	1.ATP-CP	2.Lactic	3.Oxygen	4. MIE
1.ATP-CP	-----	0.701**	0.581**	0.789**
2.Lactic		-----	0.672**	0.705**
3.Oxygen			-----	0.604**
4. MIE				-----

/BW	1.ATP-CP	2.Lactic	3.Oxygen	4. MIE
1.ATP-CP	-----	0.372	0.206	0.501**
2.Lactic		-----	0.437*	0.344
3.Oxygen			-----	0.173
4. MIE				-----

/LBM	1.ATP-CP	2.Lactic	3.Oxygen	4. MIE
1.ATP-CP	-----	0.387	0.233	0.539**
2.Lactic		-----	0.496**	0.447*
3.Oxygen			-----	0.267
4. MIE				-----

$(*; p < 0.05, **; p < 0.01)$

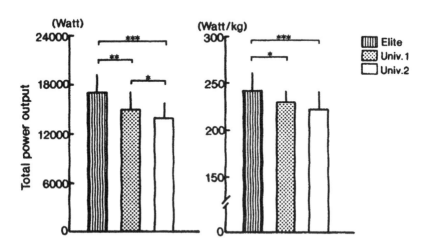

Fig. 1. Comparison of the sum of peak power during the
"MIE" in the three groups.

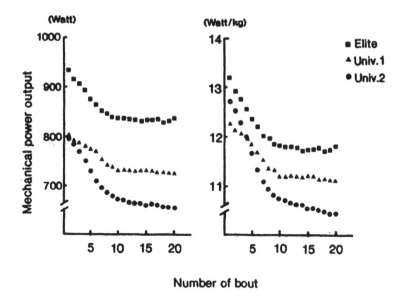

Fig. 2. Comparison of peak power curves obtained during the "MIE" in the three groups.

in a soccer match. It is known that the ATP-CP system is mobilized at the initial stage, and the glycolytic system is mobilized during a maximal continuous effort. But during intermittent exercise, the mobilized anaerobic system is mainly ATP-CP system (Margaria et al., 1969; Essen et al., 1977; Yamamoto and Kanehisa, 1989). The blood lactate level of the subjects showed 9.9±1.3 mmol/l at the end of "MIE." This values mean that "MIE" does not mainly use the glycolytic system. Therefore, these results suggest that soccer players require the use of both aerobic and anaerobic capacities, and especially require the use of the ATP-CP system. The reason is that soccer players must immediately recover or restore their ATP and CP during a short interval in order to succeed.

These results also suggest that when the competition level of the participants' is high, the performance of the "MIE" will increase. The subjects consume their ATP or CP in their skeletal muscles during "MIE," and they restore them during the recovery period by using the oxidative pathway (Yamamoto and Kanehisa, 1989, 1990). If the subjects' aerobic capacity is low, they cannot completely recover the ATP or CP. Perhaps the subjects whose results decreased abruptly were lacking in endurance capacity. In this case, the "Univ. 2" group's results decreased abruptly. However "Univ. 1" group's results did not decrease as rapidly when compared to the "Univ. 2" group during the 20 bouts. Therefore, it is suggested that the "Univ. 1" group had more endurance capacity when compared to the "Univ. 2" group. The "Elite" group appeared high in mechanical power output in each of the 20 trials and did not decrease in comparison to the "Univ. 2" group. It may be regarded that their regular training specifications helped them to maintain this high level of mechanical power. Players at a low performance level and young soccer players seem to lack muscle training, but they do seem to have adequate endurance training. As the players' level is raised or as players get older, they usually include more endurance, plus muscular strength training in their everyday practice. Therefore it may be this regular training influenced the performance of the "MIE."

In conclusion, after investigating the need for aerobic and anaerobic energy delivery systems, in connection with maximal intermittent exercise, we found that not only were those systems necessary, but also that the ATP-CP system was particularly important. It was further found that by measuring this intermittent exercise power, the physical fitness of soccer players could be estimated.

5 References

Ekblom, B. (1986) Applied physiology of soccer. **Sports Med.**, 3, 50-60.

Essen, B., Hagenfeldt, L. and Kaijser, L. (1977) Utilization of blood-borne and intramuscular substrates during continuous and intermittent exercise in man. **J. Physiol.**, 265,489-506.

Kirkendall, D. T. (1985) The applied sport science of soccer. **Physician Sportsmed.**, 13, 53-59.

Margaria, R., Oliva, R.D., DiPrampero, P.E. and Cerretelli, P. (1969) Energy utilization in intermittent exercise of supramaximal intensity. **J. Appl. Physiol.**, 26, 752-756.

Nakamura, Y., Mutoh, Y. and Miyashita, M. (1985) Determination of the peak power output during maximal brief pedalling bouts. **J. Sports Sci.**, 3, 181-187.

Reilly, T. (1986) Fundamental studies on soccer. **Sportwissenschaft und sportspraxis**, 57, 117-120.

Saltin, B., Essen, B. and Pedersen P. K. (1976) Intermittent exercise :its physiology and some practical applications. In :Advances in exercise physiology. **Med. Sport.**, 9, Karger, Basel, pp. 23-51.

Yamamoto, M. and Kanehisa, H. (1989) Endurance capacity of intermittent exercise: in relation to three energy delivery systems. **Hiroh to Kyuyo no Kagaku**, 4, 87-96.

Yamamoto, M. and Kanehisa, H. (1990) Mechanical power outputs of maximal intermittent exercise;in relation to anaerobic and aerobic working capacities. **Jap. J. Sports Sci.**, 9, 526-530.

CHANGE WITH AGE OF CARDIOPULMONARY FUNCTION AND MUSCLE STRENGTH IN MIDDLE AND ADVANCED-AGED SOCCER PLAYERS

T. Kohno, M.D., N. O'Hata, M.D., T. Shirahata, M.D., N. Hisatomi,
M.D., Y. Endo, M.D., S. Onodera, M.D., M. Sato, B.A.
Department of Sports Medicine, The Jikei University School of
Medicine, Tokyo, Japan

1 Introduction

At the first Congress in 1987 we delivered a presentation on the
topic 'Can senior citizens play soccer safely,' (Kohno et al., 1988)
in which we made five suggestions for safe and fun soccer playing by
senior citizens:

   (a) Play 20 minute halves
   (b) Use a small sized ball
   (c) Play on a regular pitch
   (d) Substitute freely
   (e) Only play opponents of the same age

   In order to determine whether soccer can be a lifetime sport for
senior citizens, we have conducted follow-up studies from a sports
medicine point of view. Here we will report on the changes in cardiopulmonary function and muscle power we found in these follow-up
studies over the past four years.

2 Subjects and Methods

The subjects in the 1986 study were 31 males aged from 54 to 77 years
old, with 62.9 years being the average age. At the time of the study
they were all company executives, who worked very hard, but still
enjoyed playing six twenty mintute soccer matches each Sunday.
   In 1990, four years after the first set of examinations, 11 of the
31 subjects were given follow-up examinations. These 11 ranged from
57 to 69 year old, with an average age of 62.3. All had continued
playing soccer for about two hours a week during the four years
between tests.
   The items on the two sets of examinations were identical, and are
listed in Table 1. Exercise tests were performed in a load-
incremental method, using a treadmill, with ECG and blood pressure
being determined both during and after exercise. At the same time the
maximum oxygen uptake was determined with an automatic metabolic
measurement system.
   Treadmill testing began at a 3% grade and a speed of 4 km/h. The
grade was held constant and the speed was increased 0.6 km/h every
minute. This protocol is special for senior citizens (see Figure 1).
   In determining when to stop the exercise tests, we used symptoms
including reported changes in self-awareness, exercise ECG, expected
maximum pulse rate, and oxygen uptake. For the measurement of knee

Table 1. Elements of the medical check-up given to subjects

At rest	Exercise Test
Blood examination	Exercise ECG
Urinalysis	Maximum oxygen uptake
Respiratory function	Muscle strength
X-ray examination	
ECG	
Blood pressure	
Anthropometry	

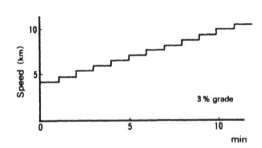

Fig.1. Protocol of treadmill testing .

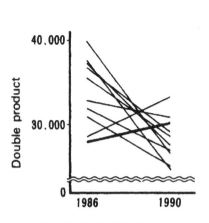

Fig.2. Individual changes
in double product.
(N = 11)

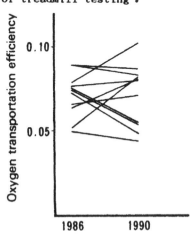

Fig.3. Individual changes in
oxygen transportation
efficiency. (N = 11)

extension and flexion strength, a Cybex II+ was used in the low range of 1.05 rad/s and at the moderate range of 3.14 rad/s.

3 Results

Data about the double product are shown in Figure 2. The double product is calculated by multiplying the maximum systolic blood pressure by the highest heart rate, and is a parameter indicating the oxygen demand of the myocardium. Eight of the eleven subjects showed a decrease in the double product from the first to the second testing.

Oxygen transportation efficiency, a value obtained by dividing the double product by the oxygen uptake, is shown in Figure 3. On comparing the two examination times, no change in the oxygen transportation efficiency was observed in eight cases. Thus the preparatory strength of coronary arterial circulatory function and

Table 2. Comparison of exercise ECG findings

| Heart Rate | First examination | | | | Second examination | | | |
| | ST-depression | | Arrhythmia | | ST-depression | | Arrhythmia | |
	No.Ss	%	No.Ss	%	No.Ss	%	No.Ss	%
Rest	0	–	0	–	0	–	0	–
to 119	1	9.1	1	9.1	3	27.3	2	18.2
120-139	6	54.5	2	18.2	4	36.4	1	9.1
140-up	7	63.6	1	9.1	3	27.3	1	9.1
After	6	54.5	2	18.2	3	27.3	4	36.4

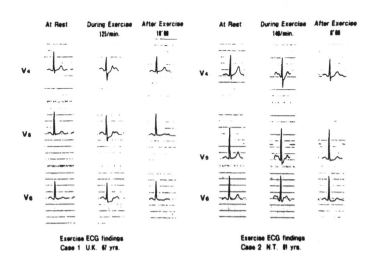

Fig.4. Exercise ECG findings – two individual cases.

peripheral vascular circulatory function were maintained during the
four years as was the resultant coronary arterial circulation.

Table 2 charts the changes in ECGs of the eleven follow-up subjects
over the four years. In terms of a decrease in ST, while the second
examinations as a whole showed a reduction as compared with the earlier data, only two cases showed evidence of severe ST-T depression.
Case 1 had a decrease in ST of 3 mm at 110 beats/min heart rate, and
the exercise test was terminated at that point (see Figure 4). Case 2
showed a decrease in ST of 2 mm when his heart rate surpassed 140
beats/min, lasting until eight minutes after the end of the exercise
period. These two subjects were given a coronary vasodilator and
exercise prescriptions were made according to their heart rates.

In terms of the change in V̇O2 max, the mean of the subjects in the
first test was 37.7 ml/kg/min, and in the second test was 33.5
ml/kg/min. Thus a decrease of about 11.2% was observed during the four
years. When individual cases were examined 7 cases showed a decrease
between the two times of testing (see Figure 5).

The results of the knee extension and flexion strength testing done
with the Cybex II+ are shown in Figure 6. Measured at 1.05 rad/s,
knee extension strength was 125.0 Nm in 1986 and 114.5 Nm in 1990, an
8.4% decrease. No change in flexion strength measured at 3.14 rad/s
was observed between these two times of testing. This means that muscle strength in the middle range had been maintained through playing
soccer once a week.

4 Discussion

Knowing how long you can continue to safely play the sport you love is
important for leading a healthy and enjoyable life. This is especially important for middle and advanced aged people, because physical
strength decreases with age. Sports suitable to their age become
limited. Kubota mentioned walking and golf as sports fitted for the

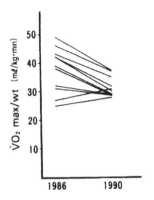

Fig.5. Individual changes in maximum oxygen uptake (N = 11).

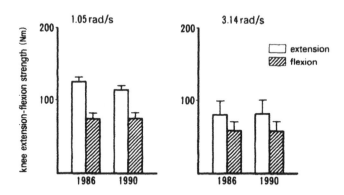

Fig.6. Changes in knee extension-flexion strength (Cybex II+).

middle and advanced aged. This is because low dynamic and low static
sports are suitable to this age group. To reverse this statement,
lowering of cardiopulmonary functioning and muscle power occurs with
aging, so sports that are too dymanic or static are not suitable.
However, there are those who want to continue to play the sports they
like after they become middle aged. For these people medical assessment as to whether to continue their sport and the prescription of
safe exercise limits are necessary.

Basically we found that it is possible for middle and advanced aged
people to play soccer safely as long as they keep some rules: They
should limit the intensity of exercise so that their pulse rates during exercise stay below 140 beats/min and they should get regular
medical check-ups. In this study we conducted a four year follow-up
study of middle and advanced aged soccer players. As a result of
their weekly soccer exercise we found improvement in double product
and oxygen transportation efficiency. Since it is vitally important
for this age group to improve coronary circulatory function it can be
said that the middle and advanced aged group can continue playing soccer safely. There were some who were judged as needing caution in the
exercise test. For these the exercise prescription was changed.

In playing sports, the most unfortunate incident is sudden death
during play (Tokutome, 1986). Sudden death can take place in any age
group and any sport, but fortunately none occurred among our cases.
Also, with ageing, lowering of physical strength becomes an obstacle
to continuing to play sports. The subjects of our study showed
slightly lowered endurance and low-range muscle power but not to the
exent of it becoming an obstacle to continuing to enjoy soccer. They
were able to maintain their mid-range muscle power as a result of
playing soccer.

5 Conclusions

Comparing the data from the four year follow-up tests with the initial tests, there was an increase in the oxygen transportation efficiency and a decrease in the oxygen demand of the myocardium. Therefore it appears that there is no major safety problem for continuing to play soccer. However, there were two subjects who showed some possibilities for ischaemic heart disease in the exercise test. Thus, soccer playing for men in this age range in not 100% safe, and regular medical check-ups are indicated.

Maximum oxygen uptake decreased by about 11.2% over the four years We found that the muscle power of knee extension and flexion was maintained. By playing soccer once a week we learned that it was possible to maintain the muscle power necessary to play sports.

Soccer is a moderate to highly dynamic and low static strength sport and may seem unsuitable for those of middle and advanced years. The results of the present study show soccer to be a sport which can be played safely by persons of middle and advanced years.

6 References

Kohno, T., O'Hata, N., Morita, H., Shirahata, T., Onodera, S., and Sato, M. (1988) Can Senior citizens play soccer safely? in Science and Football (eds T. Reilly, A. Lees, K. Davids and W.J. Murphy), E.& F.N. Spon, London, pp. 230-236.

Kubota, K. (1984) Sports and Brain Function, Tsukijishokan, Tokyo, pp. 127.

Tokutome, S. (1986) Actuality of sudden death during exercise. Medical Progress, 137, 442-444

A FITNESS EVALUATION OF GAELIC FOOTBALL CLUB PLAYERS

B. KIRGAN and T. REILLY
Centre for Sport and Exercise Sciences, Liverpool Polytechnic,
Liverpool, L3 3AF, England.

1 Introduction

Gaelic football is the national game in Eire and is played also in
countries with a sizeable population of first, second and third gen-
eration Irish immigrants. These include the United Kingdom, U.S.A.,
Australia and now European Community countries. The game was formally
organised at about the same time the other football codes were being
regulated and the first All-Ireland Championship was played in 1887.

Gaelic football calls on a variety of skills - kicking, passing
with hand or foot, catching, running, jumping, solo-runs, tackling,
blocking and so on. The full-size game is 15-a-side within a pitch
that is 130-145 m in length and 80-90 m wide. The game may flow
quickly from end to end and scores (points and goals) are frequent.
There is little published information about the fitness profiles of
Gaelic football players and whether the game has distinguishing
anthropometric and physiological characteristics among its participants. Consequently the aims of this study were to:

   (i) describe anthropometric and physiological profiles of an
       English club standard Gaelic football team;
  (ii) compare the characteristics with a reference group of games
       players of a corresponding competitive level.

2 Methods

Fifteen players (mean age ± S.D. = 20.6±1.5 years) from the
Lancashire County League (John Mitchell's Club) acted as subjects.
The reference group comprised 15 subjects (aged 22.3±1.6 years), all
of whom were in the Liverpool Polytechnic soccer squad.

A comprehensive test battery was applied to both groups. This
included anthropometry, body composition, "explosive leg strength"
anaerobic and aerobic power. The anthropometric variables were
height, body mass, ponderal index, somatotype (Heath and Carter,
1967), body composition (Durnin and Womersley, 1974). Vertical and
broad jumps were employed as measures of explosive leg strength
(Clarke, 1967) and both a stair run test (adapted from Margaria et
al., 1966) and the Wingate Test (cycle ergometer) as measures of
anaerobic power.

Maximal aerobic power ($\dot{V}O_2$max) was measured during a graded
incremental test on a motor-driven treadmill. During the test the

$\dot{V}O_2$ was computed on-line every 60 s using an automatic gas analyser (P.K. Morgan, Rainham).

Results for the two groups were formally compared using a series of t-tests. A P value of 0.05 was taken to indicate a significant difference.

3 Results and Discussion

The Gaelic footballers players had similar anthropometric profiles to the soccer players except for the lower mesomorphy. The estimated percent body fat values were compatible with sports participation in both groups (Table 1). The lower muscularity of the Gaelic footballers was reflected also in their poor performances in some of the muscular power tests. These included jumping ability (for distance), the stair run and mean power on the cycle ergometer (Table 2).

Table 1. Anthropometric profiles of the Gaelic football players and the reference group

	Gaelic Players (n=15)	Reference Group (n=15)
Height (cm)	174($\pm$5)	176($\pm$8)
Body mass (kg)	73.3 ($\pm$9.3)	79.7 ($\pm$9.3)
Ponderal Index	12.4$\pm$0.5	12.4$\pm$0.2
Body Fat (%)	14.5$\pm$2.2	15.9$\pm$2.5
Σ4 skinfolds (mm)	35.6$\pm$5.9	40.0$\pm$7.4
Somatotype:-		
Endomorphy	3.0$\pm$0.7	3.3$\pm$0.8
Mesomorphy	3.1$\pm$0.8	4.2$\pm$0.8 **
Ectomorphy	1.6$\pm$1.6	1.6$\pm$0.6

**Indicates P<0.01

Table 2. Fitness profiles of the Gaelic football players and the reference group

	Gaelic Players (n=15)	Reference Group (n=15)
Wingate Test:		
Mean Power (W)	518$\pm$59	683$\pm$99 **
(W/kg)	6.8$\pm$0.9	8.9$\pm$1.3 **
Peak Power (W)	838$\pm$88	864$\pm$99
(W/kg)	11.2$\pm$1.4	10.7$\pm$1.0
Stair Run (W)	1049$\pm$99	1196$\pm$85 **
Vertical Jump (cm)	48.6$\pm$4.7	51.0$\pm$5.5
Broad Jump (cm)	210$\pm$8	235$\pm$20 **
$\dot{V}O_2$max (ml/kg/min)	47.6$\pm$5.3	48.9$\pm$4.4

**Indicates P<0.01

The Gaelic footballers' performances matched those of the soccer players in vertical jumping; this may be due to the need to contest high catches among all outfield players. The groups were also comparable in peak power output: this ability could be important in the course of the acceleration required in both games to run with possession of the ball or run off-the-ball.

Both groups had $\dot{V}O_2$max values compatible with sports participation at club level. The mean values of 48 and 49 ml/kg/min failed to single them out as aerobically well trained or well endowed. Indeed, the aerobic power of the Gaelic footballers is likely to have had little influence from physical training since participation in the game in the United Kingdom tends to be motivated by cultural rather than fitness factors. Consequently a programme of systematic training for competitive match-play would enhance the performance capabilities of these Gaelic players.

At Club level it seems that Gaelic football players competing in English county games do not demonstrate distinguishing fitness adaptations. Besides, they would seem to lack the anthropometric requirements for high level play, being smaller and lighter than the successful All-Ireland inter-county finalists (Reilly, 1990). Their muscle power performances were not as well developed as soccer players at a comparable level, although the groups were similar in most other features. Results suggest that in the absence of a systematic training programme specific to match-play demands, Gaelic football club players have no extraordinary anthropometric or physiological characteristics.

4 References

Clarke, H.H. (1967) **Application of Measurement to Health and Physical Education.** Prentice-Hall, New York.

Durnin, J.V.G.A. and Womersley, J. (1974) Body fat assessed from total body density and its estimation from skinfold thickness: measurements on 481 men and women aged 16 to 72 years. **Brit. J. Nutr.**, 32, 77-97.

Heath, B.H. and Carter, J.E.L. (1967) A modified somatotype method. Amer. **J. Phys. Anthrop.**, 97, 57-74.

Margaria, R., Aghemo, P. and Rovelli, E. (1966) Measurement of muscular power (anaerobic) in man. **J. Appl. Physiol.**, 21, 1662-1664.

Reilly, T. (1990) **Football, in Physiology of Sports** (eds T.Reilly, N.Secher, P.Snell and C.Williams). E. and F.N. Spon, London, pp.371-425.

A COMPARATIVE ANALYSIS OF SELECTED MOTOR PERFORMANCE VARIABLES IN AMERICAN FOOTBALL, RUGBY UNION AND SOCCER PLAYERS

WERNER KUHN
Free University of Berlin, Germany

1   Introduction

The study was conducted to compare general motor performance variables of players from different football codes under standardized conditions. So far studies that have been carried out have tended to concentrate on one specific code (Reilly et al., 1988). Each football code is highly specific from a technical, tactical and conditioning standpoint. Besides, playing position places specific demands on players. Therefore, there are very few top players who have switched codes or have excelled in two or more football codes. Because of the high degree of specific factors (Douge, 1988), differences in general motor performance variables can also be expected. The aim of the study was twofold:
i)   to determine whether any differences in a general motor fitness test battery exist between American Football, Rugby Union and soccer teams;
ii)   to examine differences with regard to position in each code.

2   Methodology

2.1 Performance tests
All three teams were tested within four weeks during the final stage of their respective competitive season. A standardized warm-up was used before administering the tests: 5 min run on the treadmill at a speed of 2.5 m/s and 5 min of individual stretching exercises. The performance tests incorporated skinfold thickness, anticipation, coordination, flexibility, muscle strength and endurance tests.

Skinfold thickness was recorded at three sites: triceps, abdominal and suprailiac, using skinfold calipers. A composite score (in mm) was taken.

Visual anticipation was tested with a Bassin anticipation timer 2.88 m in length. Constant Error (CE), absolute error (Abs E) and variability error (Var E) were computed over 12 trials using different speeds (2 miles/h, 4 miles/h, 6 miles/h, 8 miles/h). Only eye-hand coordination was tested.

For agility a modified Herzberg (1968) test was used. The subject performed an obstacle course in which jumping, rolling and bending movements as well as different changes of direction were demanded. Time (s) was taken.

For visual-spatial orientation the test by Hirtz (1985, p. 133) was modified. The subject had to jump down from a 0.90 m high box and come as closely as possible to a target line with his heels. The average deviation of both heels was measured. The CE, Abs E and Var E were computed.

For dynamic balance the test by Hirtz (1985, p. 138) was modified. The subject had to hold in his extended right arm a little ball and touch his ear with his left arm, circling the right arm. The subject had to balance in this position over a beam (10 cm high and wide), kick down a medicine ball at the turning-point and balance back to the starting line. Time (s) and number of ground touches with one or two feet were registered.

For flexibility of the hip flexors, the subject had to bend down from the waist with his knees locked. Deviation from the 0 line was measured (in cm).

For flexibility of the hamstring muscles, the subject lay in a supine position, with one leg extended, the other elevated. The angle between the two legs was measured.

For explosive strength of the legs, two consecutive horizontal jumps from a standing position were performed. Both measurements (metres) were taken. The subject was instructed to minimize floor contact at take-off to the second jump.

Maximal strength (in kg) for the dominant and non-dominant hand grip muscles was tested with a hand dynamometer. Strength differentiation for the dominant and non-dominant hand grip muscles was determined. Thirty seconds after testing the maximal strength, the subject was asked to press with 50% of his maximal strength. The undershooting/overshooting was registered in percentages of the actual value (equals 100%).

Various strength measurements for leg extensors and flexors were taken with a computerized strength testing machine (Schnell company). Isometric, concentric and eccentric strength scores (Nm) were registered. The Schnell machine is driven by an electric motor that moves the training bar of the training arm via a connecting rod. Continuous pressure can be applied on the training bar. This pressure is registered through a torque measuring device as net torque [Nm]. Manually or by means of computer software, precise speeds of the training arm can be described. When used for dynamic testing and training, the training arm travels with a defined speed from a low to a high turning-point and vice versa. In the middle of the amplitude approximate isokinetic movement speeds are obtained. For static strength testing and training the training arm can be stopped at any angle.

Aerobic capacity was measured by an anaerobic threshold test on a treadmill. The speed (m/s) at the 4 mM lactate threshold (V-4 mM) was registered.

2.2 Subjects

Three teams were selected from the Berlin area on the basis
of three regular work-outs per week during the competitive
season. The American Football and Rugby Union teams are
members of the highest national league in Germany, whereas
the soccer team belonged to the top amateur league in
Berlin at the time of the study.

3   Results and discussion

An overview of team data with regard to position, age,
height and body mass for each football code is given in
Table 1. There are marked differences in age, height and
body mass. In the samples we used, American Football and
Rugby Union players were younger, taller and heavier than
soccer players.

The differences in body-size, indicated by height and
body mass, are as expected considering the fact that
American Football and Rugby Union are typical contact
games. There was a pronounced specificity of position in
these basic measurements. The average playing experience
was 4.86 (SD = 1.52) years for American Football, 9.41 (SD
= 2.33) years for Rugby Union and 15.73 (SD = 2.23) years
for soccer. These figures reflect to a certain extent the
tradition of each code in Germany.

Table 1. Team and position data (X̄, SD) for each football
code

Football	Position	Age		Height		Body Mass	
Code		X̄	SD	X̄	SD	X̄	SD
American Football (n = 22)	Attack Line	22.2	4.7	184.4	3.9	99.3	7.9
	Attack Ball	21.1	1.4	178.9	7.1	80.6	12.5
	Defence Line	21.0	1.6	184.5	2.5	109.5	18.8
	Defence Ball	22.0	3.0	184.1	3.7	84.6	8.7
	Total	21.6	2.8	182.6	5.3	91.8	15.9
Soccer (n = 15)	Defence	22.6	4.1	177.5	9.5	73.6	8.6
	Midfield	23.8	4.4	173.7	9.3	71.9	8.0
	Attack	25.5	6.4	178.3	8.1	73.3	9.6
	Total	23.5	4.2	176.1	8.8	72.8	7.9
Rugby Union Football (n = 17)	Attack	23.0	3.0	188.3	5.3	99.7	9.8
	Defence	22.4	3.5	180.3	5.0	77.9	6.3
	Total	22.7	3.2	184.1	6.5	88.2	13.7

An overview of results (X̄, SD) for all performance
tests of the three codes over all positions is given in
Table 2. One-way analyses of variance (ANOVA) were employed
to assess the differences between the teams. Statistical
analyses for the positional factor within each code were
not conducted due to the small number of subjects.

Table 2. Overview of results (X ± SD) for all performance tests of the three codes over all positions

	American Football	Soccer	Rugby Union Football
Skinfolds	51.1 ± 22.4	27.1 ± 7.5	45.5 ± 25.2
Anticipation (CE)	-0.2 ± 0.2	-0.1 ± 0.4	-0.1 ± 0.2
Anticipation (Abs E)	0.3 ± 0.1	0.4 ± 0.1	0.3 ± 0.1
Anticipation (Var E)	0.3 ± 0.1	0.3 ± 0.1	0.2 ± 0.1
Agility	7.8 ± 0.9	7.5 ± 0.7	8.0 ± 0.6
Visual-spatial orientation (CE)	-4.5 ± 5.7	-0.9 ± 4.1	-3.2 ± 3.1
Visual-spatial orientation (Abs E)	4.9 ± 5.4	3.4 ± 2.3	3.7 ± 2.4
Dynamic balance	7.5 ± 3.6	7.0 ± 2.8	7.3 ± 2.2
Flexibility (hip flexors)	7.5 ± 6.0	7.3 ± 3.9	4.8 ± 7.7
Flexibility (hamstrings dominant)	84.5 ± 7.5	87.4 ± 7.1	83.8 ± 13.2
Flexibility (hamstrings non-dominant)	88.0 ± 11.8	88.5 ± 10.5	86.3 ± 9.2
Standing broad jump (1st jump)	2.2 ± 0.2	2.1 ± 0.2	2.1 ± 0.2
Standing broad jump (2nd jump)	2.5 ± 0.3	2.5 ± 0.2	2.5 ± 0.2
Hand grip strength (dominant 100%)	61.2 ± 10.9	52.8 ± 7.7	63.8 ± 9.9
Hand grip strength (dominant 50%)	35.5 ± 10.7	34.1 ± 8.2	41.3 ± 11.4
Hand grip strength (non-dominant 100%)	61.1 ± 10.2	53.3 ± 9.8	61.2 ± 9.3
Hand grip strength (non-dominant 50%)	37.5 ± 10.6	33.2 ± 6.7	40.1 ± 10.3
Absolute isometric strength (extensors, dominant)	336.8 ± 62.4	262.0 ± 42.1	327.7 ± 75.2
Absolute isometric strength (extensors, non-dom.)	344.5 ± 72.8	269.3 ± 45.4	337.1 ± 69.2
Absolute isometric strength (flexors, dominant)	172.3 ± 33.5	144.7 ± 40.0	172.4 ± 24.9

	American Football	Soccer	Rugby Union Football
Absolute isometric strength (flexors, non-dom.)	174.1 ± 33.1	144.7 ± 39.1	161.2 ± 30.2
Relative isometric strength (extensors, dominant)	3.7 ± 0.6	3.6 ± 0.4	3.7 ± 0.5
Relative isometric strength (extensors, non-dom.)	3.8 ± 0.6	3.7 ± 0.6	3.8 ± 0.6
Relative isometric strength (flexors, dominant)	1.9 ± 0.3	2.0 ± 0.4	2.0 ± 0.3
Relative isometric strength (flexors, non-dom.)	1.9 ± 0.3	2.0 ± 0.4	1.8 ± 0.3
Absolute isometric strength (extensors non-dom./dominant)	1.0 ± 0.1	1.1 ± 0.3	1.0 ± 0.1
Absolute isometric strength (flexors non-dom./dominant)	1.0 ± 0.1	1.0 ± 0.1	0.9 ± 0.1
Absolute isometric strength (dominant, flexors/extensors)	0.5 ± 0.1	0.6 ± 0.1	0.6 ± 0.1
Absolute isometric strength (non.-dom., flexors/extensors)	0.5 ± 0.1	0.5 ± 0.2	0.5 ± 0.1
Absolute concentric strength (extensors)	478.1 ± 115.0	332.8 ± 83.4	452.5 ± 112.4
Absolute eccentric strength (extensors)	655.0 ± 155.7	554.7 ± 128.8	645.7 ± 154.0
Absolute isometric strength (extensors)	671.4 ± 137.7	504.0 ± 102.5	655.3 ± 160.8
Absolute concentric strength (flexors)	254.6 ± 50.8	207.2 ± 59.2	263.4 ± 44.1
Absolute eccentric strength (flexors)	330.2 ± 57.8	286.2 ± 85.6	331.6 ± 56.6
Absolute isometric strength (flexors)	306.4 ± 52.7	268.0 ± 74.4	290.6 ± 54.8
Anaerobic threshold (speed m/s)	3.1 ± 0.5	3.9 ± 0.3	3.4 ± 0.4

An overview of the composite scores of the skinfold measurements for each code and position is provided in Figure 1. The F-ratio ($F_{2,51}$ = 6.35) was significant (P $\leq$ 0.01). Newman-Keuls post-hoc test revealed that soccer players had significantly lower skinfolds than American (P $\leq$ 0.01) and Rugby Union Football (P $\leq$ 0.05) players. Except for soccer there were marked positional effects.

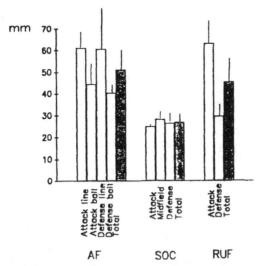

Fig. 1. Composite scores of the skinfold measurements for each code and position.

For visual anticipation, the F-ratios were significant for the Abs E and Var E ($F_{2,51}$ = 3.96 respectively 3.64, P $\leq$ 0.05), not for the CE ($F_{2,51}$ = 2.15). A post-hoc test showed that Rugby Union players performed significantly better than soccer players (P $\leq$ 0.05). A possible explanation is that the test situation favoured the Rugby players since the response button had to be pressed manually.

The F-ratios for the three tests of coordination were not significant (Agility: $F_{2,51}$ = 1.36; visual-spatial orientation: $F_{2,51}$ = 2.77, 0.80 and 1.85 for CE, Abs E and Var E; dynamic balance: $F_{2,51}$ = 0.13). There were large differences between positions in American Football. The defensive linemen in particular had relatively low scores in visual-spatial orientation and dynamic balance.

None of the F-ratios for the two tests of flexibility reached significance: $F_{2,51}$ = 1.06 (hip flexors), $F_{2,51}$ = 0.63 and 0.20 (dominant and non-dominant hamstrings). Overall, flexibility of these two muscle groups was poor.

All F-ratios for the absolute scores of dominant and non-dominant maximal hand grip strength, of dominant and non-dominant maximal isometric, concentric and eccentric

strength of upper leg extensors and flexors were
significant ($P \leq 0.05$; $P < 0.01$). American and Rugby Union
Football players had significantly higher absolute upper
leg strength scores than soccer players. However, all three
codes did not differ in their relative strength scores.

The F-ratios for the quotient upper leg flexors/upper
leg extensors were not significant ($F_{2,51}$ = 0.81 and 1.43).
All codes displayed a more or less pronounced functional
imbalance of strength in the upper leg. A quotient of 0.66
for knee flexors to knee extensors is generally considered
as a safe guideline. The F-ratios for explosive strength of
the legs were not significant for jump 1 and 2 ($F_{2,51}$ =
0.42 and 0.12).

In hand grip strength differentiation, subjects on the
average overshot the prescribed goal of 50% of their
maximal strength. Overall, American Football players
reproduced significantly (5%) better for the dominant hand
($F_{2,51}$ = 3.51). This result was not confirmed for the non-
dominant hand ($F_{2,51}$ = 2.21). Positional differences were
pronounced in American Football.

A significant ($P \leq 0.01$) F-ratio was obtained for the
team factor ($F_{2,51}$ = 14.47) in aerobic capacity. A post-hoc
test revealed that soccer players reached the 4 mM
threshold at a significantly higher speed than the other
two teams. Further, Rugby Union players differed
significantly from American Football players (Figure 2).
This finding can be explained by the demand profile of each
sport. American and Rugby Union Football can be
characterized as typical stop and go games, whereas soccer
is a relatively continuous game, requiring a higher degree
of aerobic power. In American Football specificity of
position was again high. The ball-oriented defence
displayed speeds at the V-4mM threshold that almost
equalled those in soccer.

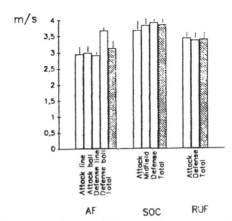

Fig. 2. Treadmill speeds (m/s) at the anaerobic
threshold for each code and position.

4 Conclusion

Based upon the conditions of this study it was concluded that there were differences between the three football codes with regard to constitutional factors (height, body mass), skinfold thicknesses, visual anticipation, various absolute strength measurements (hand grip, upper leg) and the aerobic capacity. There were no differences with regard to several coordination factors, flexibility, explosive leg strength and the corresponding relative strength measurements.

Specificity of player position was particularly pronounced in American Football, to a much lesser extent in Rugby Union Football and soccer.

5 References

Douge, B. (1988) Football: The common threads between the games, in Science and Football (eds T. Reilly, A. Lees, K. Davids and W.J. Murphy), E. and F.N. Spon, London, pp. 3–19.

Herzberg, P. (1968) Testbatterie zur Erfassung der motorischen Lernfähigkeit. Theorie und Praxis der Körperkultur, 17, 1066–1078.

Hirtz, P. (1985) Koordinative Fähigkeiten im Schulsport. Berlin: Volk und Wissen.

Reilly, T., Lees, A., Davids, K. and Murphy, W.J. (eds) (1988) Science and Football. E. and F.N. Spon, London, pp. 145–210.

The Liverpool Polytechnic ▮

● **OUR NAME . . .**

from **September 1,**

Liverpool John Moores University

School of Human Sciences

Diploma in Science and Football
1 year full-time
M.Phil, Ph.D part-time and full-time research

The Centre for Sport and Exercise Sciences at Liverpool John Moores University now runs a one year full-time course leading to a Diploma in Science and Football. The focus of the course is on the application of science to an understanding of the game. Association football (soccer) in particular is the field of study. The city of Liverpool is ideally suited for this specialisation, being the home of two leading soccer clubs, Everton and Liverpool.

The Centre has a good academic basis for this unique development: it initiated a B.Sc (Hons) degree course in Sports Science in 1975. Students on the Diploma course have access to laboratory facilities and other teaching resources used by the B.Sc (Hons) and M.Sc (Sports Science) students. The Centre hosted the First World Congress of Science and Football in 1987. It also offers opportunities for M.Phil and Ph.D research (part-time and full-time) on topics related to football. Students on the M.Sc (Sports Sciences) course may choose football for a research topic in their dissertation.

The Diploma course is the first of its kind in the world, is interdisciplinary and includes physiology of training; match-play; nutrition; fitness testing and evaluation; injury prevention; psychology of soccer; football violence; motivation; skills analysis; talent identification; management of players; club resources; computerised match-analysis; patterns of play, biomechanics of football skills, football surfaces. Elements of the course are conducted in collaboration with professional clubs. Additionally, students on the Diploma course have the opportunity to gain formal coaching qualifications.

Applications are invited from individuals with a practical background in association football. They should be able to demonstrate an ability to cope with academic work at an advanced level.

Further particulars and application forms are available from:

Admissions, Science and Football, Centre for Sport and Exercise Sciences, School of Human Sciences, Liverpool John Moores University, Byrom Street, Liverpool, L3 3AF, UK

PART THREE

Physiology of Training

COMPUTER-CONTROLLED ASSESSMENT AND VIDEO-TECHNOLOGY FOR THE DIAGNOSIS OF A PLAYER'S PERFORMANCE IN SOCCER TRAINING

WALDEMAR WINKLER
University of Goettingen, Goettingen, Germany

1 Introduction

The aim of using diagnostic means and methods in soccer is to obtain the highest degree of objectivity in the evaluation of a player's performance during training and in matches. New technology now enables coaches and physical education experts to make more exact and more complete assessments of a player's performance with regard to fitness, motor skills, or the realization of tactical abilities. This will be demonstrated by giving examples of how such technology has been applied in the area of physical conditioning. Actual results of a test study done in training with a Junior A-team (17-18 year olds) are presented in the form of computer print-outs. Finally, the implications of using video technology in training and game analysis are briefly discussed.

2 Computer-controlled assessment-systems for testing important physical fitness factors in soccer training

Physical fitness factors such as sprint velocity, jumping strength, and aerobic endurance have always been considered to be the basis for playing soccer successfully. A number of recent studies have helped to shed light on the actual physical demands placed upon a soccer player and have, as a result, also been useful in the development of valid tests to measure a player's physical performance. Analyzing the movements of all players (excluding the goal-keepers) at the same time during a game with the aid of a Dual-Video-System (Winkler, 1991), we obtain insights into the demands made on each player. At the same time we gain important input with regard to the structuring of basic conditioning tests. This is necessary because many endurance tests have distinct disadvantages. Some of these tests have little to do with soccer e.g. an ergometer test in a laboratory. Others are not standardized or require trained personnel to be implemented and/or evaluated. This has obvious financial implications. An example of the latter type is any test in which blood samples are taken to determine lactate levels. Such tests are therefore of little use to the average trainer as are tests like the "Cooper-Test" which gives - without measuring blood lactate at the same time - rather inexact information on the endurance capabilities of soccer players (Gerisch, 1990).

All the endurance tests which have to be implemented in a laboratory as well as tests which measure only linear movement and/or tests in which players have to run at a steady speed, must make way for tests geared to the actual situation of the soccer player. "The first step in this direction" could be Probst's (1988) "Interval Test".

As my studies have also revealed, it is imperative that sprint velocity over a distance of at least 30 metres be measured at certain intervals. Thus it is possible to recognize precisely any weaknesses players may have as far as their ability to accelerate is concerned.

The significance of physical strength can be observed in connection with skills such as jumping (to head the ball), passing, or shooting. Because the physical requirements of jumping are so great, it also makes sense to include a test which measures vertical jump.

Therefore, in a diagnosis program we need at least **three tests** which, if applied correctly (especially under "standard situations") during training, can produce objective and exact assessments of a player's performance with regard to his physical conditioning.

i)   **30-Metre Sprint-Test** to measure the sprint velocity.

A player starts on his own from an electronic starting mat. His times are measured by light barriers after 5, 10, 15, 20 and 30 m. These times are then fed into a computer (another type of measuring system makes it possible to feed the times directly into a computer). Through application of a special computer program all times are ranked according to the 30 m time of each youth soccer player and then printed out in this order (Table 1).

This allows differentiated judgements concerning the performances of all players to be made.

ii)   **Vertical Jump-Test** to measure the jump-time "t" and compute the jump height as an indication of vertical jump.

It is important that this kind of vertical jump is always performed under the same standard conditions mentioned above. A player, wearing sneakers, stands with both feet on an electronic jump-mat lying on a hard, flat surface. Then he jumps straight up 3 times without using his arms (both arms on the lower back) and then 3 times using his arms. As he jumps, the player should extend his legs and feet completely. He should land using the same technique. The rest between the jumps should be at least 20 s. The jump height "h" is computed with the formula: $h = 1/8 \times g \times t^2$ ($g = 9.81$ m/s^2). All values are fed into the computer which calculates the average of the two best

Table 1. Results of the 30 m Sprint

INTERVALS in meters (m), interval-times in seconds,
RK = rank, IDN = identity number, YOB = year of birth,
SUM = sum of all interval-times, JUDGE = judgement.

RK	IDN	YOB	INTERVALS (m) 0- 5	5- 10	10- 15	15- 20	20- 30	SUM	JUDGE
1	372	73	1.00	0.72	0.63	0.58	1.14	4.07	+++
2	377	74	0.97	0.73	0.65	0.61	1.14	4.10	+++
3	368	72	1.01	0.74	0.65	0.60	1.16	4.16	++
4	378	72	0.98	0.73	0.65	0.61	1.20	4.17	++
5	379	73	1.01	0.73	0.66	0.62	1.19	4.21	+
6	375	72	0.99	0.76	0.67	0.62	1.19	4.23	+
7	371	73	1.04	0.75	0.66	0.61	1.18	4.24	+
8	373	73	1.01	0.76	0.67	0.63	1.19	4.26	+
9	369	73	1.03	0.76	0.67	0.64	1.21	4.31	0
10	376	74	1.05	0.77	0.67	0.63	1.20	4.32	0
11	370	73	1.05	0.77	0.68	0.63	1.21	4.34	0
12	374	72	1.10	0.80	0.68	0.64	1.23	4.45	-
	mean		1.02	0.75	0.66	0.62	1.19	4.24	

Scale of judgement:

excellent	+++	≤ 4.10 s
very good	++	≤ 4.20 s
good	+	≤ 4.30 s
average	0	≤ 4.40 s
below average	-	≤ 4.50 s
weak	--	≤ 4.60 s
very weak	---	› 4.60 s

Table 2. Results of the Vertical Jump

RK = rank, IDN = identity number, YOB = year of birth, JUMP
HEIGHTS without/with = jump heights without/with use of
arms, DIF = jump difference without/with use of arms,
JUDGE = judgement, WT = weight, HT = height.

RK	IDN	YOB	JUMP HEIGHTS without cm	with cm	DIF cm	JUDGE without	WT kg	HT cm
1	372	73	49.0	56.0	7.0	++	60	168
2	378	72	44.0	49.0	5.0	+	74	178
3	379	73	40.5	47.0	6.5	0	70	181
4	377	74	40.0	48.0	8.0	0	72	175
5	376	74	40.0	46.5	6.5	0	66	179
6	368	72	40.0	44.0	4.0	0	74	182
7	375	72	38.0	45.0	7.0	0	74	176
8	371	73	34.0	36.0	2.0	-	64	166
9	369	73	33.5	37.5	4.0	-	67	175
10	373	73	33.0	35.0	2.0	-	76	181
11	374	72	32.5	41.5	9.0	-	80	187
12	370	73	28.0	32.0	4.0	--	65	172
	mean		37.7	43.1	5.4		70	177

Scale of judgement:

excellent	+++	≥ 51.00 cm
very good	++	≥ 46.00 cm
good	+	≥ 41.00 cm
average	0	≥ 36.00 cm
below average	-	≥ 31.00 cm
weak	--	≥ 26.00 cm
very weak	---	‹ 26.00 cm

jumps of both types for each athlete and then ranks the players according to the height they reached. The data obtained can be interpreted with the aid of a performance scale based on results of previous tests or even better "norm-data". Table 2 shows the results of this vertical jump-test with the aforementioned youth team. By comparing the results of the two types of jumps, the difference between them will be obvious. In the first case we measure the jump height without using the arms which is an indication of "pure" jumping ability and in the second case a combination of strength and coordination (as the arms are also used). Both in the sprint test and the vertical jump test the trainer obtains a differentiated picture of his players' performance; at the same time he establishes a rank order among his players. If these tests could be administered to a representative sample of players in a country, a trainer would have optimal performance comparisons.

Having made such an exact diagnosis, the trainer can then design a training programme to fit the individual needs of each player.

iii)   **Endurance-Test** (Interval-Field-Test) to determine the "anaerobic threshhold" of a soccer player.

The field-test developed by Probst (1988) has the following advantages:

-   It is more closely related to the reality of soccer, for it includes quick acceleration and deceleration phases as well as quick changes of direction. Each double round is followed by a 30 s resting period.
-   It is more practical and economical because the trainer can implement it on his own without extra personnel. The results are available immediately and without laboratory costs.
-   Because no blood samples are taken a possible psychological barrier is avoided.

The following equipment is required:

-   14 cones which are placed 10 m apart in the form of a slalom (Figure 1)
-   1 measuring tape
-   1 PC with an interface and the HRCT-software
-   1 UNILIFE/seca Trainingscomputer (e.g. Sporttester PE 4000) for every player participating in the test
-   1 microphone
-   1 amplifier
-   1 loudspeaker
-   1 printer.

Test Implementation and Results

Up to 14 players can run the course at once. Following a 20 min warm-up period, each player starts from a cone and runs the 140 m slalom course twice per turn at a speed acoustically given by a PC and loudspeaker. After each turn the player rests for 30 s. The initial speed is 10.8 km/h (= 3 m/s) which is increased by 0.6 km/h per turn.

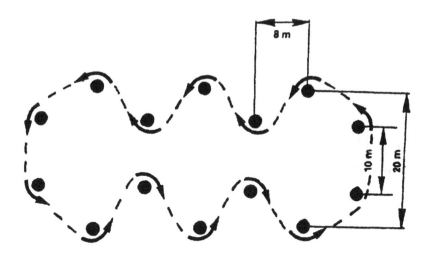

Figure 1.   The interval-test of Probst (1988).

If a player is unable to maintain this speed, he loses his
turn. Each **UNILIFE/seca** Trainingscomputer measures and
stores the pulse rate of a player as he runs. With the aid
of an interface and the HRCT-Software one obtains print-
outs of the heart rate in two different ways. Figure 2
(the bottom half) shows the pulse rate of an 18 years old
player in relation to testing-time (in minutes). In the
top half we see points which represent the pulse-rate at
the end of each turn in relation to velocity (km/h).
We can see in the lower diagram that this player has
difficulty recovering from his seventh turn (which is
actually his eighth because the print-out starts with turn
0) and subsequent turns. The top diagram shows that during
these turns he is no longer "in synch" with the "Conconi
linear graph". In this case point number 6 is therefore
called the "deflection point". The corresponding "velocity
deflection" (vd) is 14.4 km/h (= 4 m/s), as one can see
reading down from this deflection point to the x-axis. At
this velocity, according to Probst, a player has reached
his "anaerobic threshold".
In making recommendations for training the intensity of
running should be established with reference to the pulse
rate. A trainer determines this rate for each player as a
certain   percent   of   the   deflection   velocity   and   the

77

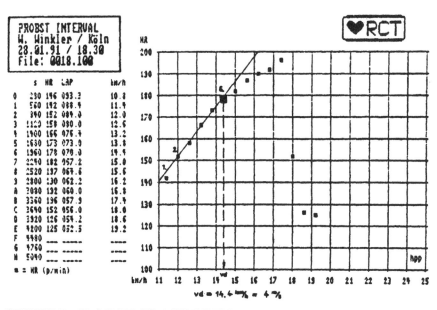

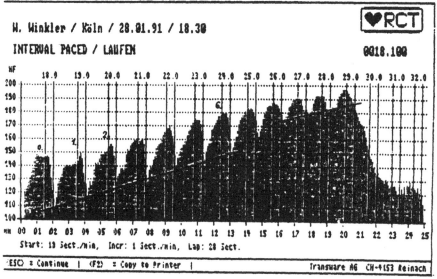

Figure 2. Pulse rate of an 18 year old soccer player.

corresponding pulse rate (which he obtains by reading from this velocity to "Conconi's linear graph" and then horizontally to the y-axis). If it is the aim, for example, to improve the endurance of a player so that he can run the same distance faster with the same pulse rate after approximately 6 weeks of training, the player should run 3 to 4 times per week. Hereby, he should have a pulse rate which is reached when he runs 90-97% of the deflection velocity for about 20-30 minutes. In a 30-40 minute session he should run at 85-90% speed (see Probst 1988). With this method the aerobic endurance can be improved by increasing the deflection speed, thus pushing the "Conconi-linear-graph" to the right. Many players feel that running at the 85% speed rate is too slow, thus giving this pace a recuperative character. The importance of this kind of recovery training has been widely accepted since Liesen's findings (1983).

Various parallel studies using Probst's approach and the "blood sample method" based on a "4 mmol/l lactat threshold conception" often produced similar results but it should be noted that neither this interval-test nor the "4 mmol/l blood sample test" can determine the exact "anaerobic threshold" of all individual athletes. This is especially true for the latter test when players at both extremes of the performance scale are tested (Braumann et al., 1991). The Probst Interval-Test must thus be considered to be an important tool in closely estimating an athlete's "anaerobic threshold". The UNILIFE/seca Trainingscomputer and the corresponding HRCT software can be recommended as a useful means for implementing this test and for controlling aerobic endurance training.

3   Computer-Controlled Video-Technology in Training and Match-Play

The construction of Dual-Video-Systems (DVS) has extended the possibilities of match analysis enormously and made both training- and match-analysis more efficient. A "two second action sequence from the 1988 World Cup qualification-match between W.Germany and the Netherlands (Munich, October 19, 1988)" was presented in the form of double-pictures made by a video-graphic-printer (Winkler, 1991). The match was recorded and evaluated by a DVS with SONY equipment. This example illustrates how important it is that players away from the ball also continue to anticipate what situations could develop. By viewing such scenes, players can be made aware of this necessity. It is clear that such analyses using single or dual video systems need not be restricted to matches. They should also be used in day to day training (Winkler and Freibichler, 1991). In order to take full advantage of this computer controlled video technology, it is important

that the trainer carefully selects the time for the video
viewing as well as the order and frequency of the scenes
to be shown. This facilitates the viewers' ability to
evaluate the scenes effectively and efficiently. By
applying such a cognitive approach together with audio-
visual materials, a trainer can lay the foundation for
long term improvement of a player's performance.

4 Conclusion

Feedback obtained both through the evaluation of match
play as well as training helps a trainer not only to
design and implement his training sessions more
effectively, but also to prepare his team optimally for
game situations. In addition, this diagnostic process
helps to make a trainer a better team leader by increasing
his credibility and offers him an objective tool for
deciding who plays in the next match and who does not. A
trainer is, therefore, well-advised to make use of such
diagnostic aids in basically all areas of his training and
coaching.
I have tried, with examples, to demonstrate that
diagnostic measures play an important role in controlling
and guiding the training process and in influencing match
play. This is accomplished by, among other things,
minimizing mistakes and helping the trainer to make wise
decisions.

5 References

Braumann, K.M., Tegtbur, U., Busse, M.W. and Maassen, N.
    (1991) Die "Laktatsenke" - Eine Methode zur Ermittlung
    der individuellen Dauerleistungsgrenze. Dtsch. Z.
    Sportmed., 6, 240-246.
Gerisch, G. (1990) Der Cooper Test. Fußballtraining, 5/6,
    61-63.
Liesen, H. (1983) Schnelligkeitsausdauertraining im
    Fußball aus sportmedizinischer Sicht. Fußballtraining,
    5, 27-31.
Probst, H.P. (1988) Intervall-Test für Fussballer.
    Magglingen, 11, 20-22.
Winkler, W. (1991) Match analysis and improvement of
    performance in soccer with the aid of computer-
    controlled dual-video-systems (CCDVS). Science and
    Football, 4, 6-10.
Winkler,W. and Freibichler, H. (1991) Leistungsdiagnostik
    beim Fußballspiel. Leistungssport, 2, 25-31.

PHYSIOLOGICAL CHARACTERIZATION OF PHYSICAL FITTNESS OF FOOTBALL PLAYERS IN FIELD CONDITIONS

E. J. MALOMSOKI
National Institute for Sports Medicine, Budapest, Hungary

1 Introduction

The aim of our work was to increase the physical fitness by the determination of the optimal training intensity. In the physiological examination of ball-orientated games, the intermittent characteristic of the efforts is apparent. As football is a good example of that, we applied an intermittent exercise protocol, based on Mader's method (1980) developed for swimmers, for the longitudinal examination of footballers' physical fitness. Moreover, we studied the connection between the aerobic and anaerobic metabolism as well as the intensity of efforts.

2 Method

In the five month measurement period, eleven footballers were examined three times.(The number of players examined was between eighteen and twenty on every occasion, but only eleven players were the same in all the three tests). They were from different positions within a single team.

The exercise test was an application of Mader's two-step method used with swimmers (Mader et al., 1980). In the case of footballers, this test was developed into an interval-type exercise. The footballers ran 30 m fifteen times and they had a 5 s break after each 30 m. After the fifteenth sprint the heart rate was measured by palpation and a blood sample obtained from an ear-lobe to establish the lactate level. The footballers had to choose the speed of the first fifteen sprints so that they were approximately in the aerobic zone, which in practical terms is equal to a warm-up of medium intensity. It represents the inflexion point of the multi-step lactate curve. About 30 min later, the players repeated the running exercise at maximum intensity. After that the heart rate was measured and blood taken again.

The first work-rate level took 3.5 to 4 min and the speed was between 2.5 and 3.5 m/s. At the second level, the exercise took 2 to 3 min and the speed was between 6 and 7 m/s.

The lactate and heart rate values obtained during the interval-type test were compared to the aerobic power, the running time and the heart rate observed earlier on the laboratory treadmill. To measure the aerobic power, we used automatic equipment (Jaeger Company).

The footballers continued on a normal training routine between each of the testing sessions. The trainer prescribed the training intensity relying upon the results of the physiological examinations.

3 Results

The lactate values measured at different points of time are shown as a function of performance (Figure 1). The results of every player are indicated for the first examination which was carried out in September, 1990. We considered the advantage in physical fitness of those footballers who could reach a relatively good performance at a moderate lactate level.For these players the "anaerobic threshold" coincided with a higher speed, and the rise of the curve, which is shown by dLas, was more moderate than for the team-average. Therefore, for these players we advised an increase in the training intensity: for example for players number 2, 6, 8, 10 and 11. It appeared that the process of anaerobic metabolism provided much less opportunities for an increase in the training intensity than for others, for example players number 1, 4 and 5. Line number 9 indicates the values for the goalkeeper. It is obvious that his performance - lactate relation as well as his physical fitness was much different from the outfield players' values.

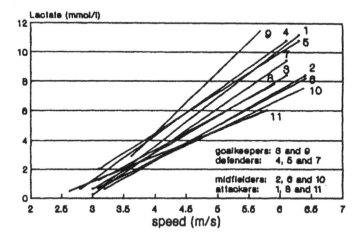

Fig.1. Lactate -speed curves of individual players.

Only the average values are presented from the examinations carried out later, in November and February (Figure 2). The running speed increased (statistically significant) during the period of study, while the lactate level decreased first, and later on, was practically unchanged. It seems that the performance of the subjects improved and if the training-intensity was still increased further improvement could be expected. In other words, the aerobic metabolism had developed favourably.

The degree of the changes can be seen in Table 1. The changes in heart rate characterize the adaptation of the cardiorespiratory system, although the changes did not run completely parallel with the development in the lactate responses.

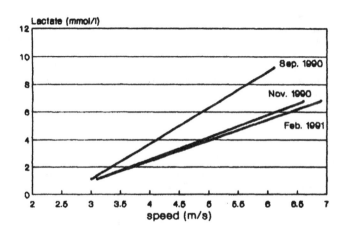

Fig.2. Lactate - speed curves of average values.

Table 1. Changes in the values for the interval running tests. ∗ = indicates $p < 0.05\%$

	Loads	Sep.-Nov.	Nov.-Feb.	Total
Speed (m/s)	1	+ 0.09	- 0.05	+ 0.04
	2	+ 0.48	+ 0.29	+ 0.77*
Lactate	1	+ 0.07	- 0.12	- 0.05
(mmol/l)	2	- 2.26	- 0.07	- 2.33*
Heart Rate	1	-10	- 7	-17
(beats/min)	2	+15	-22	7*
V-4mM (m/s)		+ 0.72	+ 0.20	+ 0.92*
dLas		- 1.54	- 0.21	- 1.75*

In table 1, dLas = dLa/(dv.a), a = sum(m)/100.
Practically, the dLas value means the amount of lactate
increase falling on unit speed increase, i.e. the
quotient shows the efficiency of the anaerobic metabolism
during the exercise.

Table 2. Average values gained on the treadmill

	Sep.	Nov.	Feb.
$\overset{\bullet}{V}O2$ ml/kg/min	59.7 ±6.5	60.0±7.2	62.7±5.2
Running time(min-s)	6-18±1-02	6-33±1-17	6-48±0-56
Heart Rate (max) (beats/min)	188 ±9	181±4	184±5

The average values of the aerobic power, the running time
and the heart rate are presented as a function of the
date of the examination in Table 2. We established that
the changes are in accordance with the anaerobic
parameters: the oxygen-uptake and the duration of the
exercise increased, while at the same time the heart rate
decreased. The changes in a physiological sense, however,
are more moderate than those measured for the anaerobic
parameters, which means that the sensitivity of the
method is moderate.

4 Discussion

By using the training intensity chosen on the basis of
the applied interval-type test, we managed to improve the
footballers' performance remarkably, or rather to create
advantageous metabolic conditions for further
improvement.
   There was some correlation between the aerobic power
measured on the treadmill and the parameters of the
anaerobic metabolism established after the interval-test
in the field. The parameters which are linked with the
lactate level expressed the increase of the performance
more sensitively than the aerobic parameters.
   It may be supposed that there are two reasons for that.
On the one hand, the aerobic power enabled a relatively
quick lactate-elimination in the breaks between the
sprints, regardless of the fact that the five-second
breaks seem relatively short for that. On the other hand,
in the case of a good aerobic power, the lactate
production was more moderate than in the case of a lower
aerobic power.
   The results can be understood in the following way,
too. For individuals with a great aerobic power, the
maximum steady state is obviously at a higher level than
for those with a small aerobic power. On the basis of
the results presented, it turns out that footballers

should have good aerobic and anaerobic metabolic characteristics. Observations on players participating in other ball-oriented games, referred to the fact that the same applies to more or less all such games (Malomsoki and Ekes, 1984).

If we accept that physical fitness plays an important role in game performance, this method of examining physical fitness can be recommended.

5 References

Mader, A., Madsen, O. and Hollmann, W. (1980) Zur Bedeutung der laktaciden Energiebereitstellung für Trainings- und Wettkampfleistungen im Sportschwimmen. Teil 1 und 2. Leistungssport 4-5, 263-279 and 408-418.
Malomsoki, J. and Ekes, E. (1984) A study of the anaerobic threshold of ball-players. Finn. Sports Exerc. Med., 3, 145-151.

THE INFLUENCE OF A SPECIAL ENDURANCE TRAINING ON THE AEROBIC AND ANAEROBIC CAPACITY OF SOCCER PLAYERS TESTED BY THE SOCCER TREADMILL METHODS

P.E. NOWACKI and M. PREUHS
Institute of Sportsmedicine, Justus-Liebig-University Gießen,
Germany.

1 Introduction

For determining the aerobic and anaerobic capacities a non-professional team was tested twice over a period of 6 months by the standard method of bicycle ergometry, the so-called Gießener model described by Nowacki et al. (1988). The third and last test was a special, intermittent treadmill ergometry for soccer players. This test was developed to verify a new method by comparing its results with the well known standard bicycle method. Further, we wanted to demonstrate that the intermittent load of soccer matches could be transferred in a laboratory test.

To achieve a high training standard and to improve the sport specific performance capacities, it is necessary to know the starting level of each player and the physical and metabolic requirements during the match. Only if these two factors are known can an optimal training programme be planned. Therefore we tested the metabolic reactions and requirements of the players during 3 official league matches and integrated the results in a special training programme.

2 Methods

Prior to each exercise test the soccer players (n = 15 players of the highest non-professional German league) had to undergo an intensive internal and orthopaedic examination, which included ECG at rest, lung function and blood pressure measurements. The anthropometric data of the soccer team showed the following mean values: age: 25.4 ± 4.2 years; body mass: 74.8 ± 7.7 kg; height: 182 ± 5.4 cm.

2.1 Bicycle ergometry
The soccer players were twice tested on the electrically braked universal bicycle ergometer "Ergotest" (E. Jaeger, Würzburg) with increasing work load according to the Gießener loading test (1 W/kg body weight) to the individual point of exhaustion. This traditional bicycle test distinguishes between trained and untrained subjects and evaluates the physical performance capacities from highly trained to pathological. The particular worth of this method is substantiated by the sharp separation between trained and untrained physical performance capacity at the transition from 3 to 4 watt/kg body weight.

2.2 Treadmill
In contrast to other treadmill tests this intermittent, special test for soccer players is characterized by a variation of the slope and

the speed of the treadmill. The interval variation of short rest
periods and increased load until individual exhaustion simulates the
typical load of a soccer match in a treadmill test in the laboratory.
As shown by Fig. 1, the speed was kept at 9 km/h for the first 15 min
and then was raised to 12 km/h. The slope, which starts at 0%,
reached the 15% summit after a 10 min duration of exercise and a
speed of 12 km/h. For this treadmill test the "Laufergotest" (E.
Jaeger, Würzberg) was employed. The physical performance capacities
can be classified on a range from very good to weak.

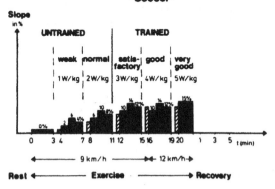

Fig. 1. Criteria for evaluation of the physical performance
         capacity following exhausting intermittent treadmill
         exercise.

The heart rate was electrocardiographically registered and simultaneously displayed on the screen of the oscilloscope by using the tri-
recorder "Cardiomat" and the oscilloscope "Servomed", both made by
Hellige (Freiburg). The respiratory data were registered in an open
system by the oxygen analyser "Oxycon" (Mijnhard, Holland). For
analysing the blood lactate concentration, the blood samples were
enzymatically treated with the "Laktat-Test" (Boehringr, Mannheim)
and spectrophotometrically investigated with a fixed wave length
(Eppendorf, Hamburg).

3 Results and discussion

After determining the starting level of each soccer player by bicycle
ergometry, the players had to take part in a 6 months intensive
programme of aerobic endurance training. The alteration of the
performance capacities was determined at the end of this training
period by the standard bicycle method, which was exactly the same as
at the first test.
     Comparing the result during exhaustive bicycling exercise the
significant improvement of the aerobic capacity data as a result of

the intensified endurance training could be shown to be impressive.
The development of the performance capacities is demonstrated by the
four most essential parameters: heart rate, relative oxygen uptake,
lactate response and physical performance capacity.

3.1 Heart rate

The improved reaction of the cardiovascular system is responsible for
the average 10 beats/min lower heart rates during the exercise at the
second test. Although progression of both curves is almost identical, the cardiac response of the second test showed significant
differences at all exercise levels. For example, at a submaximal
work load the heart rate decreased from 145 to 136 beats/min. Even
the heart rate after 5 minutes of recovery showed significant
differences. By dropping 5 beats/min from 110 to 105 beats the
players reached a very good cardiovascular recovery at the second
test.

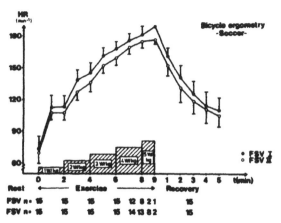

Fig. 2. Reaction of the heart frequency during and following
exhausting bicycle ergometry before (FSV I) and after
(FSV II) endurance training.

3.2 Relative oxygen uptake

The relative oxygen uptake as the most important parameter for the
cardiorespiratory system demonstrates the same development. The
higher average data as a result of an improved ventilation and an
increased aerobic power represent the enlarged performance
capacities. The mean values of the maximum relative oxygen uptake
increased from 49.3 to 55.2 ml/kg/min – that means, the amateur
soccer team reached nearly the level of the German National teams
(World Cup 1974 54.6; World Cup 1982 59.4 ml/kg/min.)

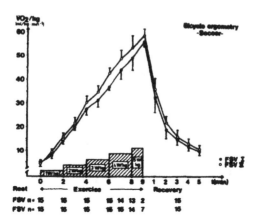

Fig. 3. The relative oxygen uptake during and following exhausting
bicycle ergometry before (FSV I) and after (FSV II) endurance
training.

3.3 Physical performance capacity
The physical performance capacity increased too. The average of the
absolute (1403 to 1545 Watt/min respectively), the relative work load
(18.9 to 21.2 Watt/min/kg) and the duration of exercise (7.42 to 8.12
min) reached a significantly (P < 0.01) higher level at the second
test. According to the criteria for evaluation of the physical
performance capacity, at the first test only one player could be
tested for 1 min at 5 Watt/kg and only seven for 2 min at 4 Watt/kg.
At the second test eleven players reached 2 min at 4 Watt/kg and two
players 1 min at 5 Watt/kg.
    The much higher values on the treadmill test (2736 Watt-minutes
absolute work load; 37.9 Watt/min/kg relative work load and 20.02 min
duration of exercise) are substantiated by the prolonged duration of
this method. The curves of the oxygen uptake demonstrate the
excellent adaptation of the cardiorespiratory system to the typical
variation in stress during soccer matches. The maximum relative
oxygen uptake increased to a mean value of 57.4 ml/kg/min.

3.4 Blood lactate
The variation in the blood lactate level between the two tests
represented improved aerobic capacities. After 6 months of intensive
endurance training, blood lactate started to accumulate much later in
the test. This could be seen by the prolonged duration of exercise
until the 4 mmol/1 aerobic/anaerobic threshold was reached (162 to
218 seconds). Even the significantly lower average data at a
submaximal load (5.3 to 4.4 mmol/1) represent improved aerobic
capacities. In addition the higher data at the third minute of
recovery (14.8 to 15.5 mmol/1) signifies the increased anaerobic
performance capacities.

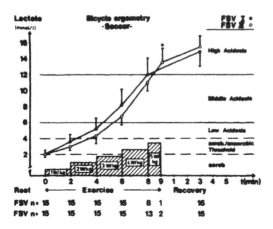

Fig. 4.   The blood lactate response during and following exhausting
          bicycle ergometry before (FSV I) and after (FSV II)
          endurance training.

3.5 Match metabolism

The average of the blood lactate data, which settled in the region of
low acidosis during the match and in the region of the aerobic/
anaerobic threshold at the end of each half-time, showed the predominant aerobic character of the match stress.   This means that the
aerobic alactacid energy productiion and the oxidative restitution
mechanisms are dominating.   This is done by the reduction of the
energy substrates ATP and creatinphosphate.   The average values of
5.3 and 5.5 mmol/1 during the match indicate that even the lactacid
restitution processes should be considered.

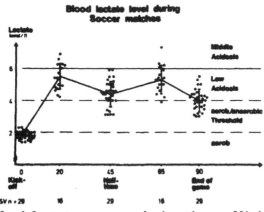

Fig. 5   The blood lactate response during three official championship
         matches.

90

4 Resume

The endurance parts of the soccer training programme should be intensified to obtain an optimal preparation for competition and
- to improve the glycogen substrate and oxygen uptake level
- to receive a quicker regneration and
- to save glycogen for high intensive physical loads by consuming fats.

Therefore it is necessary to reduce the speed endurance and strength training elements of the programme which now predominate.

As the comparison of the blood lactate response during the matches and the special interval treadmill test represent, the characteristic slow increase of blood lactate and its prompt increase at high loads are similar to the predominating aerobic requirements during league matches. Taken together with the 20 percent higher performance data of the other parameters, it could be stated that the intermittent special treadmill test for soccer players achieved a much better simulation of the load and stress of soccer matches than other ergometry methods.

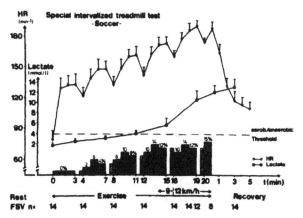

Fig. 6. Reaction of the heart rate and lactic acid production during and following the special treadmill test for soccer players.

5 References

Hollman, W. and Liesen, (1973) H. Über die Bewertbarkeit des Lactats in der Leistungsdiagnostik; Sportarzt u. Sportmed. 8, 175-182.

Novacki, P.E., Cai, D.Y., Buhl, C. and Krümmelbein, U. (1988) Biological Performances of German Soccer players (Professional and Juniors) tested by special treadmill methods, in: Science and Football (eds T. Reilly, A. Lees, K. Davids and W.J. Murphy), E. and F.N. Spon, London, pp.145-157.

Preuhs, M. (1990) Die Bedeutung des sportartspezifischen Ausdauertrainings für die aerobe and anaerobe Kapazit von Fußballspielern; Inaug. Diss. Med. JLU-Gießen.

HIGH SPEED KNEE EXTENSION CAPACITY OF SOCCER PLAYERS AFTER DIFFERENT KINDS OF STRENGTH TRAINING.

P. AAGAARD, M. TROLLE, E.B. SIMONSEN[*], J. BANGSBO, K. KLAUSEN
August Krogh Institute and [*]National Institute of Occupational Health, Copenhagen-DK

1 Introduction

The football kick involves knee extension velocities of 14-16 rad/s reached just before ball impact (Miller and Nelson, 1973). In contrast, the maximal angular velocity applied in isokinetic strength measurements has generally not exceeded 4.36 rad/s (250 °/s). Therefore a non-isokinetic method was developed to determine muscle moment, muscle power and joint angular velocity during very fast movements. One purpose was to obtain the moment-velocity and power-velocity relations of the knee extensors during slow to very fast knee extensions. Another purpose was to examine the effect of different kinds of strength training on these relations. Finally, the functional significance of the different kinds of strength training was examined.

2 Methods

Twenty four elite soccer players participated in an strength training programme involving knee extension-flexion's with either high resistance (HR), low resistance (LR), loaded kicking movements without ball (FU) or served as controls (CON). All training activity was surveyed and controlled.

The dynamic knee extension strength was measured with a modified Hill flywheel. Muscle moments due to inertial acceleration and to oppose gravity were calculated and added to the moment imposed by the flywheel. All signals were sampled into a computer with a time resolution of 1 ms. The knee joint angle was measured with a non-rigid type of goniometer and the signal lowpass filtered with a digital 4th order Butterworth filter at 4-11 Hz cut off frequencies. Angular velocity and acceleration at the knee joint were derived with a finite element method, $dt = 2ms$. The following mechanical parameters were determined: peak moment (M_{peak}), moment at 50° knee extension (M_{50}), peak power (P_{peak}), power at 50° (P_{50}) and peak velocity (V_{peak}) as well as the corresponding moment, power and velocity at each parameter. $0° =$ fully extended leg.

Since moment, power and corresponding velocity varied throughout the movement, exponential polynomials were fitted to the recorded data ($r \geq 0.9$ in all cases), in order to allow comparison at standardized velocities. Functional kicking performance was estimated by measuring ball velocity at standardized maximal soccer kicks by means of a Doppler radar. For statistical evaluation the Kruskal-Wallis analysis of variance and Wilcoxon signed rank test were used.

3 Results

Maximal recorded knee joint velocity, -moment and -power ranged 8.36-17.98 rad/s (479-1030°/s), 157-323 Nm and 573-2580 W among all subjects with no significant differences observed after training.

Only the HR-group increased performance at all mechanical parameters after the training: M_{peak} increased 10-26% at the standardized velocities 0, 4.18 and 5.24 rad/s, M_{50} increased 9-14% at velocities 0 and 0.52 rad/s, and P_{peak} and P_{50} increased 5-29% at velocities above 3.14 rad/s. Moment and power exerted at the instant of V_{peak} increased 24-42% and 18-32%, respectively, at standardized V_{peak} values above 5.24 rad/s. The moment-velocity and power-velocity curves for the HR-group are shown in Fig.1 and Fig.2.

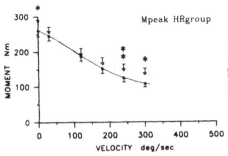

Fig.1 The moment-velocity relation (M_{peak}) before (full line, filled triangles) and after strength training. * $p < 0.05$, **$p < 0.01$.

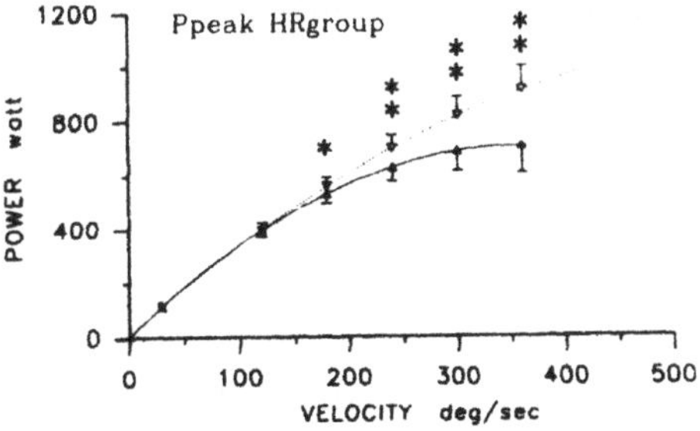

Fig.2 The power-velocity relation (P_{peak}) before (full line, filled triangles) and after strength training. * $p < 0.05$, **$p < 0.01$.

For the FU-group M_{peak} increased 7-13% at velocities 0.52, 2.09 and 3.14 rad/s, M_{50} increased 9-14% at velocities 0 and 0.52 rad/s, P_{peak} increased 7% at 4.18 rad/s and P_{50} increased 9-12% at velocities 0.52, 2.09 and 3.14 rad/s. In the LR-group M_{peak} increased 9% at 2.09 rad/s.

No change in ball velocity was observed in any of the groups after training.

4 Conclusion

Muscle moment was enhanced at low knee extension velocities by the high resistance (HR) strength training and at moderate velocities by the functional (FU) and low resistance (LR) training. The training velocity in the FU-group transiently shifted between 0 and 8.72 rad/s (0-500 °/s), and maximal external load on the knee extensors was estimated to occur at a velocity of 1.75-4.36 rad/s (100-250 °/s). Thus, the increases in dynamic muscle strength were in general observed at the specific velocities used in the different training protocols, in line with previuos findings (Kaneko et al., 1983). Unexpectedly, the high resistance strength training increased muscle force and power also at the high knee extension velocities. Possible changes in neural and morphological factors could, hypothetically, explain these findings (increases in rate of force development, increases in muscle mass, increases in angle of fibre pennation). Another possibility for the improvements could also be a somewhat low pre training level at these particular speeds. However, no significant differences were observed between the groups.

In the present study the shape and magnitude of the power-velocity curves closely resembled previous reports on isokinetic knee extension power, at the rather low velocities where comparison was possible (Ivy et al., 1981). The specificity of training velocity and load on the improvement in power seemed not quite clear. In the FU-group, increases in muscle power were seen at the velocities involving the highest external load. This is in line with other studies in which the improvement of peak power was located to the specific velocity of training (Kanehisa et al., 1983; Tabata et al., 1990). In contrast, the muscle power was increased at high knee extension velocities following the high resistance training with low velocity. Kicking performance was not improved by any of the groups. This lack of transfer from the gain in muscle force and muscle power into enhanced functional performance could be due to the hip muscles being more important in kick performance than the quadriceps muscle (Robertson & Mosher, 1983; Narici et al., 1988). Furthermore, a succesful soccer kick depends on a precisely coordinated action of the leg muscles (deProft et al., 1988) rather than on isolated muscle strength. Neural coordination should apparantly be trained extensively in order to improve the kicking performance of elite soccer players.

5 Acknowledgement

This study was supported by the Team Denmark Elite Sports Organization, The Danish Research Council for Sports and The National Institute of Occupational Health.

6 References

de Proft, E., Clarys, J.P., Bollens, E., Cabri, J. and Dufour, W. (1988) Muscle activity in the soccer kick, in **Science and Football** (eds T. Reilly, A. Lees, K. Davids and W.J. Murphy), E. and F. N. Spon, London, pp. 434-440.

Ivy, J.L., Withers, R.T., Brose, G., Maxwell, B.D. and Costill, D.L. (1981) Isokinetic contractile properties of the quadriceps with relation to fiber type. **Eur. J. Appl. Physiol.**, 47, 247-255.

Kanehisa, H. and Miyashita, M. (1983) Effects of isometric and isokinetic training on static strength and dynamic power. **Eur. J. Appl. Physiol.**, 50, 365-371.

Kaneko, M., Fuchimoto, T., Toji, H., Svei, K. (1983) Training effects of different loads on the force-velocity relationship and mechanical power output in human muscle. **Scand. J. Sports. Sci.**, 5, 50-55.

Miller, D. and Nelson, R. (1973) **Biomechanics of Sports.** Lea & Febiger, Philadelphia.

Narici, M.V., Sirtori, M.D., and Mognoni, P. (1988) Maximum ball velocity and peak torques of hip flexor and knee extensor muscles, in **Science and Football** (eds T. Reilly, A. Lees, K. Davids and W.J. Murphy), E. and F. N. Spon, London, pp. 429-33.

Robertson, D.G. and Mosher, R.E. (1983) Work and power of the leg muscle in soccer kicking. **Biomechanics IX-b**, pp. 533-542.

Tabata, I. Yoriko, A. Kanehisa, H. Miyashita, M. (1990) Effect of high intensity endurance training on isokinetic muscle power. **Eur. J. Appl. Physiol.**, 60, 254-258.

EFFECTS OF STRENGTH TRAINING ON KICKING PERFORMANCE IN SOCCER.

M. TROLLE, P. AAGAARD, E.B. SIMONSEN[*], J. BANGSBO, K. KLAUSEN
August Krogh Institute and [*]National Institute of Occupational Health, Copenhagen-DK

1 Introduction

When muscles contract at increasing velocity the muscle force decreases. For excised muscle a hyperbolic relation exists between the force developed and the velocity of contraction (Hill, 1938). Conflicting results have been reported on the moment-velocity relations obtained during isokinetic knee extensions in humans (Perrine and Edgerton, 1978; Thorstensson et al., 1976). Moreover, only few reports exist for the effect of different training regimens on the force-velocity relation of the knee extensors. The purpose of the present study was to examine the effect of different strength training regimens on the force-velocity relation of the human knee extensors, and describe the effect on kicking performance.

2 Methods

Twenty four male elite soccer players participated in the study. The players, all free from previous knee injury, were recruited from football teams ranked within the 20 best teams in the national league. The players performed either hydraulic strength exercise at high resistance (HR) or low resistance (LR), or trained functionally (FU) in a loaded kicking movement without ball. The last group served as controls (CON). The training consisted of 36 sessions over a period of 12 weeks. At each training session 4 sets of 8RM (group HR), 24RM (group LR) or 16RM (group FU) knee extension movements, respectively, were performed. All training sessions were surveyed in order to assure a maximal training intensity. No ball practice took place during the training period.
Isokinetic and isometric knee extension strength was measured with the use of a Kin-Com dynamometer. Peak moment and constant-angle moment were measured at knee extension velocities of 0, 0.52, 2.09 and 4.18 rad/s (0,30,120 and 240 °/s). All moments obtained were corrected for the effect of gravity on the lower leg, the foot and the ankle-pad. In order to reduce the influence from hamstring strain on this gravity correction, the reference gravity moment was not determined at 0 ° but at 10 ° knee joint flexion (0 ° = knee fully extended).
Maximal kicking performance was estimated by ball velocity obtained during a standardized indoor soccer kick. The velocity was measured by means of a custom-built Doppler radar, with the players shooting towards a handball goal from a distance of 11.3

m. At least 20 shots were performed by each subject.

Non-parametric statistics were used, with the level of significance set to 5%.

3 Results

Only high resistance training (group HR) resulted in significant improvements in knee extension strength (Fig. 1). At the velocity of 0.52 rad/s a 14% increase in peak moment was observed (from 271.7 Nm to 310.4 Nm), as well as a 14-28% increase in constant-angle moment at all angles 20-70 °. Isometric extension moment was increased 14-23% at 50, 60, and 70 ° knee flexion. Group mean values increased from 202.2, 236.7, 254.6 Nm to 247.9, 282.8, 290.2 Nm at 50, 60, 70 °, respectively.

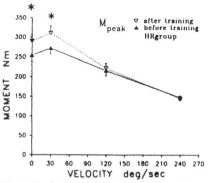

Fig.1 Peak knee extension moment (M_{peak}) at 0,30,120 and 240 °/sec. * $p<0.05$.

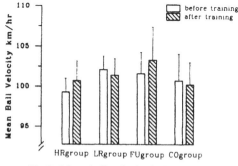

Fig.2 Mean ball velocity in km/hr (mean of five best trials).

No significant change in ball velocity was observed for any of the groups (Fig. 2). Mean ball velocity of the individual groups was in the range of 99.3-103.6 km/h and 99.6-105.9 km/h before and after training. Peak ball velocity ranged from 85 km/h to 115 km/h among all subjects.

4 Conclusion

In contrast with previous findings (deProft et al., 1988a) kicking performance was unaffected by the different kinds of strength training. Obviously none of the training regimens was ideal for inducing a better kicking performance in highly trained football players. Factors such as timing and motor control are probably more important. Furthermore, the hip flexor muscles play a more dominant role in kicking performance than the knee extensors (Narici et al., 1988). Eccentric action of the knee flexors and hip extensors also seem to be of importance, as indicated by electromyograhic (deProft et al., 1988b) as well as kinematic (Luhtanen, 1988) studies. However, our subjects had excellent kicking abilities prior to the training and the training regimens could possibly have better effects on less skilled subjects. Another major finding was that only the high resistance strength training (HR group) improved peak- and constant-angle moment. The improvements were seen in the velocity range from 0 to 0.52 rad/s, which was close to the actual training velocity 0.34-0.85 rad/s (20-50 °/sec). This influence of velocity and load used during the exercise on the gain in muscle strength is in line with previous studies (Moiffroid & Whipple, 1970). In contrast with previous studies there was no effect of the training with low resistance (high velocity, LR group). In the present study the effects of learning were minimal since different training- and measuring devices were used. Thus, it appears that only high resistance strength training induces increases in isokinetic muscle strength in the absence of learning effects.

In all groups a levelling off was observed for the moments measured at low velocities (≤ 0.52 rad/s) compared to the hyperbolic Hill curve. In previous studies such a plateau in knee extension moment has been proposed to be due to inhibitory tension-limiting factors (Perrine and Edgerton, 1978; Wickiewicz et al., 1984). However, numerous factors can be suggested to explain the discrepancy between the force produced by excised muscle and the force exerted at a joint in vivo. Among those are the level of neural activation, change in muscle moment-arm as well as change in angle of pennation of the muscle fibres with change in joint angle, muscle synergism and antagonist co-activation.

5 Acknowledgements

This study was supported by the Team Denmark Elite Sports Organization, The Danish Research Council for Sports and The National Institute of Occupational Health.

6 References

de Proft, E., Cabri, J., Dufour, W. and Clarys, J.P. (1988a) Strength training and kick performance in soccer players, in **Science and Football**, (eds T. Reilly, A. Lees, K. Davids and W.J. Murphy), E. and F. N. Spon, London, pp. 108-113.

de Proft, E., Clarys, J.P., Bollens, E., Cabri, J. and Dufour, W. (1988b) Muscle activity in the soccer kick, in **Science and Football**, (eds T. Reilly, A. Lees, K. Davids and W.J. Murphy), E. and F. N. Spon, London, pp. 434-440.

Hill, A.V. (1938) The heat of shortening and the dynamic constants of muscle. **Proc. R. Soc. London Ser.B.**, 126, 136-195.

Luhtanen, P. (1988) Kinematics and kinetics of maximal instep kicking in junior soccer players, in **Science and Football**, (eds T. Reilly, A. Lees, K. Davids and W.J. Murphy), E. and F. N. Spon, London, pp. 441-448.

Moffroid, M. and Whipple, R. (1970) Specificity of speed of exercise. **Phys.Ther.**, 50, 1692-1699.

Narici, M.V., Sirtori, M.D. and Mognoni, P. (1988) Maximum ball velocity and peak torques of hip flexor and knee extensor muscles, in **Science and Football**, (eds T. Reilly, A. Lees, K. Davids and W.J. Murphy), E. and F. N. Spon, London, pp. 429-433.

Perrine, J.J. and Edgerton, V.R. (1978) Muscle force-velocity and power-velocity relationship under isokinetic loading. **Med. Sci. Sports**, 10, 159-166.

Thorstensson, A., Grimby, A.G. and Karlsson, J. (1976) Force-velocity relations and fiber composition in human knee extensor muscle. **J. Appl. Physiol.**, 40, 12-16.

Wickiewicz, T.L., Roy, R.R., Powell, P.L., Perrine, J.J. and Edgerton, V.R. (1984) Muscle architecture and force-velocity relationships in humans. **J. Appl. Physiol.** 57, 435-443.

THE INFLUENCE OF MAXIMAL STRENGTH TRAINING OF LOWER LIMBS OF SOCCER PLAYERS ON THEIR PHYSICAL AND KICK PERFORMANCES

F. Taïana, J.F. Gréhaigne and G. Cometti.
UFR-STAPS Université de Bourgogne, France.

1 Introduction

Exercises aimed at developing soccer players' strength are often used with utmost caution in training programmes (Gréhaigne, 1989). Fixture lists are often so full that one hesitates planning muscle strengthening exercises during the season as they require a lot of effort. The solution most frequently opted for consists of arranging for strength development outside competition periods, particularly at the beginning of the season. Possible strength gains thus acquired are thereafter maintained by sprinting, jumping and kicking exercises and possibly plyometrics performed throughout the season.

The aim of our study was to analyse the influence of a ten week muscle development programme for young soccer players designed to gain maximal lower body strength.

2 Methods

2.1 Subjects

The experiment was carried out on 15 Fourth Division players at the *Institut National du Football de Clairefontaine* (age 18.1 ± 0.3 years; body mass 67 ± 5.8 kg; height 173.3 ± 6.3 cm). The group consisted of a goalkeeper, 5 defenders, 5 midfielders and 4 forwards.

2.2 Training programme

The programme was solely aimed at improving the lower body strength. The sessions were made up of three parts :
- squatting exercises
- triceps surae exercises
- leg swinging exercises.

Maximal strength training for soccer players should be approached with caution, so exercises which combine pre-fatigue and isometrics are most suitable. Also built into the sessions were simple plyometric situations as well as ball exercises in order to prevent the excessive alteration of motor-skills in the subjects.

Each maximal strength training session was based on the model in Fig.1 and each participant does the sequence 3 to 6 times.

The sequence of the session was as follows :
- the dynamic exercises (hurdles) or ball exercises (heading, kicking) remain the same ;
- only the exercises with weights were modified mainly by changing the mode of contraction (Fig. 2)

2.3 Performance tests

In order to evaluate the relevance of this programme and some possible progress made by the players, a number of tests were set up.

2.3.1 Kick performance

The test took place facing a wall upon which there was a chalk drawn square target (100 cm x 100 cm). The ball was placed 10 metres from the wall, just behind the beam of a photo-electric cell (TAG HEUER HL 2-11 ™) which triggers off a stopwatch as soon as the ball crosses it. The stopwatch is stopped by a microphone (TAG HEUER HL 556 ™) situated at the foot of the wall. The average ball speed is calculated by a SPEEDMETER 510 (TAG HEUER ™) from the time elapsed between the two impulses.(Fig. 3).

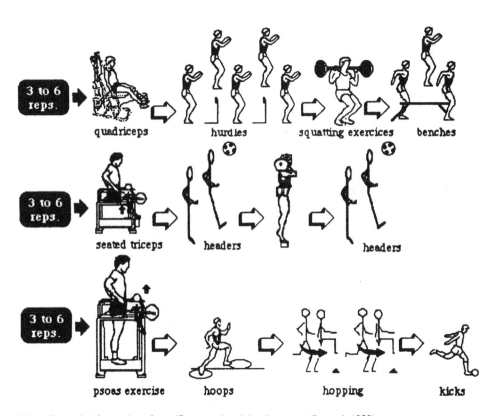

Fig. 1. Example of a session of specific strength training in soccer (Cometti, 1989).

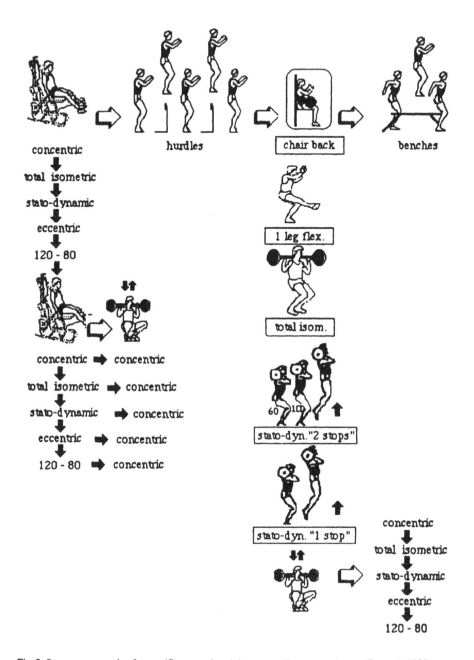

concentric

total isometric

stato-dynamic

eccentric

120 - 80

hurdles

chair back

benches

1 leg flex.

total isom.

concentric ➡ concentric

total isometric ➡ concentric

stato-dynamic ➡ concentric

eccentric ➡ concentric

120 - 80 ➡ concentric

60   100

stato-dyn. "2 stops"

stato-dyn. "1 stop"

concentric

total isometric

stato-dynamic

eccentric

120 - 80

Fig. 2. Sequence example of a specific strength training course for soccer players (Cometti, 1989).

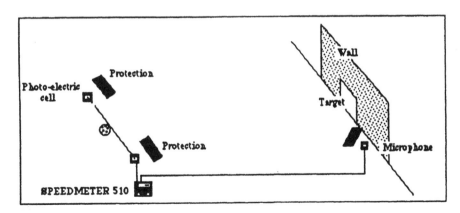

Fig. 3.The kick test.

The subjects took their run up as they wished so as to kick the ball as hard as possible and try and hit the target. They each had five kicks using whichever foot they wished. The results are displayed automatically in km/h.

2.3.2 Sprint test
The subjects had to run a distance of 30 metres on a synthetic track as fast as they could wearing soccer kit. The start was given by starting pistol and the photoelectric cells were positioned 10 and 30 metres from the starting line and linked to a CHRONOPRINTER 500 (TAG HEUER ™). The subjects had two attempts.

2.3.3 Jump tests
Three performance tests according to Bosco et al. (1983) were included to evaluate the explosive power of the leg extensor muscles. An ABALAKOV ™ belt was used to obtain maximum precision. That is a reel of thread fixed to the floor and attached to the subjects belt which unwinds during vertical jumps. The apparatus displays the length of thread unravelled and thus the elevation of the jumper's centre of gravity.

In a Squat Jump (S.J.), the subject jumps vertically from a squatting position, legs bent at 90°, without using his arms.

In a Counter-Movement Jump (C.M.J.) the subject jumps vertically from a standing position, without using his arms.

In a "With Arms Movement Jump" (W.A.M.J.) he jumps vertically from a standing position, using his arms.

3   Results

3.1 Kick performance
The subjects were tested twice. Their performance ranged from 72.96 km/h to 108.95 km/h.
The average performance for the group was 96.02 km/h with a standard deviation of 9.06 km/h. These results are comparable to those obtained by Poulmedis (1985) with Greek First Division players (Table 1.).

Table 1. Comparison of results obtained from different kick tests

	Mean	S.D.	Min. perf.	Max. perf.
POULMEDIS (1985)				
11 D.1 Greeks: 25.5 ± 3years	97.48	4.74	91.4	106.52
TAIANA Present study				
15 Jun.2 INF:18.1 ± 0.3years	96.02	9.06	72.96	108.95

101

After 10 weeks of muscle development exercises, all subjects had progressed. The progress variation is + 0.09 km/h to + 17.9 km/h (+21 %) and was very different from one person to another. The average improvement for the group was 6.59 km/h (Table 2.). These improvements were significant (P< 0.05).

Table 2. Kick test results and progress achieved

	TEST 1: Mean ± SD	TEST 2: Mean ± SD	Progress: (km/h)
Max. kick	94.51 ± 6.07	101.10 ± 4.82	6.59 ± 5.53

It is likewise to be noted that, on the average, forwards and defenders kick harder than midfielders (Table 3.). The differences between the groups were non-significant (P < 0.05).

Table 3. Best kicks made by the subjects in relation to their team position

Defender:		Midfielder:		Forward:	
1	101.40	5	95.19	8	108.95
2	100.42	7	96.9	9	100.94
4	101.83	11	92.2	10	99.26
6	94.04	14	108.95	12	96.75
13	105.46	15	95.37	X̄	101.48
X̄	100.63	X̄	97.72	S.D.	5.27
S.D.	4.15	S.D.	6.50		

3.2 Sprint test
All the subjects tested improved in the 10 metres and 30 metres tests.

Table 4. Sprint test results and progress achieved

	TEST 1: Mean ± SD	TEST 2: Mean ± SD	Progress: (s)
10 m	2.07 ± 0.20	1.99 ± 0.36	0.08 ± 0.02
30 m	4.56 ± 0.03	4.48 ± 0.15	0.07 ± 0.15

Over 10 metres the smallest improvement was 0.06 s (+2.9 %) and the most substantial 0.12 s (+5.8 %) whereas the average was 0.08 s (+ 3.8 %). Over 30 metres the same margin of progress was found, which indicates that progress was achieved particularly in the 10 metres test.

3.3 Jump tests
The performances obtained in the squat jump ranged from 42 cm to 48 cm. They are close to those obtained by Bosco (1985) using the ergojump apparatus with the Italian national team (31cm ±5 cm).

The counter-movement jump (C.M.J.) performances range from 51 cm to 55 cm and are inferior to those obtained by Gauffin et al. (1989) with senior Swedish players (56.8 cm ±6.2 cm).

The C.M.J. -S.J. differences reveal, according to Bosco (1985), the elasticity potential of the subjects tested.

The With Arms Movement Jump (W.A.M.J.) performances ranged from 63 cm to 71 cm.

Table 5. Jump test results and progress achieved

	TEST 1: Mean ± SD	TEST 2: Mean ± SD	Progress: (cm)
Squat jump	45.00 ± 2.16	45.33 ± 2.05	0.33 ± 3.09
Counter mov. jump	53.33 ± 1.24	50.33 ± 4.11	-3.00 ± 2.94
CMJ - SJ	8.33 ± 1.24	5.00 ± 5.10	-3.33 ± 5.73
With arms mov. jump	65.33 ± 2.05	67.66 ± 3.39	2.33 ± 2.62

At the end of the muscle development programme of exercises, an appreciable progress in the With Arms Movement Jumps test was noted where the second test performances were 3.44 % better than the first test results. This observation is reassuring as the test situation is much closer to match conditions.

In the squat jump, progress was slight and a regression of -5.6 % in the counter-movement jump was found. It can be noted that the C.M.J.-S.J. differences (on average 6.7 cm) reveal - contrary to what is usually thought about soccer players - good use of their elastic muscular potential.

4   Discussion.

The progress achieved was above all been obtained in the most explosive exercises and those which are closest to skills required in soccer. The whole group progressed significantly in the kick test : + 6.59 km/h ± 5.53 (P < 0.05). Even though there was no statistically significant difference between team positions, it was noted that forwards and defenders, on average, kick harder than midfielders. The goalkeeper's performances have not been taken into account.

Progress was considerable in the 10 and 30 metres. The subjects gained, on the average, nearly a tenth of a second.

Over the whole range of jumping tests mixed results were obtained. Performances clearly improved in the W.A.M.J. and, to a very slight degree, in the S.J. On the other hand, they diminished in the C.M.J. The differences between C.M.J. and S.J. indicated good use of subjects' elastic muscular potential.

So the programme of muscle development exercises has proved fruitful, even though the subjects did only one session per week. It should nevertheless be pointed out that this programme was carried out during the competition period and that it would not have been wise to have more than one training session per week. This may seem insufficient for us to claim to develop maximal strength, the extra fatigue caused by this training was taken into account in such a way so as not to be detrimental to the players' performances in the matches they had to play.

Tuesday appeared to be the most appropriate day of the week for training sessions. The players had recuperated from the fatigue of the weekend match and still had four days to prepare for the next one.

So, with a little hindsight, it appears preferable to carry out this kind of training at the beginning of the season or during mid-season breaks, rather than during competition periods. The possible gains in strength thus acquired can then be maintained throughout the season by sprinting, jumping and kicking exercises as well as perhaps plyometrics.

This study was limited by the lack of a control group, but there were not enough people to form one. The aim then was simply to experiment with the spin-offs of a maximal strength training programme with soccer players.

5   References.

Bosco, C.; Mognoni, P.; Luthanen P. (1983) Relationship between isokinetic performance and ballistic movement. Eur. J. Appl. Physiol., 51, 357-364.

Bosco, C.(1985) Elasticita moscolare é forza esplosiva nelle attivita fisico-sportive. Roma : Sociéta stampa sportiva.

Cometti, G.(1989) Les méthodes modernes de musculation: Données théoriques.et pratiques. Compte rendu du colloque de novembre 1988 à l'UFRSTAPS de Dijon. Ed : Université de Bourgogne.

Gauffin, H.; Ekstrand, J.; Arnesson, L.and Tropp, H. (1989) Vertical jump performance in soccer players. A comparative study of two training programmes. J. Human Movement Stud., 16, 215-224.

Gréhaigne, J.F. (1989) Football de mouvement. Vers une approche systémique du jeu. Thèse (nouveau régime). Université de Bourgogne. Ronéo.

Poulmedis, P. (1985) Isokinetic maximal torque power of Greek elite soccer players.
J. Orth. Sports Phys. Therapy, 5, 293-295.

INVESTIGATION OF PLYOMETRIC TRAINING IN RUGBY LEAGUE PLAYERS

M. DOYLE and T. REILLY
Centre for Sports and Exercise Sciences, Liverpool Polytechnic,
Liverpool, L3 3AF, England.

1 Introduction

Plyometric training describes exercises that utilise stretch-short-ening cycles of muscle actions. Training regimens that employ plyometric drills - such as bounding, hopping and drop-jumping - are employed by specialists in sprinting, jumping, gymnastics and other sports that engage the involved muscles eccentrically prior to forceful concentric actions. Due to the stretch-shortening loads employed during intense actions such as sprinting and jumping during games play, it is thought that plyometric training would be of benefit to football players. As repeated eccentric muscular actions cause delayed onset muscle soreness which peaks 2-3 days following execution of plyometric drills (Boocock et al., 1988), it is not clear whether this form of training would have any advantage when introduced during the competitive season . This study aimed to investigate the efficacy of a regimen of plyometric drills using professional Rugby League players within their competitive season.

2 Methods

Subjects (n=14) were professional players for Swinton Rugby League club, aged 21-30 years. They agreed to participate in the study after being informed about the rationale and organisation.

Players were randomly assigned to an experimental group and a control group (both n=7). Members of the experimental group incorporated plyometrics into their training twice a week for 8 weeks. The programme consisted mainly of repeated single-leg and double-leg bounding drills and jumps: it was supervised by one of the authors (M.D.) and progressively increased during the period of investigation. The normal fitness training consisted of 15 min warm-up with touch Rugby followed by 5 min stretching. Circuit training, comprising 3 circuits of 12 stations, each exercise being performed for 25 s on the first circuit and 20 s on subsequent circuits, then followed. The plyometric training at first consisted of 2 x 20 m double leg hops, 2 x 20 m single leg hops and 2 x 20 m double leg bounds. High knee tuck jumps, cone work (20 s) and squat jumps were included by the second week. From then on the programme was varied from week to week but included 6-7 different drills, each performed twice. The control group substituted sprinting drills for the plyometric regimen. These consisted of 6 x 20 m in the first

week. By the third week players were doing 4 x 30 m sprints, 4 x 30 m
towing a sledge plus a "press-up walk" over 30 m twice. Some of the
sprint sessions incorporated running with the ball. Otherwise, both
groups did their normal training programme, including the circuit
weight-training and muscle power work in common. The muscle power
work generally incorporated seven separate exercises engaging arm and
shoulder muscles, trunk, and leg muscle groups.

During the experimental period muscle soreness was rated by the
subjects in the days following each training session (Boocock et al.,
1988). The effects of the training were assessed using vertical and
standing broad jump tests (Fox, 1984), a modification of the
stair-run test of Margaria et al. (1966) and the Wingate Anaerobic
test. Form measurements in both groups were obtained before and
after the experimental period.

3 Results and Discussion

The plyometric regimen produced muscle soreness in experimental
subjects which peaked 24-72 hours after the training. The highest
soreness ratings were during the second week, the training load
having been increased at this time from the initial level (Figure 1).
A significant decrease in exercise-induced muscle soreness was noted
after 5 weeks compared to peak values in Week 2, suggesting
adaptations to the training by this time. Although the soreness
continued to decrease with repeated exposures, the plyometric
training did still cause soreness after 8 weeks.

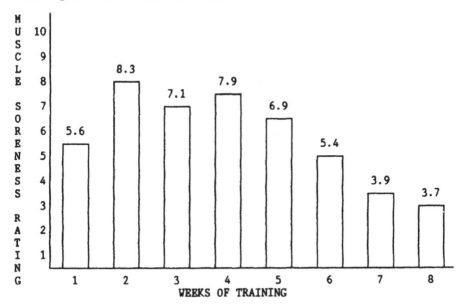

Fig.1. Muscle soreness ratings in experimental subjects over
the 8 weeks of plyometrics training.

Table 1. Muscular power performances in the control and experimental groups before and after the 8-week experimental period

Tests	Control		Experimental	
	Before	After	Before	After
Vertical jump (Power - W)	1313±146	1326±150	1398±252	1364±230
Standing broad jump (cm)	222±8	222±6	222±2	221±2
Stair run (W)	2608±352	2670±386	2729±275	2765±289
Peak power (Wingate - W)	926±113	941±102	865±71	857±104

All comparisons, before and after training and between groups are non-significant (P>0.05).

The players reported perceived benefits of the additional plyometric training and increased enjoyment. Despite these favourable subjective reactions, no improvements in muscular power were noted (Table 1). This calls into question the specific drills used, their introduction mid-way through the competitive season or their superimposition on the normal training programme. Further, the conventional tests of muscular power used in this study may have been insensitive to changes occurring within the muscular system that would be of benefit in games contexts but not necessarily in laboratory tests.

The enjoyment reported by the subjects suggests that in a modified form plyometrics may have a role to play in injecting variety into the training programme of Rugby League players. Future work should examine the efficacy of plyometrics introduced pre-season and as replacement for rather than supplemental to selected elements of the normal training prescription. A more extended period of study is recommended to evaluate both the performance enhancement and injury risk reduction of this regimen and alternative forms of plyometric training.

4 References

Boocock, M.G., Garbutt, G., Reilly, T., Linge, K. and Troup, J.D.G. (1988) The effects of gravity inversion on exercise-induced spinal loading. **Ergonomics**, 31, 1631-1637.
Fox, E.L. (1987) **Sports Physiology**. Saunders, Philadelphia.
Margaria, R., Aghemo, P. and Rovelli, E. (1966) Measurement of muscular power (anaerobic) in man. **J. Appl. Physiol.**, 21, 1662-1664.

THE EFFECT OF SEVERE EXERCISE ON FATIGUE AND ANAEROBIC ENERGY PRODUCTION DURING SUBSEQUENT INTENSE EXERCISE - THE IMPORTANCE OF ACTIVE RECOVERY.

J. Bangsbo, L. Johansen, & B. Saltin. August Krogh Institute, University of Copenhagen, Denmark

1 Introduction

A soccer player's capacity to perform repetitive high intensity exercise during a match might be crucial for the final outcome. During such exercise anaerobic energy is provided from the splitting of endogenous energy-rich phosphagens (i.e. intramuscular stores of adenosine triphoshate (ATP) and creatine phosphate (CP)) and from glycolysis which leads to lactate production even during exercise of short duration (Boobis, 1987). High blood lactate concentrations have been observed during soccer matches, and the question is whether these impair performance (Ekblom, 1986; Gerisch and Rutemoller, 1988; Bangsbo et al., 1991). Within the sports community, it is taken as a fact that lactate accumulation is the cause of the perceived fatigue during high intensity exercise. Based on several recent investigations, an exclusive role of lactate and pH may not be that obvious (Sjogaard et al., 1985; Juel et al., 1990). For soccer players the time needed to recover from high intensity exercise should be as short as possible. It is well known that low intensity exercise accelerates lactate disappearance from the blood (Hermansen and Stensvold, 1972). However, the influence of such exercise on muscle lactate concentration and on subsequent performance is not well established.

Thus, the aim of the present study was to evaluate 1) the role of muscle lactate (muscle pH) in the development of fatigue, 2) the effect of previous intense exercise on the anaerobic energy production, 3) the effect of low intensity exercise on muscle lactate disappearance and muscle performance. The exercise model chosen was the one-legged knee-extensor exercise, which allows for precise and quantitative metabolic evaluation, as well as for the establishment of relationships between these metabolic events and exercise performance (Bangsbo et al., 1990).

2 Methods

Six male subjects exercised in a supine position with the knee-extensors of one limb at a supramaximal work load (mean: 59 W; frequency: 60/min) to exhaustion (EX1). This was followed by 1) 10 min of recovery, 2) intense intermittent exercise (7 x 15 s exercise (90 W) and 15 s recovery) and 3) a 2.5 min recovery period. Then, the exhaustive exercise was repeated at the same power output (EX2). During all recovery periods the leg either rested (Passive-P) or performed low intensity exercise (Active-A). After a rest period of 1 h the other leg carried out the same exercise protocol, but with the opposite pattern of activity during the recovery periods. The choice of legs was randomized. Prior to and immediately after each exhaustive exercise bout a muscle biopsy was taken from m. vastus lateralis of the active muscle for lactate, glycogen, CP, ATP and pH analysis.

Catheters were placed in the two femoral veins and in one femoral artery. Measurements of leg blood flow and arterial-venous difference for oxygen and lactate were performed before and regularly during the supramaximal exercises and the recovery period after EX1. For references to the methods and calculations of leg oxygen uptake, muscle lactate production, and leg oxygen deficit, which has been shown to express the total leg anaerobic energy production, see Bangsbo et al. (1990). Part of the data have been published elsewhere (Bangsbo et al., 1992a).

3 Results

Prior to EX2-P muscle lactate of 13.1 mmol/kg w.w. was higher (P<0.05) than before EX1, and muscle pH of 6.85 was lower (P<0.05) the prior to EX1 (Fig. 1). Immediately after EX2-P muscle lactate tended to be lower and muscle pH tended to be higher than at the end of EX1 (Fig. 1).

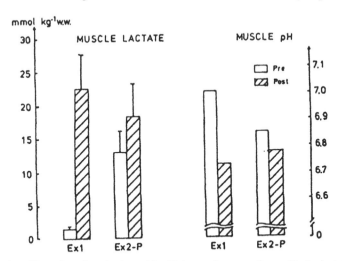

Fig. 1. Muscle lactate (left) and muscle pH (right) before (open bar) and immediately after (hatched bar) EX1 and EX2-P (modified from Bangsbo et al., 1992a).

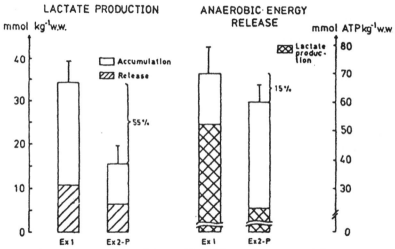

Fig. 2. Lactate production (left) and anaerobic energy production (right) during EX1 and EX2-P (modified from Bangsbo et al., 1992a).

The exercise time for EX2-P was reduced by 45 s or 20% compared to EX1 (3.73 min). Muscle glycogen was 94.1 mmol/kg w.w. prior to EX2-P, which was about 30% lower than before EX1. Glycogen depletion during EX2-P was reduced by 6.6 mmol/kg w.w. or 26% of EX1, and the lactate production was reduced by 55% (Fig. 2).

Limb oxygen uptake increased at the same rate during EX1 and EX2-P, and a similar peak value was reached. The estimated oxygen deficit for EX2-P was 22% lower (P<0.05) than for EX1 (Fig. 2), but this reduction (17 mmol ATP/kg w.w.) was less than the difference in release of ATP (28 mmol ATP/kg w.w.) due to the lowered lactate production during EX2-P. The actual depletion of ATP and CP amounted to about 17 mmol/kg w.w. and it was similar in EX1 and EX2-P (Table 1). This represented 23 and 28% of the total anaerobic energy production, respectively.

<u>Table 1</u>. Muscle CP and ATP concentrations (mmol/kg w.w.) before (PRE-) and after (POST-) the exhaustive exercise bouts. Means SE are given.

	EX1		EX2-P		EX2-A	
	PRE-	POST-	PRE-	POST-	PRE-	POST-
CP	19.75	3.63	15.46	3.32	16.40	3.11
	0.43	0.36	1.81	2.76	2.26	1.29
ATP	6.15	5.06	4.90*	3.99*	4.96*	3.57*
	0.42	0.63	0.65	0.72	0.53	0.60

*: Significant difference (P<0.05) from EX1.

Active recovery.

The net muscle lactate removal rate during the active recovery was larger (P<0.05) than during the passive recovery. Thus, prior to EX2-A muscle lactate of 9.9 mmol/kg w.w. was lower (P<0.05) than before EX2-P. During EX2-A, muscle lactate increased to 20.4 mmol/kg w.w., which was similar to EX2-P. The muscle pH during EX2-A was reduced from 6.84 to 6.76 or similar to EX2-P.

Time to exhaustion for EX2-A was lowered from 3.46 (EX1) to 3.00 min or by 13%, which was slightly less than the difference between EX1 and EX2-P. Prior to EX2-A, muscle glycogen concentration was 97.2 mmol/kg w.w. Muscle glycogen utilization by EX2-A was depressed compared to EX1, but the reduction amounted to only 3.4 mmol/kg w.w. or 13%. Lactate production was smaller in EX2-A compared to EX1, and the difference was in the order of 16.5 mmol/kg w.w. or 52% (P<0.05) which was similar to the alteration in EX2-P.

When the light exercise was performed during recovery leg blood flow and oxygen uptake were at a higher level at the start of EX2-A. Thus, the rate of utilization of the oxygen deficit during the first minute of EX2-A was about two-third that of EX1. This resulted in a 28% lower oxygen deficit (P<0.05) in EX2-A compared to EX1. Depletion of ATP and CP was similar for EX1 and EX2-A, and amounted to 16.7 and 18.5 mmol/kg w.w., respectively (Table 1).

4 Discussion

The high blood lactate concentrations observed during soccer play indicate that muscle lactate and H^+ concentrations can be high during a match (Ekblom, 1986; Gerisch and Rutemoller, 1988; Bangsbo et al., 1991). The question is how does that influence performance during the intense periods of a soccer match? Based on the findings in the one-leg experiment the effect of elevated muscle lactate and lowered pH appears not to be very dramatic. Muscle lactate concentration and muscle pH at exhaustion varied markedly between subjects, and muscle pH tended to be higher at the end of the second exercise bout, although muscle pH was lowered prior to this exercise. These findings are in agreement with data from Sahlin and Ren (1989) showing that, despite a persistently high muscle lactate (probably lowered muscle pH), contraction force was completely restored 2 min after intensive isometric muscle contractions.

It appears that other factors caused fatigue and impaired performance in the second exercise bouts. Lack of available ATP seems not to be among these, since in every case muscle ATP at exhaustion was only slightly lower than the level prior to exercise (less than 20%). This conclusion was supported by a lower anaerobic energy production during the second exercise bout after the active recovery when the initial oxygen uptake was elevated compared to the EX2-P. Thus, the exercise was terminated before the anaerobic capacity was utilized. It appears that the elements responsible for the development of fatigue retard cross-bridge cycling and the concomitant usage of ATP, and lead to a gradual decrease in muscle tension development and ultimately to exhaustion. The same reduction in ATP concentration in each case indicates that ATP utilization is tightly matched by its rate of resynthesis.

Performance during the second exercise bout after the active recovery was less impaired in comparison to exercise followed by passive recovery. Based on the discussion above and the fact that the same muscle pH was observed prior to the two exercise bouts, it seems that the lower muscle lactate concentration prior to EX2-A cannot explain the difference in performance. Other factors involved in the development of muscle fatigue must have been influenced by the low intensity exercise.

The intense intermittent exercise prior to the second exercise bouts resulted in a lowering of the glycogenolytic rate and rate of lactate production during the subsequent intense exercise, which was not influenced by low intensity activities during the recovery periods. The question remains as to what causes these effects. The lowered muscle glycogen concentration is an unlikely candidate, since it has been demonstrated that glycogenolytic and glycolytic rates during short term intense exercise are independent of initial muscle glycogen concentration when it is above 30 mmol/kg w.w. (Bangsbo et al., 1992b).

The lowered pH prior to the second exercise bout could be a possibility, as it has been shown in vitro that elevated H^+ in the muscle inhibits phosphorylase and PFK activities, both of which are considered the key regulating enzymes of the glycogenolytic and glycolytic rates, respectively (Chasiotis, 1983). It is questionable whether the reduction in pH was large enough to inhibit these enzymes in vivo. Recent studies on the allosteric regulation of PFK within the physiological range have shown that the effect of pH is negated as long as pH is above 6.6 (Dobson et al., 1986). In addition, it was observed in a separate study that the lactate production rate was reduced even after 1 h of recovery, when muscle lactate had returned to resting level (Bangsbo et al., 1992b). Thus, it appears that the elevated H^+ concentration is not the only explanation for the reduction in glycogenolytic and glycolytic rates. Support for this notion is the finding of a tendency towards higher pH at exhaustion in the EX2 bouts. For further discussion of this topic see Bangsbo et al. (1992a).

The present study showed that previous intense exercise has a definite effect resulting in a lowering of perf-

ormance time and lactate production during a subsequent
short term intense exercise bout. Sprinting and other high
intensity exercise periods in soccer are short (Bangsbo et
al., 1991), but the energy demand of the exercising muscles
is probably higher than for the muscle in this knee-
extensor study. Thus, it is likely that changes similar to
those observed for the isolated muscle group in the present
study occur after intense exercise periods in soccer
(Boobis, 1987). This is supported by the high blood lactate
concentration often observed during soccer, which reflects
even higher muscle lactate concentrations (Jacobs and
Kaiser, 1982; Ekblom, 1986). By combining these items of
information it appears that fatigue, characterized by the
players not being able to perform maximally, could occur
after high intensity exercise periods in soccer. It is
temporary and could last for several minutes, but in most
cases it is much shorter. Nevertheless, as fatigue of a
player might be crucial for the final outcome of a match,
it is very important that the players recover as fast as
possible from the intense exercise periods. The present
study showed that active recovery reduced the impairment in
performance during subsequent exercise. This means that the
muscles reach normality faster when low intensity exercise
is performed, and that it might be advantageous for the
players to walk or jog instead of standing still after the
high intensity exercise periods during a match. By this
exercise the rate of muscle lactate removal is also
increased, but this might not be important, since factors
other than muscle lactate appear to cause fatigue in these
circumstances.

5 References

Bangsbo, J., Gollnick, P.D., Graham, T.E., Juel, C., Kiens,
    B., Mizuno, M., & Saltin, B (1990) Anaerobic
    energy production & O_2 deficit - debt relationship
    during exhaustive exercise in humans. J. Physiol., 422,
    539-559.
Bangsbo, J., N_ rregaard, L. and Thors_ , F. (1991)
    Activity profile of competition soccer. Can. J. Sports
    Sci., 16,110-116.
Bangsbo, J., Graham T., Johansen L., Strange S. and Saltin
    B. (1992a) Elevated muscle acidity and energy
    production   during exhaustive exercise in man. Am.
    J. Physiol., submitted.
Bangsbo, J., Graham, T.E., Kiens, B. and Saltin, B.
    (1992b) Elevated muscle glycogen and anaerobic energy
    production during exhaustive exercise in man. J.
    Physiol., in press.

Boobis, L.H. (1987) Metabolic aspects of fatigue during sprinting, in **Exercise: Benefits, Limits and Adaptations** (eds D. Macleod, R. Maughan, M. Nimmo, T. Reilly and C. Williams), E. & F.N. Spon, London/New York., pp. 116 143.

Chasiotis, D. (1983) The regulation of glycogen phosphorylase and glycogen breakdown in human skeletal muscle. **Acta Physiol. Scand. Suppl.**, 518, 1-68.

Dobson, G.P, Yamamoto, E. & Hochachka, P.W. (1986) Phosphofructokinase control in muscle: Nature and reversal of pH-dependent ATP inhibition. **Am. J. Physiol.**, 250, R71-76.

Ekblom, B. (1986) Applied physiology of soccer. **Sports Med.**, 3, 50-60.

Gerisch, G., Rutemoller, E. & Weber, K. (1988) Sportsmedical measurements of performance in soccer, in **Science and Football** (eds T. Reilly, A. Lees, K. Davids, and W.J. Murphy), E. & F.N. Spon, London/New York, pp. 60-67.

Hermansen, L. and Stensvold, I. (1972) Production and removal of lactate during exercise in man. **Acta Physiol. Scand.**, 86, 191-201.

Jacobs, I. and Kaiser, P. (1982) Lactate in blood, mixed skeletal muscle, and FT and ST fibres during cycle exercise in man. **Acta Physiol. Scand.**, 114, 461-466.

Juel, C., Bangsbo, J. and Saltin, B. (1990) Lactate and potassium fluxes from skeletal muscle during intense dynamic knee-extensor exercise in man. **Acta Physiol. Scand.**, 140, 147-159.

Sahlin, K. and Ren, J.M. (1989) Relationship of contraction capacity changes during recovery from a fatiguing contraction. **J. Appl. Physiol.**, 67, 648-654.

Sjogaard, G., Adams, R.P and Saltin, B. (1985) Water and ion shifts in skeletal muscle of humans with intense dynamic knee extension. **Am. J. Physiol.**, 248, R190-196.

Acknowledgments

The original data presented in this article were obtained in studies supported by grants from Team Danmark and Danish Natural Science Foundation (11-7776).

VARIATIONS IN PHYSICAL CAPACITY IN A PERIOD INCLUDING SUPPLEMENTAL TRAINING OF THE NATIONAL DANISH SOCCER TEAM FOR WOMEN

K. JENSEN and B. LARSSON
Team Denmark Testcenter, Odense and Copenhagen, Denmark

1 Introduction

Female soccer is a growing part of the Danish soccer federation's activity. At club level the players in the First Division train about 2-3 times each week. While male players selected for the national team are full time professionals and physically very well trained, this is not always the case for female players. With the intention of bringing the female team up among the best female teams in the world, supplementary physical training was induced in the group of female players from the national team. The purpose of this study was to follow variations in physical capacity in that period.

2 Methods

Body composition, maximal oxygen uptake, running capacity on a treadmill, and jumping height were monitored four times between August 1989 and November 1990 in ten players with an age of 23 (range 19-26) years, a height of 169 (159-179) cm and a body weight of 63.2 (54.6-74.1) kg. Percent body fat was estimated using skinfolds measurements according to Durnin and Womersley (1974). The players ran continuously 2-3 times 5 minutes on a treadmill at 11-15 km/h corresponding to a relative intensity from 70-95 % of maximal oxygen uptake. After 10-15 minutes rest they did a maximal test at 15 km/h with an increasing inclination of 2 %, applied after 2, 3.5, and 5 min respectively. Heart rate, maximal oxygen uptake, blood lactate concentration and total time during the "all out" session were measured. The velocity corresponding to a concentration of blood lactate of 4 mmol/l, (OBLA), was estimated according to Sjodin and Jacobs (1981). During the rest period between the submaximal and the maximal test the players performed a countermovement jump on a force platform to estimate the maximal jumping height. A supplementary training programme including general strength training and interval running was given to the players. At least every second month they reported back to the national coach the total amounth of training done during the period. The programmes were evaluated and changed according to test results and individual background.

3 Results

3.1 Laboratory test

Estimated percent body fat went down from 22.3 (20.1-28.3)% to 20.1 (17.5-25.0)%, (P<0.005). According to this, body weight was reduced by 1 kg. The running velocity on a treadmill correspondent to a blood lactate concentration of 4 mmol/l (OBLA), was increased from 11.4 (11.0-13.3)km/h to 13.4 (11.5-15.6)km/h, (P<0.005). The maximal running time, (at 15 km/h and at increasing incrementals of +2 % submitted after 2, 3.5 and 5 min respectively) was increased from 3.87 (2.70-5.50)min to 4.57 (3.77-5.93)min (P<0.05). The maximal oxygen consumption was increased from 53.3 (48.0-60.8)ml/kg/min to 57.6 (51.5-63.8)ml/kg/min (P<0.001). The jumping height in a countermovement jump (estimated from flying time measured on a force platform) was increased from 34.0 (26.4-41.9)cm to 37.8 (30.7-45.7)cm, (P<0.05).

Table 1. Variations in antropometric characteristics of female players

N =10	Age (years)	Height (cm)	Weight (kg)	Body fat (%)
Aug 89	23.4 (19-26)	169 (159-179)	63.2 (54.6-74.1)	22.3 (20.1-28.3)
Feb 90	23.9 (20-26)	169 (159-179)	63.7 (53.7-74.0)	22.3 (18.9-27.8)
Aug 90	24.4 (21-27)	169 (159-179)	62.0 (53.6-71.1)	20.5 (18.2-23.2)
Nov 90	24.7 (21-27)	169 (159-179)	62.2 (53.9-74.1)	20.1 (17.5-25.0)

Table 2. Variations in maximal running time, velocity at OBLA, maximal oxygen uptake and jumping height

Maximal running time at 15 km/h and inclination from 0-6 % (min)	Velocity at onset of blood lactate accumulation" "OBLA" (km/h)	Maximal oxygen uptake (ml/kg/min)	Maximal jumping height (cm)
3.87 (2.70-5.50)	11.4 (11.0-13.3)	53.3 (48.0-60.8)	34.0 (26.4-41.9)
3.99 (3.00-5.33)	12.8 (11.0-14.5)	53.9 (47.2-61.6)	35.4 (29.5-44.2)
4.28 (3.00-6.00)	12.8 (11.2-14.5)	55.1 (48.2-62.9)	37.5 (31.9-47.2)
4.57 (3.77-5.93)	13.4 (11.5-15.6)	57.6 (51.5-63.8)	37.8 (30.7-45.7)

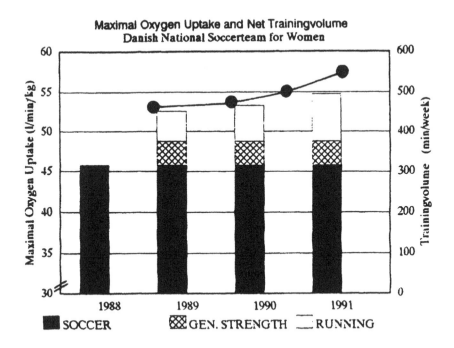

Fig. 1. Net training volume and the oxygen uptake

3.2 Supplemental Training

Supplemental training of players from the national Danish soccer team was included for a period of 15 months. In Danish soccer clubs the training of women during the season consists of 2-3 sessions of 90 min per week. The extra training of the national players consisted of running sessions (2-4 times 20-30 min per week) and general strength training (1-2 times 30 min per week). The training frequency was individually adapted according to civil work status and so on. The intensity of the running sessions was increased during the period. Typical training models in the first part of the period was steady state running, in the second part interval training (e.g. 5-4-3-2-1 min with increasing intensity), and in the third part very short intervals (e.g. 3 times 6 min with 15 sec "all out" running and 15 sec "jogging").

4 Conclusion

It is concluded that the increased physical capacity was due to the combination of supplementary training as well as to changes in the women's attitudes to physical training.

5 References

Durnin, J.V. and Womersley, J. (1974) Body fat assessed from total density and its estimation from skinfolds thickness: measurements on 481 men and women aged from 16 to 72 years. Br.J.Nutr., 32, 77-99.

Sjodin, B. and Jacobs, I. (1981) Onset of blood lactate accumulation and marathon running performance. Int. J. Sports Med., 2, 23-26.

PART FOUR

Physiology o
Match-play

WORK INTENSITY DURING SOCCER MATCH-PLAY (A CASE STUDY)

T.OGUSHI *J.OHASHI **H.NAGAHAMA ***M.ISOKAWA ****S.SUZUKI

The Dept.of Physical Education,Sophia University,Tokyo,Japan.
 *Daito Bunka University   **Asia University
***Tokyo Metropolitan University ****Seikei University

1 Introduction

Studies report that work intensity during a soccer game is approximately 75 to 80% $\dot{V}O2$ max(Ekblom,1986 and Van Gool et al.,1988). These are estimated values calculated from heart rate during the game.

The purpose of this study was to estimate work intensity during soccer match-play using actual oxygen uptake during a game.

2 Method

Two student players were chosen for this investigation.The players' age, height,body mass,$\dot{V}O2max$ and HRmax are shown in Table 1.

Subjects had a 90 min friendly match for measurement of $\dot{V}O2$ and HR during the game. They played the game wearing a mask and a 200 l Douglas bag for collecting expired gases midway through each half.

The collection time of expired gases was 141 to 168 s. The weight of the kit for collecting expired gases was 1200 g.

The HR during the game was monitored continuously with short range radio telemetry.

The distance covered during the game by each player was analysed by hand notation.

Table 1. Physical characteristics of the subjects

	Age (yrs)	Height (cm)	Body Mass (kg)	$\dot{V}O2max$ (ml/kg/min)	HRmax (beat/min)
A	21	174.5	63.0	62.5	200
B	21	173.8	62.0	62.1	194

3 Results

Table 2. The average HR and the HR during the measurement
of oxygen uptake during a game

| | Average(beat/min)(±SD) | | Under measurement(beat/min)(±SD) | |
	1st Half	2nd Half	1st Half	2nd Half
A	160.2(19.5)	159.3(16.5)	167.9(12.0)	140.8(6.9)
B	161.2(17.3)	162.1(14.4)	167.0(3.1)	164.7(11.4)

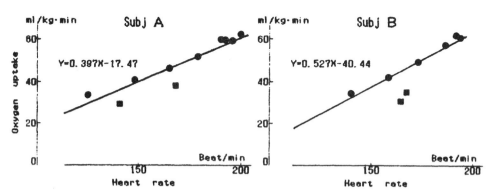

Figure 1. The relationship between heart rate and oxygen
uptake (●laboratory, ■during the game).

The $\dot{V}O_2max$ and HRmax of subjects are shown in Table 1. The
average HR and the HR during the measurement of oxygen
uptake are shown in Table 2.

The HR during the measurement of oxygen uptake was a
little higher than the average HR. The relationships
between HR and oxygen uptake obtained by the laboratory
test and field test are shown in Figure 1.

The estimated values of oxygen uptake calculated by
HR-$\dot{V}O_2$ regression lines were 47 to 49 ml/kg/min, 38 to
46 ml/kg/min for each half. These values correspond
respectively to 76 to 79% and 61 to 74% of $\dot{V}O_2max$. The
values of actual oxygen uptake during the game were 35 to
38 ml/kg/min, 29 to 30 ml/kg/min in each half. These
values also correspond respectively to 56 to 61% and 47 to
49% of $\dot{V}O_2max$.

4 Discussion

To play wearing a mask and a Douglas bag did not have much
effect on the player, because the measured HR for oxygen

Table 3. The average distance covered and distance covered under measurement of $\dot{V}O2$ (5min conversion)

	Average(m/5min)		Under measurement(m/5min)	
	1st Half	2nd Half	1st Half	2nd Half
A	755	561	685	460
B	483	603	381	610

uptake was not much different from the average HR(Table 2) and the distance covered under measurement was similar to the average distance covered during the game.(Table 3)

There are several reports concerning % $\dot{V}O2max$ during a soccer game. It is reported that approximately 75 to 80% $\dot{V}O2max$ is the work intensity during a soccer game(Matsumoto,1977; Ekblom,1986; Van Gool et al.,1988). Our predictions from HR also showed a similar result,but the values of % $\dot{V}O2max$ obtained by the actual oxygen uptake were 56 to 61% and 47 to 49% of $\dot{V}O2max$. They were 30 to 50% lower than values of % $\dot{V}O2max$ calculated by HR-$\dot{V}O2$ regression lines.It is expected that the values of % $\dot{V}O2max$ of previous reports are also 30% higher.

Soccer is said to have a high work intensity, but from this result the values are closer to moderate intensity exercise. The major component of physical load in soccer is running(Rohde et al.,1988),but the standing, walking and jogging between dash and dash make a soccer game closer to moderate intensity exercise.

We suggest that there is a large error in presuming work intensity using HR in intermittent exercise like soccer. This is due to a difference in $\dot{V}O2$ response between intermittent excercise and steady state exercise.If standard error can be made clear by gathering a large amount of data,the value of work intensity calculated by HR will be revised more accurately.

5 References

Ekblom,B.(1986) Applied physiology of soccer. **Sports Med.**, 3, 50-60.

Matsumoto,M.(1977) A study on game analysis in soccer. **J.Sport Sci.**, Fukushima University, 29, 55-65

Rohde,H.C.and Espersen,T.(1988) Work intensity during soccer training and match-play,in **Science and Football**, (eds T.Reilly, A.Lees, K.Davids and W.J.Murphy),E.and F.N.Spon, London, pp.68-75

Van Gool,D., Van Gerven,D. and Boutmans,J.(1988) The physiological load imposed on soccer players during real match-play,in **Science and Football**,(eds T.Reilly,A.Lees, K.Davids and W.J.Murphy),E.and F.N.Spon,London, pp.51-59

THE RATIO OF PHYSIOLOGICAL INTENSITY OF MOVEMENTS DURING SOCCER MATCH-PLAY

J. OHASHI[*], M. ISOKAWA[**], H. NAGAHAMA[***] and T. OGUSHI[****]
* Daito Bunka University, Saitama, Japan
** Tokyo Metropolitan University, Tokyo, Japan
*** Asia University, Tokyo, Japan
**** Sophia University, Tokyo, Japan

1 Introduction

Soccer players move in many directions and at various speeds during a match. The movements in the field are dependent on their various physiological abilities such as aerobic power, anaerobic power and so on. In order to design proper training programmes for soccer players, an estimate of the distribution of the ratios of physiological intensities is needed. Reilly and Thomas (1976) reported that the percentage of the distance covered at the individual's top speed was 11.2% of the total distance. Withers et al. (1982) reported that it was 18.8%. Mayhew and Wenger (1982) reported that 11.3% of the total match time was at the highest speed. Yamanaka et al. (1988) reported that it was between 7 and 10%. As these investigators estimated the distance covered and the time spent by the use of pre-determined modes of players' movement, such estimations seem to reduce the precision or objectivity of the data.

Ohashi et al. (1988) developed a new method of measuring movement speeds and distances covered during a match. The methodological principle was an application of a triangular surveying method which was input to a computer. This system made it possible to obtain precise measurements of the distance and the time covered at various speeds.

The purpose of this study was to estimate the ratios of physiological intensity using measurements of movement speeds during an actual match and relate these to running speeds and corresponding blood lactate concentrations obtained in a laboratory test.

2 Methods

The subjects were three university soccer players. All of them were players in the 2nd Division of the University

124

Soccer League in the Kanto area. Table 1 shows subjects'
physical characteristics.

Table 1. Physical characteristics of the subjects

Subject	age	Height (cm)	Body Mass (kg)	VO_2max (1/min)	VO_2max (ml/kg/min)
KYO(FW)	21	176.2	69.6	3.80	54.6
FJI(MF)	22	165.7	51.4	3.24	63.0
KAB(DF)	22	175.3	68.5	3.71	54.2

In order to obtain the relationships between the
running speeds and blood lactate levels, a treadmill test
was administered. Three university soccer players were
required to run on a treadmill for 4 min each at speeds of
150 m/min up to 300 m/min with the speed increased by 30
m/min. The inclination of the treadmill was constantly
maintained at zero degree throughout the run. The blood
samples were taken from the subjects' earlobes within 1 min
rest after each work period. The blood lactate
concentrations of the samples were analyzed by the
enzymatic method using a TOYOBO Diagluca lactate analyzer.
   The subjects' movement speeds during an actual match
were measured in a regular match of their university
league.
   Two VTR cameras were set up on two spots, 20 m away from
the corner flag outside the field. Each tripod which was
attached to the VTR camera was equipped with
potentiometers. A subject was always followed at the centre
of the viewfinders of two cameras;i.e. signals indicating
angles obtained by potentiometers were sequentially
converted into digital data and recorded on a data tape
recorder at an interval of 0.5 seconds(Fig.1).

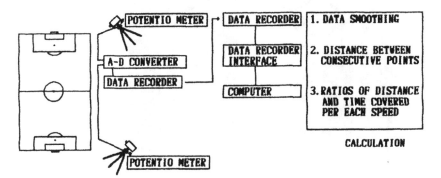

Fig.1 Measurement instruments and the data flow.

After the data were input into the computer, every X,Y
co-ordinate of a player was calculated from two-angle data
and the constant distance between the two cameras. Then,
the distance between two consecutive X,Y co-ordinates was
calculated continuously to obtain the total distance
covered(Fig.1).

In this study, each subject was interchangeably followed
up to 5 min each 6 times for 30 min during the whole period
of the match.

3 Results

In the treadmill test, the running speeds coresponding to 4
mM blood lactate level of the three subjects were 3.4, 3.7
and 3.9 m per second, respectively (Table 2).

Table 2. Running speed at 4 mM blood lactate level and the
ratio of time and distance covered above that
level during an actual match

subject	running speed at 4 mM (m/s)	above 4 mM time (%)	above 4 mM distance (%)
KYO	3.7	8.8	24.9
FJI	3.9	11.9	31.1
KAB	3.4	10.4	27.4

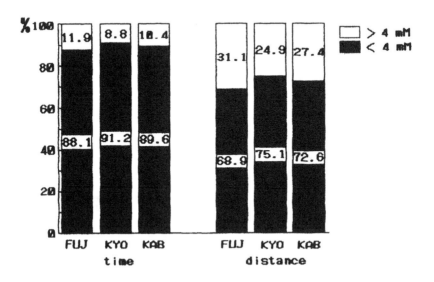

Fig.2 Ratios of movement speed at 4 mM during a match.

The distances covered in 5 min for each subject were approximately 500 to 600 m. Although there were differences in the distance covered in 5 min among the three subjects, the distance covered at below 4 m/s was approximately 400 m for all the subjects.

In this study 50 to 60 percent of the total distance was covered at below 3m/s and about 70 percent was covered below 4m/s. Also, 75 to 80 percent of the total time of motion was spent below 3 m/s and approximately 90 percent was below 4 m/s.

The ratios of distance covered at above the 4 mM lactate level were 24.9, 31.1 and 27.4 percent, for the three subjects. The ratios of time spent at the same level were 8.8, 10.4 and 11.9 percent, respectively (Table 2, Fig. 2).

4 Discussion

Estimating physiological intensity of movement in an actual soccer match is one of the most important factors for planning soccer training. The distance covered during a match can be a rough estimate of physiological intensity. Ohashi(1981) reported that Japan national team players (n=50) covered 11,529 m and Ohashi et al.(1991) reported that the world's top club team players (n=199) who took part in the Toyota European South American Cup (1980-1989) covered 9,971 m. Using published reports (Withers et al., 1982; Whitehead,1975; Reilly and Thomas,1976) Ekblom (1986) concluded that soccer players covered approximately 7 - 13 km in a match and he also indicated that 10 players in a German second division team covered an average of 9.8 km in a game of high quality. Furthermore Ekblom (1986) noted; 'it seems that the main difference between players of different quality is not the distance covered during the game but the percentage of overall fast speed distance during the game and the absolute values of maximal speed play during the game'.

Reilly and Thomas (1976) and Withers et al. (1982) respectively reported that 11.2% and 18.8% of the total distance were covered at the highest individual speed. Mayhew and Wenger (1985) and Yamanaka et al.(1988) reported that 11.3% and 7-10% of the total match time were spent at the highest speed. In these studies the individual player's actual speed was not measured during a match. The speeds in these previous studies were estimated by observing modes of players' movement. Therefore, their work intensities had a reduced objectivity.

In this study, we estimated the ratio of aerobic vs. anaerobic aspects using actual movement speeds measured during a match, using the 4 mM lactate level determined in a treadmill test for reference. The 4 mM lactate level which was termed OBLA (Onset of Blood Lactate Accumulation) by Sjodin and Jacobs (1986) is one of the predictors of the "anaerobic threshold"(AT). Although there are many other physiological views about AT, we use the 4 mM lactate level as a convenient reference parameter which is applicable to physiological testing and physical training.

In the present study, the ratios of distance covered and time spent at above the 4 mM lactate level were 24.9, 31.1 and 27.4 percent in distance covered and 8.8, 10.4 and 11.9 percent in time spent during a match, respectively (Table 2, Fig. 2). Assuming that movement speed at above the 4 mM lactate level indicates high intensity anaerobic work, it is suggested that the ratios of aerobic vs. anaerobic aspects of work during an actual match were 7:3 in the total distance and 9:1 in the total match time.

References

Ekblom, B.(1986) Applied physiology of soccer. Sports Med.,3,50-60.

Mayhew, S.R. and Wenger, H.A.(1985) Time-motion analysis of professional soccer. J. Human Mov't. Stud., 11, 49-52.

Ohashi, J. and Togari, H.(1981) Changes of moving distance in football match-play (in Japanese). The Proceedings of the Department of Physical Education, College of General Education, University of Tokyo 15, 27-34.

Ohashi, J. Togari, H. Isokawa, M. and Suzuki, S. (1988) Measuring movement speeds and distances covered during soccer match-play, in Science and Football (eds T. Reilly, A. Lees, K. David and W.J. Murphy), E. & F.N. Spon, London, pp. 329-333.

Ohashi, J. Togari, H and Takii, T. (1991) The distances covered during matches in the world class soccer players. (in Japanese)The Proceedings of the Department of Sports Sciences, College of Arts and Sciences, University of Tokyo 25, 1-5.

Reilly, T. and Thomas, V. (1976) A motion analysis of work-rate in different positional roles in professional football match-play. J Human Mov't. Stud., 2, 87-97.

Sjodin, B., and Jacobs, I. (1981) Onset of blood lactate accumulation and marathon running performance. Int. J. Sports Med.,2,23-26.

Whitehead W. (1975) Conditioning for Sport, E.P.Publishing Co. Ltd, Yorkshire, pp.40-42.

Withers, R.T., Maricic, Z., Wasilewski, S. and Kelly, L. (1982) Match analyses of Australian professional soccer players. J. Human Mov't. Stud., 8, 159-176.

Yamanaka, K., Haga, S., Shindo, M., Narita, J., Koseki, Y., Matsuura, Y. and Eda, M. (1988) Time and motion analysis in top class soccer games. in Science and Football (eds T. Reilly, A. Lees, K. David and W.J. Murphy) E. & F.N. Spon, London, pp. 334-340.

BLOOD LACTATE LEVELS IN COLLEGE SOCCER PLAYERS DURING MATCH-PLAY.

M SMITH, G CLARKE, T HALE and T McMORRIS.
West Sussex Institute Of Higher Education, College Lane, Chichester, West Sussex
PO19 4PE, England.

1 Introduction

When looking at the demand characteristics of soccer, in terms of rate and duration of energy supply, it is evident that a player must have well developed anaerobic and aerobic capacities. The energy demands associated with the repeated bursts of very intense, yet brief activity are met via anaerobic processes. Aerobic metabolism provides the ongoing energy supply which enables the player to last the duration of a game.

Time and motion studies (Whitehead, 1975; Reilly and Thomas, 1976; Mayhew and Wenger, 1985; and Ekblom, 1986) have shown that players cover between 7.5 - 13.5 km per game, with the majority of energy being supplied via aerobic processes. Mayhew and Wenger (1985) stated that football is 88% aerobic in nature. Data from previous research (Cochrane and Pyke, 1976, Ekblom, 1986) looking at the maximum aerobic power of players revealed a range of 56.1 - 66.0 ml/kg/min. Therefore the link between the need and the existence of a well developed aerobic power is clearly evident.

With the development of new technology, such as portable heart rate monitors and lactate analysers, researchers have become increasingly interested in not only evaluating the rate at which a player accumulates lactate (derived via anaerobic glycolysis) but also assessing the importance of anaerobic glycolysis in the overall supply of energy during match-play. Carli et al. (1986) measured lactate after the warm-up (just prior to kick off), at half time and at full time. During match-play blood lactate ranged between 1.5 - 4.0 mM. Rohde et al. (1988) compared blood lactate and heart rate responses recorded during training with those recorded at half time and full time in Danish first division games. Results showed work intensity to be significantly lower in training compared to matches and the authors recommended increasing the training intensity. Lactate levels recorded during match-play ranged between 3.2 and 7.8 mM (mean 4.4 mM). In a study using top German amateur teams, Gerisch et al. (1988) measured lactate at half time and full time during competitive matches to compare systems of play. Results ranged from 2.2 mM to 12.4 mM (mean 6.0 mM). They found zonal coverage systems produced lower lactate levels than "man to man" defence.

The importance of energy supplied via anaerobic glycolysis to meet the demands for a rapid rate of energy supply during match-play is therefore evident. However, there were important limitations with these previous pieces of research. The limitations related to not only the number of blood samples taken, but also, the time of sampling (pre-match, half time and full time). Consequently, a true reflection of lactate kinetics during match-play has not yet been established.

The purpose of this study was to examine blood lactate kinetics during match-play.

2 Method

Six football players (West Sussex Institute of Higher Education 1st XI) whose mean
(± S.D.) height, body mass and age were 179.5 5.5 cm, 73.98 2.67 kg and 21.2
1.3 years respectively, gave their informed consent to take part in the study.

Each subject was required to perform an exercise test for the determination of
blood lactate accumulation on a Quinton motorised treadmill. Before each test was
conducted the temperature of the physiology laboratory was recorded along with the
subject's height and body mass. The subject was fitted with a short range radio
telemeter (PE 3000 Sports tester) which allowed heart rate to be monitored.

The test began once the subject had increased his heart rate to 140 - 150 beats/min
during a 5 min warm-up. The subject was then required to complete a series of 5 min
work stages until a blood lactate concentration of 4mM had been achieved. Once the
subject had reached 4mM, the test was terminated.

During the treadmill test the speed was increased by 1 km/h every 5 min. Heart rate
(beats/min) was recorded during minutes 3 - 4. A 50 microlitre fingertip blood
sample was drawn in the fifth minute and measured for lactate concentration using a
Kontron 640 Lactate analyser.

Three days after the treadmill test the subject played in a South East England
Colleges league match. Each subject was fitted with a PE 3000 Sports tester watch
which recorded and stored his heart rate at 15 s intervals. Fifty microlitre finger tip
blood samples were drawn randomly throughout the game. The samples were taken
when the game had stopped to either retrieve the ball, for treatment of injuries or
cautions. The sampling took approximately 10 s. Both the referee and opposition
gave their consent for the subject to go off the pitch during blood sampling. Heart
rate plots were subsequently drawn post-game using a BBC Computer. Blood
samples were analysed for lactate concentration using a Kontron 640 Lactate
analyser.

Team positions among subjects varied, allowing positional comparisons to be
made.

3 Results

Data was collected during two South East England Colleges league game between
two mid-table teams. The results of the games were 0-0. Table 1 shows the range of
heart rates and lactate values recorded for each subject during match-play. All
subjects had lactate values above 4 mM with subjects PB (centre midfield) and GN
(centre forward) exhibiting the highest values, 10.52 and 11.63 mM respectively.
Also all subjects reached heart rates well above those recorded during the treadmill
test to establish the 4 mM reference point heart rate. Subject PS (left back) recorded
the highest heart rate of 200 beats/min.

Table 1: Individual subject's heart rate at the 4 mM reference point, range of heart rates and range of lactates for each of the subjects during match-play.

	Heart Rate at 4 mM (beats/min)	Match HR (beats/min)	Match Lactate (mM)
PS (LB)	175	125 - 200	2.79 - 8.49
RHO (CH)	169	97 - 185	1.84 - 5.64
PB (CM)	179	132 - 193	2.55 - 10.52
GC (LM)	166	122 - 176	2.51 - 7.68
RHA (RM)	173	134 - 189	2.29 - 7.33
GN (CF)	143	126 - 181	3.95 - 11.63

Key: left back (LB), centre half (CH), centre midfield (CM), left midfield (LM), right midfield (RM), centre forward (CF)

Figure 1 (a), (b) and (c). Heart rate, blood lactate responses and 4 mM heart rate reference points for subjects RHO (centre half), PS (left back) and PB (centre midfield), respectively.

Figure 1(a).

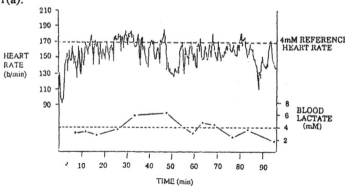

Figure 1 (b).

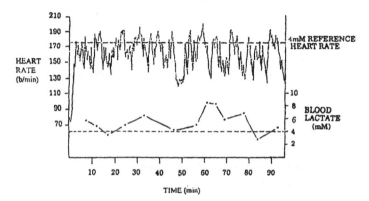

Figure 1 (c).

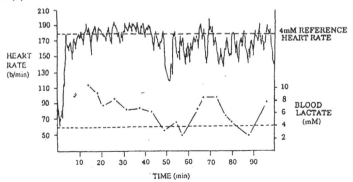

Figures 1 (a), (b) and (c) show heart rate, blood lactate responses and 4 mM heart rate reference points for subjects RHO (centre half), PS (left back) and PB (centre midfield), respectively. RHO's (Figure 1a) heart rate rarely rose above the 4 mM reference heart rate figure of 169 beats/min. A blood lactate value of 5.64 mM was the highest achieved, this occurring just prior to half time. The heart rate trace, for subject PS (Figure 1b), shows a frequent increase above the 4 mM heart rate reference value of 175 beats/min, with a highest heart rate of 200 beats/min. A blood lactate value of 8.49 mM was recorded during the second half. The lactate response shows marked fluctuations as the player adjusted to the changing energy demands experienced throughout the game. Of interest for subject PB (Figure 1c) is the contrast in physiological responses experienced between first and second half. During the first half the heart rate response was consistently near or above the 4 mM reference heart rate of 179 beats/min, with a highest lactate value of 10.52 mM. In the second half the heart rate response was much lower, with the highest lactate level being 8.70 mM.

4 Discussion

The purpose of the study was principally to examine the levels of lactate concentration a footballer experiences during match-play, and from this outline implications for individual training. Results of the study showed a range of lactate levels among the subjects of 1.84 - 11.63 mM (mean 5.23 mM). These results are higher than previous research when blood samples had been taken at half and full time (Carli et al., 1986; Gerisch et al., 1988; Tumilty et al., 1988 and Rohde and Espersen, 1988). The lactate values found in the present study were higher than those found by Bangsbo et al. (1991) who sampled at several intervals during a non-competitive match.

The most probable explanation of the higher lactate values found in this study lie in the methods used. Whereas previously blood samples have been taken during breaks in the game i.e. half and full time (except for Bangsbo et al., 1991), in the present study samples were taken at random intervals throughout the matches. This has obvious advantages over previous methods. Continual lactate sampling provided a frequent indication of the importance of anaerobic glycolysis during match-play. By being able to pull off a player randomly and evaluating the quantity of lactate produced, the truly intermittent nature of football becomes fully apparent. Lactate levels were seen to change rapidly and within a wide range for each individual. For example, subject PB (centre midfield) showed lactate responses ranging between 2.55 - 10.52 mM during a game.

Lactate and heart rate recordings highlighted different levels of stress experienced by players operating in different positions. Subject RHO (centre half) experienced the lowest lactate and heart rate responses when compared to the other players. This may be related to the system his team adopted for that particular match in that he played as part of a zone defence, marking space rather than "man to man" marking. These findings agree with Gerisch et al. (1988) who showed that zonal coverage systems produced lower lactate levels than "man to man" marking. If RHO (centre half) had been playing in a system using "man to man" marking he would have shadowed the opposing centre forward. Therefore, it would be reasonable to suggest that his heart rate and lactate responses would be different to those found in this study and he would be more likely to demonstrate similar physiological responses to those of the opposing centre forward.

An important consequence of this study is the need to highlight the importance of individual training programmes in relation to the role the player is being asked to fulfil within the team. Subject PS (left fullback) shows the characteristic stop - start nature of a position relying heavily upon anaerobic bursts of highly intense activity, be it overlapping or completing recovery runs. Subject PB's (centre midfield) heart rate response shows the importance of a well developed aerobic capacity to sustain the required level of energy supply. Even in these central positions the supply of energy from anaerobic glycolysis cannot be overlooked, with subject PB often exhibiting lactate values greater than 8.00 mM. Therefore once the demands of each position, style of play or tactics are understood, a comprehensive positional training programme can be developed to maximise performance.

5 References

Bangsbo, J., Norregaard, L. and Thorso, F. (1991) Activity profile of competition soccer. **Can. J. Sports Sci.**, 16, 110-116.

Carli, G., Bonifazi, M., Lodi, L., Lupo, C., Martelli, G. and Vita, A. (1986) Hormonal and metabolic effects following a football match. **Int. J. Sports Med.**, 2, 67-80.

Cochrane, C. and Pyke, F. (1976) Physiological assessment of the Australian soccer squad. **Aust. J. Health Phys. Ed. & Rec., 75,** 21-25.

Ekblom, B. (1986) Applied physiology of soccer. **Sports Med.**, 3, 50-60.

Gerisch, G., Rutmoller, E. and Weber, K. (1988) Sports medical measurements of performance in soccer, in **Science and Football** (eds T. Reilly, A. Lees, K. Davids and W. J. Murphy), E and F.N. Spon, London, pp. 60-67.

Mayhew, S. R. and Wenger, H.A. (1985) Time and motion analysis of professional soccer. **J. Human Mov't Stud.**, 11, 49-52.

Reilly, T. and Thomas, V. (1976) A motion analysis of work rate in different positional roles in professional football match-play. **J. Human Mov't Stud.**, 2, 87-97.

Rohde, H, D. and Espersen, T. (1988) Work intensity during soccer training and match-play, in **Science and Football** (eds T. Reilly, A. Lees, K. Davids and W. J. Murphy), E. and F. N. Spon, London, pp. 68-75.

Tumilty, D., Hahn, A.G., Telford, R.D. and Smith, R.A. (1988). Is "lactic acid tolerance" an important component of fitness for soccer ? in **Science and Football** (eds T. Reilly, A. Lees, K. Davids and W. J. Murphy), E. and F. Spon, London, pp. 81-86.

Whitehead, N. (1975) **Conditioning for Sport**. E.P. Publishing Co. Ltd. Yorks.

THE ROLE-RELATED DIFFERENCES OF SOME SERUM IRON PARAMETERS IN TOP LEVEL SOCCER PLAYERS

A. Resina , L. Gatteschi , M.G. Rubenni , L. Vecchiet .
1 Cattedra di Medicina dello Sport - Università di Firenze
2 Sezione Medica del Settore Tecnico F.G.C. - Firenze

1 Introduction

Several studies have reported that physical training may affect iron related haematological parameters (Clement and Sawchuk, 1984; Newhouse and Clement, 1988). The most common finding is a decrease of serum ferritin, a parameter which reflects tissue iron stores (Siimes and Dallmann, 1974). This decrease is considered the first stage in developing iron deficiency and is referred to as prelatent iron deficiency. The next stage is a decrease of serum iron with an increase of total iron binding capacity, called latent iron deficiency (Clement and Sawchuk, 1984). This has been observed especially in endurance runners, and the iron cost of training seems to be mainly related to the exercise load (Clement and Sawchuk, 1984; Colt and Heyman, 1984; Newhouse and Clement, 1988).

Many studies have described a decrease of iron related indices in other athletes such as cross-country skiers, cyclists, swimmers (Dufaux et al., 1981) and female hockey players (Diehl et al., 1986).
Running plays an important role in soccer training (Ekblom, 1986), but little is known about iron status of soccer players (Resina et al., 1991). It is also known that the metabolic load of playing soccer differs according to positional roles (Reilly and Thomas, 1976).

The purpose of the present study was to evaluate in a group of top level soccer players if the positional role influences some indices of iron status.

2 Methods

Nineteen professional soccer players from an Italian First Division team gave their informed consent to participate in this study. The players had been training regularly 4-5 times a week during the previous 9 months. Based on their role they were divided into 4 groups: 2 Goalkeepers (G), 7 Defenders (D), 6 Midfielders (M) and 4 Forwards (F).

The blood sample was taken after an overnight fast, and three days from the last match or training session. Iron status was evaluated by assessment of Serum Iron (SI), Total Iron Binding Capacity (TIBC), Transferrin Saturation (TSat), Serum Ferritin (SFe), and Serum Haptoglobin (SHpt). Serum iron and serum total iron-binding capacity were measured spectrophotometrically by the colorimetric method (Boehringer Mannheim). Transferrin saturation was calculated by dividing serum iron concentration by serum TIBC. Serum ferritin was measured by Enzymum Test Ferritin (Boehringer Mannheim). Serum haptoglobin was measured by radial immunodiffusion (Nor-Partigen Haptoglobin, Behring). The values were expressed as mean plus standard deviation. Data were analyzed by the non-parametric Kruskall-Wallis test. The significance level was set at $P < 0.05$. We have evaluated in each group the number of players who showed values below the normal range for SI, SHpt and TIBC; we have also established the number of players who showed SFe below 64 ng/ml and below 10 ng/ml, respectively indicative of iron depletion (Heinrich et al., 1977) and diagnostic of iron deficiency (Fairbanks and Beutler, 1990). Because of the small number of players in each group we have not statistically evaluated these percentages. After the warm-up and running, the goalkeepers followed a specific role-related training, and therefore they were not considered for the statistical evaluation of serum parameters.

3 Results

The groups did not show significant differences for mean values of SFe, SI, and TSat (Table 1). Mean TIBC was higher in the defender's group than in forward ($P<0.05$). Six defenders (85%), three forwards (75%) and six midfielders (100%) showed SHpt below the normal range. Two midfielders (33%) and two defenders (28%) showed SFe below 64 ng/ml; one midfielder (16%) had SFe below 10 ng/ml, and he showed also the lowest SHpt level (0.22 g/l).

4 Discussion

The aim of this study was to establish if positional role exerts an influence on some serum iron parameters. A decrease of body iron occurs when the balance between iron intake and loss is negative (Fairbanks and Beutler, 1990). Moreover, several studies suggest that exercise may cause an increased intravascular haemolysis (Dufaux et al., 1981; Eichner, 1985; Selby and Eichner, 1986), due mainly, but not only, to footstrike trauma (Clement and Sawchuk, 1984; Miller, 1990), and it provokes a decrease of serum haptoglobin that binds the so-released haemoglobin (Bunn, 1972; Hershko, 1975).

Table 1. Values of some iron status indices in the four groups of soccer players

	SI (umol/l)	TIBC (umol/l)	TSat (%)	SFe (ng/ml)	SHpt (g/l)
Normal Range	7.5–25	50–70	30%	20–200	1–3
Goalkeepers n=2	29.53+1.77	55.40±3.66	53.5±6.74	201.5±112	.71±.31
Defenders n=7	18.29±2.61	64.81±12.97	29.31±7.6	79.57±44.4	.64±.03
Midfielders n=6	19.26±2.79	57.36±2.90	33.76±6.0	79.16±57.1	.46±.25
Forwards n=4	19.93±2.23	54.89±3.32	32.73±4.0	78.5±12.1	.75±.48

Our results about SI, TIBC and SFe suggest that these soccer players are not prone to iron deficiency. The high prevalence of low SHpt values leads us to argue that in these players the amount of intravascular haemolysis might not be neglegible.

The positional role seems to exert an influence only on SHpt. Low levels of SHpt may indicate an increase of intravascular haemolysis.

The Hb-Hpt complexes are taken up and metabolized almost exclusively by liver parenchymal cells (Bissel et al., 1972). This may lead to a shift of the red cells' catabolic pathway and to a redistribution of iron stores among tissue compartments (Magnusson et al., 1984; Resina et al., 1988).

These soccer players belonged to the same team. They were exposed to the same matches and training sessions, but with different workloads in relation to their role. Our midfielders' group showed the lowest SHpt levels. All the midfielder's showed SHpt below the normal range and three of them showed also SFe below 64 ng/ml, indicative of iron depletion. Low ferritin levels occur especially in athletes like runners, often related to the load of training (Clement and Sawchuk, 1984); low serum ferritin levels may be due also to an increase of intravascular haemolysis, because of the redistribution of iron between tissue stores, and running is an important factor in provoking intravascular haemolysis (Clement and Sawchuk, 1984, Miller, 1990).

In a soccer game or training session the greatest distances are covered by midfielders (Reilly and Thomas, 1976); so both the higher percentage of SFe values below 64 ng/ml and the lowest values of SHpt might be related to the different amount of running in their training session.

Actually physical conditioning holds an important role also in team sport, and so these kind of players had undertaken a greater amount of non-specific workloads like running.

Our results seem to suggest that evaluation of iron metabolism in soccer players needs to take into account both the amount and the type of training.

5 References

Bissel, D.M. Hammaker, L. and Schmid, R. (1972) Hemoglobin and erythrocyte catabolism in rat liver: the separate roles of parenchymal and sinusoidal cells. Blood, 40, 812-822.

Bunn, H.F. (1972) Erytrocyte destruction and hemoglobin catabolism. Semin. Hematol., 9, 3-17.

Clement, D.B. and Sawchuk L.L. (1984) Iron status and sports performance. Sports Med., 1, 65-74.

Colt, E. and Heyman, B. (1984) Low ferritin levels in runners. J. Sports Med. Phys. Fit., 24, 13-17.

Diehl, D.M. Lohman, T.G. Smith, S.C. and Kertzer, R.J. (1986) The effects of physical training on iron status of female field hockey players. Int. J. Sports Med., 7, 264-270.

Dufaux, B. Hoederath, A. Streitberger, I. Hollman, W. and Assman, G. (1981) Serum ferritin, transferrin, haptoglobin and iron in middle- and long-distance runners, elite rowers and professional racing cyclists. Int. J. Sports Med., 2, 43-46.

Ekblom, B. (1986) Applied physiology to soccer. Sports Med., 3, 50-60.

Eichner, E.R. (1985) Runner's macrocytosis: a clue to footstrike hemolysis. Am. J. Med., 78, 321-325.

Fairbanks, V.F. and Beutler E. (1990) Iron deficiency, in Hematology 4rd Edition (eds W.J. Williams, E. Beutler, A.J. Erslev, and M.A. Lichtman), McGraw Hill Book Co, New York, pp. 482-505.

Heinrich, H.C. Burggemann, J. Gabbe, E.E. and Glaser, M. (1977) Correlation between diagnostic $56Fe^{++}$ absorption and serum ferritin concentration in man. Z. Naturforsch., 32, 1023-1025.

Hershko, C. (1975) The fate of circulating haemoglobin. Brit. J. Haematol., 29, 199-204.

Magnusson, B. Hallberg, L. Rossander, L. and Swolin, B. (1984) Iron metabolism and "sports anemia". II. A hematological comparison of elite runners and control subjects. Acta Med. Scand., 216, 157-164.

Miller, B.J. (1990) Haematological effects of running. A brief review.

Sports Med., 9, 1-6.

Newhouse, I.J. and Clement, D.B. (1988) Iron status in athletes. An update. Sports Med., 5, 337-352.

Reilly, T. and Thomas, V. (1976) A motion analysis of work-rate in different positional roles in professional football match-play. J. Hum. Movement Stud., 2, 87-97.

Resina, A. Gatteschi, L. Giamberardino, M.A. Rubenni, M.G. Trabassi, E. and Troni M.G. (1988) Comparison of RBC indices and serum iron parameters in trained runners and control subjects. Haematologica, 73, 449-454.

Resina, A. Gatteschi, L. Giamberardino, M.A. Imreh, F. Rubenni, M.G. and Vecchiet, L. (1991) Hematological comparison of iron status in trained top-level soccer players and control subjects. Int. J. Sports Med., 12, 453-456.

Selby, G.B. and Eichner E.R. (1986) Endurance swimming intravascular hemolysis, anemia, and iron depletion. Am. J. Med., 81, 791-794.

Siimes, M.A. and Dallmann, P.R. (1974) New kinetic role for serum ferritin in iron metabolism. Brit. J. Haematol., 28, 7-18.

AN ANALYSIS OF PHYSIOLOGICAL STRAIN IN FOUR-A-SIDE WOMEN'S SOCCER.

A. MILES, D. MACLAREN, T. REILLY, and K. YAMANAKA.
Centre For Sport and Exercise Sciences, Liverpool
Polytechnic, Liverpool. L3 3AF, England.

1 Introduction

Soccer research, like the game itself, still appears to
be male dominated. In the U.K. participation rates
amongst females has grown considerably in recent years.
In 1980 the Women's Football Association had 188
registered female clubs and this figure had, by early
1991, grown to 321 registered clubs, representing in
excess of 5,000 registered female players. The soccer
literature, however, does not mirror this increase in
popularity of the female game. This study aimed to extend
research by MacLaren et al. (1988), which looked at the
physiological strain placed upon male players in small-
sided soccer, to the female game. The purpose was to
observe the demands placed on novice female soccer whilst
playing small-sided soccer.

2 Method

Ten female novice soccer players, with mean
characteristics shown in Table 1, performed the study in
two different stages. Firstly, in the laboratory,
subjects performed an incremental run to volitional
exhaustion on a motorised treadmill. Oxygen consumption
($\dot{V}O_2$) was recorded every 20 s using a computerised gas
analysis system (Sensorimedics, Salford) and heart rate
(HR) was recorded every 15 s using a short range radio
telemetry device (Polar Sports Tester). Subjects began
exercising at 6 km/h for 2 min and this was increased by
2 km/h every 2 min until a plateau in $\dot{V}O_2$ was reached.
For each subject a regression line was drawn relating
heart rate and $\dot{V}O_2$.
    In the second session, subjects played indoor small-
sided soccer under 3 different conditions:- an All-
Female Outfield (FO) condition in which the subject
played outfield in a 4 female versus 4 female match, an
All-Female Goal (FG) condition in which the subject took

on the role of goalkeeper in a similar 4 female versus 4
female match and a Mixed Outfield (MO) condition in which

Table 1. Subject data   (n=10).

```
--------------------------------------------------------
                                 Mean        SD.
Age (Years)                      20.6        0.9
Body Mass (kg)                   63.2        5.8
V̇O₂ max ( ml/kg/min)            42.4        4.3
Maximum Heart Rate (beats/min)   200         11
--------------------------------------------------------
```

the subject played outfield in a match involving 2 males
and 2 females per team. Subjects played for a 1-hour
period on 2 occasions, separated by a period of 1 week,
and changed between the four conditions every 5 min.
Heart rate was monitored, using the short range telemetry
system, every 15 s for 5 min of each playing condition
and for a 5 min resting period. After each 5 min period
a finger prick blood sample was taken for subsequent
analysis of blood lactate levels using an Analox (London)
lactate analyser. During each of the outfield conditions
the subject was video-taped so that a work-rate analysis
could be performed in terms of the length of time spent
walking, running and stationary. From the heart rate data
collected in the games and from the regression lines
drawn, the V̇O₂ for each individual for each playing
condition was estimated.

3 Results

There were no significant differences between the mean
heart rate values for the Female Outfield condition and
the Mixed Outfield condition (Table 2). Both these

Table 2. Heart rate, predicted % V̇O₂ max and blood
          lactate for each 5 min period. (Means ± SD).

	Rest	Female Goal	Female Outfield	Mixed Outfield
Heart rate (beats/min)	88 ± 12	147 ± 17	171 ± 11	169 ± 13
% V̇O₂ max		49.7	73.6	70.7
Blood Lactate (mM)	1.9 ± 0.4	2.3 ± 0.7	4.0 ± 1.2	4.1 ± 1.4

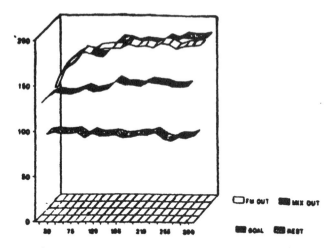

Fig. 1. Mean heart rates for each 5 min period.

conditions showed significantly higher heart rates than the Female Goal condition (P< 0.01). The mean heart rates for the Female Outfield (171 beats/min) and the Mixed Outfield conditions (169 beats/min) represented 85.7 % and 84.8% of maximum heart rate, respectively. (Figures 2 and 3).

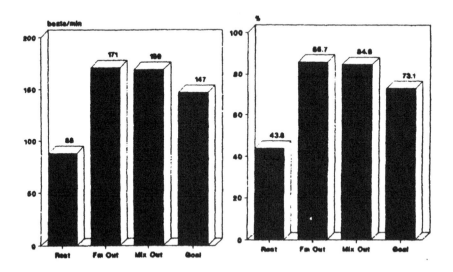

Fig. 2. Mean heart rate for each condition.

Fig. 3. Percent of the maximum heart rate for each condition.

142

The predicted oxygen consumption values represented 73.6% $\dot{V}O_2$ max for the All-Female Outfield play, 70.7% $\dot{V}O_2$ max for Mixed Outfield play and 49.7% $\dot{V}O_2$ max for the Female Goal condition (Figure 4). Significant differences existed between the Female Goal and both the Outfield conditions (P< 0.05) but no significant differences were found between the Female Outfield and Mixed Outfield conditions.

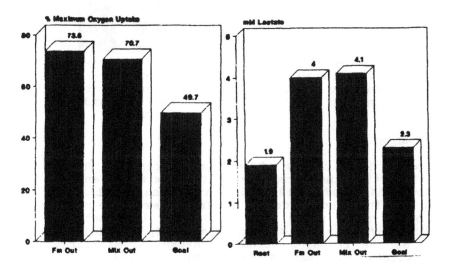

Fig. 4. Percent $\dot{V}O_2$ max achieved in each condition.

Fig. 5. Blood lactate values for each condition.

The blood lactate levels for both the Female and Mixed Outfield conditions were significantly elevated (P<0.05) over the Resting and Female Goal levels (Table 2), but there was no significant difference in blood lactate levels between the two outfield conditions (Figure 5). The analysis of work-rates (Figures 6 and 7) showed that in the Mixed Outfield condition subjects spent longer walking than they did in the Female Outfield condition (P< 0.05) but remained stationary for longer in the Female Outfield condition (P< 0.05). In the Female Outfield condition subjects ran for longer periods than in the Mixed Outfield condition (P< 0.05) but there was no significant difference between the length of time spent walking and that spent running in either condition.

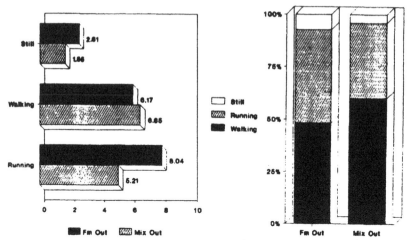

Fig.6. Mean duration of bouts of standing still, walking and running.

Fig.7. Percent time spent standing still, walking and running.

4 Discussion

The maximum heart rate of the subjects during the $\overset{\circ}{V}O_2$ max test was within the normal range for their age and sex (Åstrand and Rodahl, 1986) and the mean heart rates whilst playing soccer both as a single sex group and as part of a mixed group were above the 140 beats/min suggested by the American College of Sports Medicine (1978) as the training stimulus threshold. Similarly, these values represented in excess of 70% of the subjects' maximum heart rate, suggesting that the intensity of exercise was sufficient to induce a training effect if regular match-play was undertaken. The rise in heart rate over rest which occurred in the female playing in goal may have been due to the anxiety effect of taking that role and thus attributable in part to psychological rather than physiological factors. The values obtained when the subjects played outfield did not differ significantly whether players were in an all-female group or playing with two male players per team. This implies that the involvement of the males in the game had no effect on the overall work intensity of the females although playing patterns may well have been affected. These values for outfield small-sided soccer play compare well with the previous findings for male soccer. Work by Van Gool et al. (1983) included heart rate analysis of males in 11-a-side match-play using radio telemetry and found mean heart rates of 167 beats/min. MacLaren et al. (1988) found male players had a mean heart rate of 172 beats/min during small-sided play.

The relationship between heart rate and oxygen consumption in females has been examined by Franklin et al. (1980) who found a linear relation. This study suggests that percentage maximum heart rate values of 85.7% (Female Outfield) and 84.8% (Mixed Outfield) represent 73.6% and 70.7% $\dot{V}O_2$ max respectively. This intensity of exercise suggests an anaerobic element to the match-play of the females which is supported by the blood lactate levels recorded. The value of 4mM of lactate is widely used as a reference level and is thought to approximate the " anaerobic threshold ", and both the outfield conditions in this study produced blood lactate values at or above this 4mM level.

Work-rate analysis of the females during match-play highlights the intermittent activity in soccer. Figure 6 shows the mean duration of running and walking bouts and it can be seen that subjects ran for no longer than 8 s at a time and walked for approximately 6.5 s at a time. These short bursts of running constitute high intensity anaerobic exercise superimposed on aerobic activity and interspersed with low intensity recovery walking.

When playing as an all-female group there was no difference in the time spent walking and running. When males were introduced female participation in the match was reduced as the greater skill level of the males led to their dominating the game.

Future studies might investigate whether the heart rate and physiological strain experienced in females varies with skill level. There is also scope for looking at physiological demands of full 11-a-side matches.

5 References

American College of Sports Medicine (1978) Position statement on " The recommended quantity and quality of exercise for developing and maintaining fitness in healthy adults." **Sports Med. Bull.**, 13:1.

Åstrand, P.O., and Rodahl, K. (1977) **Textbook of Work Physiology.** McGraw-Hill, New York.

Franklin, B.A., Hodgson, J. and Buskirk, E.R. (1980) Relationship between percent maximal O_2 uptake and percent maximal heart rate in women. **Res. Quart. Exerc. Sport,** 51, 616-624.

MacLaren, D., Davids, K., Isokawa, M., Mellor, S. and Reilly, T. (1988) Physiological strain in 4-a-side soccer, in **Science and Football** (eds T. Reilly, A. Lees, K. Davids and W.J. Murphy), E. and F.N. Spon, London, pp. 76-80.

Van Gool, D., Van Gerven, D. and Boutmans, J. (1983) Heart rate telemetry during a soccer game: a new methodology. **J. Sports. Sci.,** 1, 154.

RELATIONSHIP BETWEEN MAXIMAL AEROBIC POWER AND PERFORMANCE OF A PROFESSIONAL SOCCER TEAM

G.S. ROI, E. PEA, G. DE ROCCO, M. CRIPPA, L. BENASSA, A. COBELLI and G. ROSA.
Marathon Sports Medical Center, Brescia, Italy

1 Introduction

The literature on soccer reports that professional players have values of 55 to 71 ml/kg/min for maximal aerobic power ($\dot{V}O_2$max) and it is commonly agreed that factors other than $\dot{V}O_2$max are decisive for success (Ekblom, 1986; Reilly, 1990). Furthermore the data so far published always refer to different teams; longitudinal studies analyzing the relationship between $\dot{V}O_2$max and performance are unknown. The aim of this paper was to analyze this relationship of an international level team (Atalanta BC) participating in the 1st division of the Italian national league between 1984 and 1990.

2 Methods

The $\dot{V}O_2$ was measured by a Sensor Medics 4400tc Analyzer, on 72 players, excluding the goalkeepers, during treadmill running (1% slope, 8 km/h starting velocity with increments of 2 km/h every 3 minutes until exhaustion). The value of $\dot{V}O_2$ measured in the last minute of each test was chosen as $\dot{V}O_2$max. For each season we calculated the mean value (± 1 SD) of $\dot{V}O_2$max for the team. The differences between the means were evaluated by unpaired Student's t-test. Significance was declared when $P<0.05$.

3 Results

The mean values (± SD) of $\dot{V}O_2$max and final classification of the team are shown in Table 1.

Table 1. Mean $\dot{V}O_2$max (ml/kg/min) and final position of the team from 1984-5 to 1989-90 seasons.

Season	84-85	85-86	86-87	87-88	88-89	89-90
$\dot{V}O_2$max	54.7	56.9	53.0	52.5	53.4	51.2
± SD	3.8	5.1	6.4	4.5	6.6	4.1
Class	10th	8th	15th(R)	2nd div	6th	8th

No significant differences ($P < 0.05$) in $\dot{V}O_2$max were found in the period examined. On the other hand the final classification of the team was between 6th (88-89) and the relegated position (R) to the 2nd division (86-87).

4 Discussion

The mean values of $\dot{V}O_2$max found in this study were a little lower than those reported in the literature for professional soccer players (Ekblom, 1986; Reilly, 1990). This difference may have been due to the pre-season assessment of $\dot{V}O_2$max.

It is interesting to note that the team renews some players every year and that the trainer was substituted four times in the period of this investigation.

These alterations do not affect the mean $\dot{V}O_2$max of the team, but likely they affect its performance. From that, it is impossible to state a relationship between $\dot{V}O_2$max and performance of the team considered here.

In conclusion, the results of this paper confirm the finding obtained with transverse studies demonstrating that the performance of a team depends on factors (e.g. technical and tactical) other than on $\dot{V}O_2$max alone.

5 References

Ekblom, B. (1986) Applied physiology of soccer. **Sports Med.**, 3, 50-60.
Reilly, T. (1990) Football, in **Physiology of Sports** (eds T. Reilly, N. Secher, P. Snell and C. Williams) E. & F.N. Spon, London, pp. 371-425.

PART FIVE

Match Performance Analysis in Football

NOTATION ANALYSIS IN FOOTBALL

MIKE HUGHES,
Centre for Sport and Exercise Sciences, Liverpool
Polytechnic, Liverpool L3 3AF, England.

1 Introduction

A considerable amount of research has been
devoted to establishing the need for objective forms
of analysis and their importance in the coaching
process (e.g. MacDonald, 1984; Franks and Miller,
1986). They have clearly established the
difficulties facing any single individual attempting
to analyse and remember objectively the events
occurring in complex team games. One of the main
solutions to these inherent problems has been the
use of notation analysis systems. Consciously or
unconsiously, coaches, scouts and managers have
adopted, designed and developed systems for
gathering information. Over the last three decades
these have been improved by both workers in the
field and sports science researchers, almost to the
point where the design of the systems has become an
end in itself. The aim of this work is to review not
only the data that have been produced, but also
assess the major innovations and developments in the
systems used for notation analysis.

2 Hand Notation Systems

The definitive piece of work in motion analysis
of soccer was by Reilly and Thomas (1976) who
recorded and analysed the intensity and extent of
discrete activities during match-play in field
soccer. They combined the use of hand notation with
the use of an audio tape recorder, to analyse in
detail the movements of English First Division
soccer players. Besides extending the work into a

physiological context, they were able to specify work-rates of the different positions, as well as distances covered in a game, and the relative distances covered for each position in each of the different ambulatory classifications. This work has become a standard against which other similar research projects can compare their results and procedures.

A detailed analysis of the movement patterns of the outfield positions of Australian professional soccer players was completed by Withers et al. (1982). The data produced agreed to a great extent with that of Reilly and Thomas (1976); both studies showed that players cover 98% of the total distance in a match without the ball, and were in agreement in most of the inferences made from the work-rate profiles.

An alternative approach towards match analysis was exemplified by Reep and Benjamin (1968) who collected data from 3,213 matches between 1953 and 1968. They reported that 80% of goals resulted from a sequence of three passes or less. Fifty percent of all goals came from possession gained in the final attacking quarter of the pitch. Similar work was completed by Hughes (1973) and applied to tactics in soccer. Bate (1988) explored aspects of chance in football and its relation to tactics and strategy in the light of the results presented by Reep and Benjamin (1968) and data from unpublished research by C.F.Hughes. Pollard et al. (1988) used Reep and Benjamin's (1968) method of notation in order to quantitatively assess determinants and consequences of different styles of play. A hand notation system developed by Ali (1988) attempted to ascertain whether there were specific and identifiable patterns of attack and how successful each pattern was in influencing the result of the match. Harris and Reilly (1988) considered attacking success in relation to space and team strategy, by concentrating mainly upon space in relation to the defence and overall success of an attacking sequence. This was a considerable departure from many of the systems previously mentioned which have tended to disseminate each sequence into discrete actions.

Bate (1988) presented data collected by C.F.Hughes in an analysis of international soccer in the 1980's. It was found that 94% of goals scored at all levels of international soccer were scored from movements involving four or less passes, and that 50-60% of all movements leading to shots on goal originated in the attacking third of the field.

Lyons (personal communication, April 1991) has gathered data manually, for a period of ten years, on the Rugby Union Home International Championship and has created a sound data-base. From this data-base he claimed to predict the actions in the England-Wales match in the 1986-'87 season to within 3 passes and 2 kicks.

All these hand notation systems share the same advantages of being cheap and accurate but suffer from the fact that the more sophisticated the systems are, the longer it takes to learn the codes and the application process. In addition the more complex systems produce masses of data that in turn take a long time to process.

3 Computerised Notation Systems

Using computers introduces extra problems. Data entry can be difficult, laborious and require keyboard skills - possibilities of error are increased by either operator errors, or hardware and software errors. To minimise both of these types of problems, careful and complete validation of computerised notation systems must be carried out. Computers can produce large quantities of data, so much so that it is easy to lose important aspects of the information about a particular match. Skilful management of data output can make understanding and assimilation of the data easier for the coach or player. The advances made in tackling these problems in computerised notation analysis provides a useful structure with which to explore the developments in this field.

3.1 Data entry

A fundamental difficulty in using a computer is entering information. The traditional method employs the QWERTY keyboard, but this can be a lengthy and boring task. Mayhew and Wenger (1985) used the principle ideas behind the work of Reilly and Thomas (1976) and Withers et al. (1982) and calculated the time spent by three professional soccer players in different match-play activities by computer. The work did not extend in any way the efforts of the earlier researchers.By assigning codes to the different actions, positions and players, the data entry can be eased. Hughes and Charlish (1988) used this process on a mainframe computer to record and analyse data for American football. An alternative to this approach to the problem is to use a specifically designed keyboard. Franks (1983) configured a keyboard on a mini-computer to resemble the layout of a soccer field and designed a program which yielded frequency tallies of various features of play.

Minimal consideration had been given to the number of games to be notated prior to the establishment of a recognized system of play. This is important, since any fluctuation in the patterns and profile will affect the inferences made, particularly with reference to the match outcome. Teams may also vary their system and pattern of play according to opponents, although these factors were not considered by any of the researchers mentioned above. Furthermore, the existence of patterns of play peculiar to individual players was not illustrated. It was on this area that Church and Hughes (1987) concentrated, in an attempt to identify patterns of play in a soccer team and whether any reasons could be found to explain the results. They developed a computerised notation system for analysing soccer matches using a concept keyboard. This is a touch sensitive pad that can be programmed to accept input to the computer. This permitted a pitch representation, as well action and player keys to be specific and labelled. This considerably reduced the time to learn the system, and made the data input quicker and more accurate. The system enabled an analysis to be performed of patterns of play, both at team and player levels, and with respect to match outcome. An analysis of six matches played by Liverpool during the 1985-6 season led to these main observations: a greater number of passes was attempted when losing than when winning, possession was lost more often when losing and a greater number of shots was taken when losing than when winning.

Hughes at al. (1988), used the same concept keyboard and hardware system developed by Church and Hughes (1987), but with modified software, to analyse the 1986 World Cup soccer finals. Patterns of play of successful teams, those teams that reached the semi-finals, were compared with those of unsuccessful teams, i.e. teams that were eliminated at the end of the first rounds. Lewis and Hughes (1988) extended this work, analysing attacking plays only, to examine whether such unsuccessful teams use different attacking patterns to successful teams. Partridge and Franks (1989a and 1989b) produced a detailed analysis of the crossing opportunities from the 1986 World Cup. They defined how they interpreted a cross, and gathered data on different aspects of crosses. In an attempt to transfer their results from the laboratory to field conditions, the findings were related to the design of practices to help players understand their roles in the successful performance of crossing in soccer.

Treadwell (1988) and Hughes and Williams (1988) developed software for the analysis of rugby union using a similar system of hardware to that previously used on soccer (a BBC computer and concept keyboard). Patrick and McKenna (1988) developed a similar system for the computerised analysis of Australian Rules football whilst McKenna et al. (1988) completed a computer-video analysis of activity patterns in Australian Rules Football.

The use of digitisation pads has considerably eased some of the problems of data entry, but the most recent innovation in input is the introduction of voice entry of data into the computer. Taylor and Hughes (1988) were able to demonstrate that this type of system can be used by the computer 'non-expert'.

3.2 Data output

In practical applications to sport, it is imperative that the output is immediate and, perhaps more important, clear, concise and to the point. The first systems produced tables of data, often incorporated with statistical significance tests, that were difficult for the non-scientist to understand. Some researchers attempted to tackle the problem (Sanderson, 1983), but the type of presentation was only marginally easier to understand than the tables of data. Frequency distributions across graphical representations of the playing area (Hughes et al.,1988), traces of the path of the ball prior to a shot or a goal (Franks and Nagelkerke, 1988), and similar ploys, have made the output of some systems far more attractive and easier to understand. The system developed by Hughes and McGarry (1991) specifically tackled this problem and produced some 3-D colour graphics that presented the data in a compact form, which coaches of different nationalities have found easy to assimilate. This application has been further extended for use in soccer.

3.3 Computers and video

The ability of computers to control the video image has introduced exciting pssibilities in feedback. An inexpensive IBM based system was described by Franks et al. (1989). Franks and Nagelkerke (1988) developed such a system for the team sport of field hockey. The system has recently been modified to analyse and provide feedback for ice-hockey and soccer.

3.4 Future developments

There are several developments that will extend notation analysis over the next few years. The first will be the development of 'all-purpose', generic software. Work in some centres has almost reached this point now. Another technological advance that will make computerised notation more easily handled by the non-specialist will be the introduction of "voice-over" methods of data entry. Taylor and Hughes (1988) have demonstrated that this is possible now, but relatively expensive at present.

The integration of both these technological developments with computerised-video feedback will facilitate both detailed objective analysis of competition and the immediate presentation of the most important elements of play. As these systems are used more and more, and larger data-bases are created a clearer understanding of each of the football codes will follow. The use of subjective qualitative data together with accurate statistical analyses, typified by Eom (1989), will make these systems more accurate and more relevent to football with their predictions.

4 REFERENCES

Ali, A.H. (1988) A statistical analysis of tactical movement patterns in soccer, in **Science and Football**, (eds T.Reilly, A.Lees, K.Davids & W.J.Murphy), E. & F. Spon, London, pp. 302-308.

Bate, R. (1988) Football chance: tactics and strategy, in **Science and Football**, (eds T.Reilly, A.Lees, K.Davids & W.J.Murphy), E. & F. Spon, London, pp. 293-301.

Church, S. and Hughes, M.D. (1987) Patterns of Play in Association Football - A computerised Analysis. **Communication to First World Congress of Science and Football**, Liverpool, 13th-17th April.

Eom,H (1989) Computer-aided recording and mathematical analysis of volleyball. Unpublished Master's Thesis. University of British Columbia, Vancouver.

Franks, I.M. (1983) An analysis of the 1982 World Cup of association football. **Communication to the British Association of Sports Sciences Conference**, Liverpool, 12-16th September.

Franks, I.M., & Miller, G. (1986) Eyewitness testimony in sport. **J. Sport Behavior**, 9, 39-45.

Franks, I.M. & Nagelkerke, P. (1988) The use of computer interactive video technology in sport analysis. **Ergonomics**, 31, 1593-1603.

Franks, I.M., Nagelkerke, P. & Goodman, D. (1989) Computer controlled video: an inexpensive IBM based system. **Computers Educ.**, 13, 33-44.

Harris, S. & Reilly,T. (1988) Space, teamwork and attacking success in soccer, in **Science and Football**, (eds T.Reilly, A.Lees, K.Davids & W.J.Murphy), E. & F. Spon, London, pp. 322-328.

Hughes, C. (1973) **Football Tactics and Teamwork**, E.P. Publishing Co. Ltd., Wakefield.

Hughes, M. & Charlish F. (1988) The development and validation of a computerised notation system for American football. **J.Sports Sci.**, 6, 253-254.

Hughes, M. & McGarry, T. (1991) The development of 3D graphics to illustrate data presentation from a computerised analysis of squash, **Proceedings of Computer Graphics in Sport**, Sheffield, 10-12th April.

Hughes, M. & Williams, D. (1988) The development and application of a computerised Rugby Union notation system. **J. Sports Sci.**, 6, 254-255.

Hughes, M., Robertson, K. & Nicholson, A. (1988) An Analysis of 1984 World Cup of Association Football, in **Science and Football**, (eds T.Reilly, A.Lees, K.Davids & W.J.Murphy), E. & F. Spon, London, pp. 363-367.

Lewis, M. & Hughes, M. (1988) Attacking play in the 1986 World Cup of association football. **J. Sport Sci.**, 6, 169

MacDonald, N. (1984). Avoiding the pitfalls in player selection. **Coaching Sci. Update**, 41-45.

Mayhew, S.R. & Wenger, H.A. (1985) Time-motion analysis of professional soccer. **J. Human Movement Stud.**, 11, 49-52.

McKenna, M.J., Patrick, J.D., Sandstrom, E.R. & Chennells, M.H.D. (1988) Computer-video analysis of activity patterns in Australian rules football, in **Science and Football**, (eds T.Reilly, A.Lees, K.Davids & W.J.Murphy), E. & F. Spon, London, pp. 274-281

Partridge, D. & Franks, I.M. (1989a) A detailed analysis of crossing opportunities from the 1986 World Cup. (Part I) **Soccer Journal**, May-June, 47-50.

Partridge, D. & Franks, I.M. (1989b) A detailed analysis of crossing opportunities from the 1986 World Cup. (Part II) **Soccer Journal**, June-July, 45-48.

Patrick, J.D. & McKenna, M.J. (1988) CABER - a computer system for football analysis, in **Science and Football**, (eds T.Reilly, A.Lees, K.Davids & W.J.Murphy), E. & F. Spon, London, pp. 267-273.

Pollard, R., Reep, C. & Hartley, S. (1988) The quantitative comparison of playing styles in soccer, in **Science and Football**, (eds T.Reilly, A.Lees, K.Davids & W.J.Murphy), E. & F. Spon, London, pp. 309-315.

Reep, C. & Benjamin, B. (1968) Skill and chance in association football. **J. Royal Stat. Soc.**, Series A, 131, 581-585.

Reilly,T. & Thomas, V (1976) A motion analysis of work-rate in different positional roles in professional football match-play. **J. Human Movement Stud.**, 2, 87-97.

Sanderson, F.H. (1983) A notation system for analysing squash. **Phys. Educ. Rev.**, 6, 19-23.

Taylor, S. & Hughes, M. (1988) Computerised notational analysis: a voice interactive system. **J. Sports Sci.**, 6, 255.

Treadwell, P.J. (1988) Computer aided match analysis of selected ball-games (soccer and rugby union), in **Science and Football**, (eds T.Reilly, A.Lees, K.Davids & W.J.Murphy), E. & F. Spon, London, pp. 282-287.

Withers R.T., Maricic, Z., Wasilewski, S. & Kelly, L. (1982) Match analyses of Australian professional soccer players. **J. Human Movement Stud.**,8, 158-176.

COMPUTER-ASSISTED SCOUTING IN SOCCER

W. DUFOUR
Institute for Physical Education, Free University of Brussels,
Belgium.

1 Introduction

Sport like every form of game tends by itself to find more logical,
rational and effective forms. It is autoformal. The coach's task is
precisely to accelerate this immanent process through the collecting
of the greatest number of objective data in order to evaluate his
players and, if possible, to look for an eventual correlation between
peculiar parameters and their consequences. As soccer is a very
aleatory sport and much dependent on chance - only 1% of attacks ends
with a goal - this task is quite complex. In spite of these
restrictions it is evident that conscious elimination of factors of
hazard is the ostensible goal of every game form. Modern computer
technology gives new possibilities of collecting and treating
observations on a large number of parameters.

The joint observation of physical efforts, technical elements and
tactical movements enables the observer to collect and analyse
information on:
  - i) the evolution of those parameters during the match for the
    whole competition or the year (historical or diachronical
    perspective);
  - ii) the level of the player in relation to the average level of
    the team (comparative or synchronical perspective);
  - iii) the level of the team in relation to other ones (diachronical
    or synchronical perspective).

All these elements have to be interpreted by the coach in order
to:-
  - i) evaluate the players and the team in the three given fields;
  - ii) plan the training and cope with deficiencies;
  - iii) discover if possible, the inherent structure of soccer;
  - iv) situate soccer in a more general game theory.

2 Observation of physical activity

2.1 Technique of scouting : Tape recorder and computer
Through the input of three electrical signals, differing in intensity
(low, medium, high) into a portable recorder, it is possible to
follow one player in his running (slow, tempo, sprint) and to
evaluate his efforts through:
  - i) the profile of his physical efforts during the match, the
    whole competition in training and so on;

160

ii) the comparison of that profile with the average of the team or of his own line (defence or attack) or over the year;
iii) the distribution pattern of his efforts related to the instructions of the coach;
iv) statistics for the pattern of the efforts (type and frequency) in order to estimate physiological demands and to plan adequate training;
v) comparison of level and pattern of the efforts of the opposing team and tactical conclusions;
vi) evulation of a talented young player's physical condition;
vii) analysis of the intensity of efforts which is afterwards compared with the blood level of lactate (for example) in order to establish the techniques of physical preparation which are physiologically justified.

2.2 Some observations are as follows

In 90 minutes of a game, there are about 60 minutes of play. The players are running for 20% to 40% of the effective time. In 1954 players ran 4.5 km, in 1986 7 km. In addition to the running activities, they walk for about 3 km.

Approximately 61% of efforts are aerobic (60-70% of $\dot{V}O_2$max) (3 to 10 km/h). It is estimated that 24% of efforts take place at the "anaerobic threshold" depending on the physical capacity of the player (about 80% of $\dot{V}O_2$max) (10 to 17 km/h).

About 14% of short sprints are for 2 s and call for alactic capacity (18-27 km/h). The number of short sprints (10-15 m - 2 or 3 s) per game is on the increase - in 1947 : 70; in 1970 : 145; in 1985 : 185; in 1989 : 195. Despite the high number of sprints blood lactates rarely go above 5 mmol/l.

Since 1880 defence had been progressively reinforced (1-1-8; 2-3-5; WM; 4-2-4; 4-4-2). More and more attacks and defences involve the complete team and in 1990 many teams applied a constant aggressive "pressure" everywhere which requires a very good physical condition.

Modern football requires every player to be active for about 30% to 35% of the total time. About 50% of the efforts last between 1 and 3 s (7-20 m) (alactic metabolism).

Nevertheless some teams playing "pressure football" make 12% efforts of 10 s (40-50 m) and more at a high tempo. Good players still play in aerobic conditions. Their "anaerobic threshold" corresponds to about 16.5 km/h. A "libero" is still an exception with activity taking up only 17% of the effective time.

Despite a tendency towards homogeneity two types of players are still observed. These are analogous to long distance endurance runners and "explosive" sprinters.

Success in modern collective football requires a homogeneous team of athletes who possess a good work capacity. They should be able to run 3200 m in 12 min, and to transport about 65 to 70 ml/kg/min ($\dot{V}O_2$max), Their "anaerobic threshold" should be at about 16 km/h (80 to 85% of $\dot{V}O_2$max). This supposes a long, permanent, individualised and heavy training programme for development of the aerobic capacity (30 min every day).

They also need a musculature similar to sprinters with a very good alactic capacity in order to repeat about 180 explosive sprints of 15 to 20 m at a great speed (27 km/h). Strenuous efforts longer than8 s must be avoided because they produce high blood lactate levels which destroy technical competencies and restrain recuperation. Long efforts dependent upon lactic metabolism happen only rarely in normal matches.

The comparison of data issued from scouting endeavours with physiological measures on the field will allow an individual training programme to be linked with collective training.

3 Observation of technical elements

The goal is to collect information on all the technical elements possible. It may be necessary to conduct factor analysis of these data and through multiple regression try to find a correlation between the game elements and the result of the match.

Since 1966 we have worked with new equipment made of three connected machines (a Summigraphics digital panel, a BBC concept-keyboard and an IBM computer). The team of scouts consists of two trained persons: Scout A watches the match, comments on the actions around the ball and digitizes their places on the panel with a stylus (X-Y) while Scout B notes at the same time these actions on a keyboard with 127 sensors, according to an algorithm we developed (the number of the player, the game-actions and their tactical values).

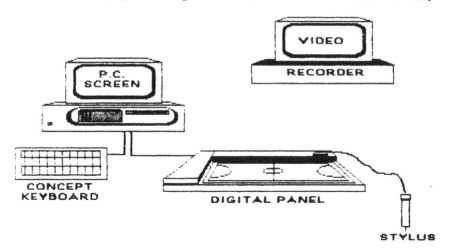

Fig. 1. The computer system's configuration.

In a cadence of 10 actions/min we can reconstruct "the story of the ball". We observe 900 actions and 6 bits per action or 5400 data points. The reliability reached 95% with trained observers.

Of course the coordination of the two scouts, who simultaneously input the two sources of data, requires about 10 hours of training. They can input a whole match with less than 5% mistakes in two hours.

Immediately after the input of the data, all the required statistical results asked by the coach are obtained and treated "a la carte". The observations have been reduced to 10 parameters. These are the top game actions, touches of the ball, playing time, passes, interceptions, duels, shots and goals, feet or head, centres and offside.

4 Quantitative analysis of technical actions

In 65% of the cases, the team which has got the ball wins. An active player touches the ball 60 to 120 times and this action normally lasts for 2 s. In 1990 aggressive pressure football forced the players to play only one touch. Maradona, for example, was under constant pressure (48 fouls in the World Cup finals). Only 4.3 dribbles of more than 25 m/match were noted.

More than 55% of the time is played without a ball. For the remaining part one notes the following distribution: interception : 50.6%; passes : 22.4%; controls : 18.7%; tackling and duels : 4.5%; shots : 2.4%; other actions : 1.4%. Altogether 62% of winning teams play longer with the ball than do the losing teams.

Depending on the tactics of the team we record important variations in the number of passes:- Antwerp -230, Anderlecht -420. South American teams choose progression with relatively more short passes, British teams prefer "kick and rush". But the risk of missing a pass depends on its length. A total of 75% of passes are short, only 10% of them fail; 15% are semi-long, 20% of them fail; 10% are long and 50% fail!

As the number of goals is inversely proportional to the number of passes, we may conclude as follows:

A short pass avoids risk but pays little.

One long pass of two fails ... or creates a goal.

The more you pass, the less you surprise.

Up to 80% of the goals are made after 0, 1 or 2 passes.

About this, the discussion gets animated between the "Possession football", ended by a sudden short acceleration (Rinus Michels) or, the "Kick and rush" approach with 4 long passes coming from the defence.

In the 1974 World Cup, Beckenbauer started 68% counter-moves from far away in the defence whereas Cruyff preferred the midfield in 53% of cases. In 1982 80% of the goals were made with 4 passes (Bate, 1988). In 1990 only 12% of attacks happened with counters with a good efficiency of 12% and 88% of attacks were developed in a slow way but with a low efficiency of 7%. Germany, the winners, was highly efficient in long passes (65%) but Scotland missed all passes in depth (15), Egypt 44/51.

For interceptions Talaga (1976) noted that the Poles intercepted 126 Italian passes (in 1972) through the following actions : 58 missed by the passer himself - 35 anticipations - 19 tackles - 16 by individual pressure. The Italians made 120 interceptions : 8 in the defence zone, 70 in the midfield, 44 in the attack zone.

The number of duels in modern soccer has grown to about 200/match in the 1990 World Cup. In 1990 Germany had the best average of +33%, Belgium -0.8, Korea the worst -30.3.

The number of duels in heading has also grown to 40.5 per match and the average won is important for victory. The British Isles teams fought 101 duels in a match. It is much easier in defence than in attack: none of the 24 teams had a positive average in attack in

1990. Germany won 102 out of 138 duels in defence and lost only 2 of 18 in the final.

For shots at goal 90% of attacks end without a shot. Of the remaining 10% only 1% enters the opposing goal because 45% are diverted, 45% pass sideways, 8 to 12% give a score.

In the 1982 World Cup 54% came from the penalty zone with an efficiency of 11%, 46% came from more than 22 m with an efficiency of 0.5%. In 1990 80% of goals came from the penalty zone and resulted from 50% of all the shots with an efficiency of 10%. Shots from 5.5 m have an efficiency of 15%, from 30 m = 0%.

During the World Cup in 1982 Piecniczk (1983) noticed the goals scored came from:-

45% on a stopped phase (10 s - 3 passes);
27% on a fast attack (5 s - 4 passes);
28% after a slow progression;
40% come from a direct shot, heading or volley;
24% follow a slalom or an individual penetration.
During the World Cup in 1990 Loy (1990) noted that:-
30% came from a stopped phase;
rapid counters represented only 12% of all attacks;
88% were slowly built up.

The higher frequency of shots does not warrant success. The team with most shots wins in only 56% of cases. The quality of shots is much more determinant: 65% of goals happen at the beginning or the end of the second half. Loss of concentration by defenders or poor physical condition explains this fact.

Starosta (1988) reported among 134 finalists of the 1978 World Cup a total of 452 shots. Of these:

225 (55%) with a right foot gave 24 goals (9.5%);
131 (28%) with a left foot led to 6 goals (4.58%);
69 (15%) with the head led to 8 goals (11.5%).
In 1986, the same author confirmed his results : 42.3% of the 26 best shooters prefer the left foot and have a better efficiency. But the real stars such as Platini, Maradona, Alofs, Butrageno, Ceulemans play with both feet.

In 1990 the headers represented 16% of shots and brought 25% of the goals (29). The efficiency is also about 12% because of the short distance : 5 to 11 m.

About 25% of the goals come from a centre in spite of a total efficiency of only 2%! More than 70% of the centres give no effect because of a bad direction or an interception, and only 10% give an opportunity for a shot from 11 m which has a high efficiency of 21%. Good centres are very difficult (the Russians lost 40/52) but also very effective. Centres from the left side are much more effective (probability of 1/29) than from the right side (1/54) but are less frequent (40%).

During an analysis of the European Nations Cup in 1984, we counted 313 offside actions; an average of 22.5 a match. Only 55% of them were correctly executed. Of those only 29% were correctly estimated by the referee, whereas 26% were unjustly whistled. But 9% of incorrect offside movements were nevertheless granted. In short, only 38% of the traps prove effective. The judgement of the referee here is very important. Van Meerbeek et al. (1988) reported that the best referees at the 1986 World Cup Finals whistled about 17.4% wrong decisions.

These statistical elements may be used for two purposes. They may a comparative study of teams (or players) during the season or with their opposing players in order to correct the bad points. Secondly they may be employed in fundamental research on the game structure in order to help to find the pertinent parameters, that is to say those with a decisive influence on the result of the game itself. Until now the description of these 10 parameters gives an orientation but none is decisive and none gives a solid correlation with the match result.

Using the 10 parameters, it is possible to make an evaluation of the technical capacity of the teams or the players. Some examples of possible applications may be cited.

During the 15 matches of the European Nations Cup 1984, not any significant difference and hence not any correlation was found concerning the 10 parameters. Nevertheless it is possible to derive a partial quotient (for every player) of successful or lost actions and a selective quotient of effectiveness in attack or defence (player or team) compared with the average of the moment or with past games. A technico-tactical profile may also be generated in relation to an ideal profile which corresponds with the player's place and function in the team.

The computer prints, when asked, graphic pictures of field zones where the player was active, positions and directions and length of passes. Decisive actions are produced graphically.

A sociogram measures the frequencies of the passes of players among one another and induces the types of relations and the privileged ways of communication between the players. This may be computer-operated.

Quotients of relative effectiveness - shots to the goal/attacks - goals/shots - shots/defensive phases and so on - may also be produced. Basketball coaches realize a quite precise formula of effectiveness of a player. They even help to modify the composition of the team during the match at the moment when a player's coefficient is seen to drop. This undisputed formula does not yet exist in football.

Establishing a logical formula meets a series of difficulties. Which parameters are we to choose and why? Which specific weight has to be given to every parameter? Has a pass backward less value than a long pass forward? Is a shot more valuable than a decisive pass? How do we try to measure the creativity of an attacker?

5 Observation on tactics

The most important criticism of the types of observations which are only focussed on the "history of the ball" is that the collective actions and the movements of players without the ball are missed. To collect this global information we need another algorithm which is the result of a scientific approach of detectable tactical elements and of their mutual correlations.

6 Conclusions

i) The correct interpretation of those numerous data needs a
dialogue between the scout and the coach in order to compare
their conclusions. The statistical observation tries to
correct subjective judgements.

ii) These statistical treatments demonstrate how much the
inherent structure of the game on the one hand and technical
elements on the other are situated in a dialectic relation.
A game-theory, a strategic innovation on the blackboard, can
lead to a deduction of new techniques or tactical movements.
Alternately, the invention of an intuitive and gifted
technician can also induce unexpected tactics and game
structures.

In that difficult debate it should be possible to determine
by means of a computer the invariants which give the game its
internal coherence. It is not at all sure that this
coherence is a static structure, which would admit no
evolution. A phenomenological approach is here the only
valuable (but the most difficult) way to combine objective
measurements and subjective interpretations.

iii) Because of the great facility of interception, which makes
soccer so aleatory, the final problem is to know to what
extent it is possible to reach a complete objective knowledge
of a game. For the moment, the result of a match is still
too much determined by the surprising creativity of an
inventive player who in an illogical irrational way, develops
an action, which revises all the principles. This action is
certainly elaborated at a sub-cortical level and guided with
a sort of driving intuition.

How indeed do we measure and mathematically foresee what has been
referred to by Merleau-Ponty as "a speaking body"? Maybe this is the
impossible challenge of this research.

7 References

Bate, R. (1988) Football Chance : Tactics and Strastegy, in Science
and Football (eds T. Reilly, A. Lees, K. Davids and W.J. Murphy),
E. and F.N. Spon, London, 11. 293-301.

Loy, R (1990) Entwicklungstendenzen im Weltfussball.
Fussballtraining, 9, 23-31.

Piecniczk, A. (1983) Preparation of football teams for Mundial
Competition in 1986. Communication to 9th UEFA course for
National Coaches and Directors of Coaching of the Member
Associations (Split).

Starosta, W. (1988) Symmetry and assymetry in shooting demonstrated
by elite soccer players, in Science and Football. (eds T. Reilly,
A. Lees, K. Davids and W.J. Murphy), E. and F.N. Spon, London, pp.
346-355.

Talaga, J. (1976) Fussbaltraining. Sportverlag, Berlin.

Van Meerbeek, R., Van Gool, D. and Bollens, J. (1988) Analysis of
the refereeing decisions during the World Soccer Championship in
Mexico, 1986, in Science and Football (eds T. Reilly, A. Lees, K.
Davids and W.J. Murphy), E. and F.N. Spon, London, pp. 377-382.

COMPUTER- AND VIDEO-AIDED ANALYSIS OF FOOTBALL GAMES

G. GERISCH and M. REICHELT
DEUTSCHE SPORTHOCHSCHULE KÖLN, KÖLN, GERMANY

1   Introduction

Transforming theoretical insight into advice which can be utilized in practice is a major aim of a practical approach to sports science. However, scientists frequently fail in this intention, not only because of the complexity of the material but especially due to the chosen forms of presentation. In addition to collecting and interpreting the data, the scientist must find the means to communicate his findings to trainers and athletes without burdening them with large, intricate tables of figures and complicated graphs. The method of analysis introduced here is oriented towards practical needs particularly as far as its presentation is concerned. The large amount of data collected is separated and transferred into several diagrams, each depicting a certain aspect of the available information (cf. Bisanz and Gerisch 1988; Gerisch and Reichelt 1991; Harris and Reilly 1988; Loy 1989a, 1989b; Reichelt 1990; Reichelt and Gerisch 1991, Winkler 1985).

2   Methods

The objects of analysis are the one-on-one-situations of a soccer game. The two semi-final matches of the European Cup between Bayern Munich and Red Star of Belgrade (10. and 24.04.91) were analyzed, but only selected results of the first game are shown here as examples. On the basis of video-tapes (TV or own recordings), all situations of the match in which one player is pitched against an opposing player are evaluated. The following categories are distinguished:

- **time** (elapsed playing time in minutes and seconds, as shown on the display of the videorecorder; this was recorded at the completion of the one-on-one-situation in question, i.e. when it can be determined whether player A or player B has fulfilled his situational aim and thus won or lost the duel);

- **player** (the player of team A - in the case of this study, Bayern Munich -, identified by his number; players' names are inserted in the graphics);
- **action**: **headers • fouls • possessions won/lost • intention reached/failed** – the category mentioned last contains all one-on-ones not allotted to any of the former categories (it is determined whether the attacker or the defender has fulfilled his situational aim, such as making/blocking a centre, making/blocking a shot, outplaying an opponent/preventing him dribbling, etc.). These one-on-ones are further separated into **offensive** and **defensive** actions;
- **zone** (defence, midfield, offence - left, centre, right);
- **won / lost** (general definitions are:
  • in the category of **headers**, the player who touches the ball is considered to have won the duel; if both players reach the ball, the player deflecting it in the direction of his intent is registered as the winner;
  • in the category of **fouls**, the player being fouled is regarded as the winner, the player committing the foul the loser of the one-on-one; situations are only registered as fouls if the referee interrupts play;
  • a player is considered to have won a **possession** if the ball was held by the other team before the one-on-one and is clearly in his own team's possession after the duel;
  • in all other one-on-ones, it is determined whether player A or player B has reached his situational **intention** (see above under "action");
- **opposing player** (the player of team B - in the case of this study, Red Star of Belgrade -, identified by his number; players' names are inserted in the graphics).

The raw data thus obtained (on average, between 200 and 270 one-on-one-situations per game) are organized into tables, calculated and the results transferred into graphics which are designed to give immediate feedback about one or more aspects of the player's or team's performance, often emphasizing key situations resulting in fouls, goals, or chances. The information gained should serve as an enhancement to the trainer's personal analysis (live and by video). The trainer as well as the players profit from the more objective data about the performances as far as one-on-one-situations are concerned. The data are also utilized as the basis for further research (cf. Reichelt and Gerisch 1991).

3   Results and discussion

In the first game, Munich's players won half of the one-on-one-situations (125:125). These figures do not, however, provide any information about the course of the game. For this purpose, the distribution of the one-on-ones in time and zones of play must be evaluated.

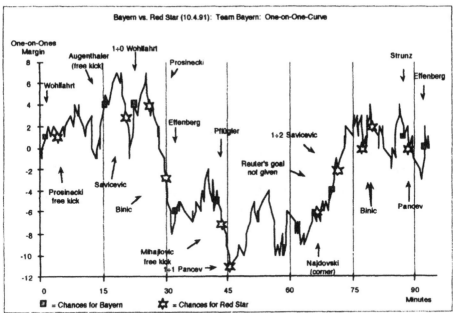

Fig. 1. FC Bayern Munich vs. Red Star of Belgrade (Game 1 on 10.04.91): One-on-one-curve from the point of view of FC Bayern Munich.

The one-on-ones are plotted as a cumulative value on the time axis so that stronger or weaker phases with respect to one-on-one-situations can be determined from the upward or downward angle of the curve. Figure 1 shows the "one-on-one-curve" for both teams from the point of view of Bayern Munich. It is evident that Bayern's performance – after a strong opening phase with the goal by Wohlfahrt – suffered a decline. This period of weakness lasted almost without interruption until half-time, leading to four good chances for Belgrade and the equalizing goal by Pancev. After the break, Bayern tried to recover from that goal by increasing the pressure on the opponents. They could not immediately force any chances. Only after approximately 60 minutes playing time did they mount more dangerous attacks, and Reuter scored a goal which was, however, disallowed. Almost immediately afterwards and during the team's strongest phase, Bayern conceded a goal scored by Savicevic as the result of a classical counter-attack after a turnover due to a misplaced pass by Effenberg. Both teams had chances for further goals in the remaining time. Our one-on-one analysis points out two vital causes for Bayern's defeat:

- the period of weakness between the 30th and 45th minutes of play;
- the failure to capitalize on their phase of dominance (when Bayern was on the offensive and won significantly more one-on-one-situations), when the Yugoslavs even managed to score the winning goal against Munich's exposed defence.

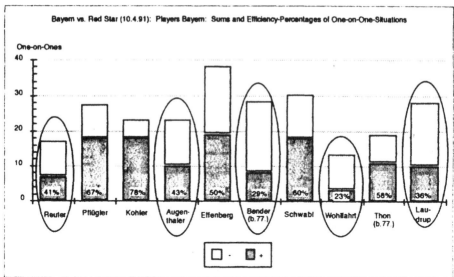

Fig. 2. *FC Bayern Munich vs. Red Star of Belgrade (Game 1 on 10.04.91): Sum totals and efficiency percentages of one-on-one-situations for FC Bayern Munich.*

The score of 125 to 125 one-on-ones was not divided evenly among individual players. Some players in key positions had a notably low success quota in one-on-ones – this applies in particular to the strikers Wohlfahrt and Laudrup, sweeper Augenthaler and the two outside players Reuter and Bender (Fig. 2).

Further deductions regarding possible causes for the defeat can be made from the distribution of the one-on-one-situations into the zones of the field. The action was divided disproportionately between the two sides of the field, with almost twice as many one-on-ones on Bayern's left side rather than on the right. The opposite wing was thus neglected by both teams, although both have outstanding players (internationals Mihajlovic and Reuter) on that side. The distribution described was particularly one-sided in the first half.

Individual players could not sufficiently recover from the increased loads to which they were exposed in the specified zones. This can be demonstrated from the example of midfielder Bender, who had a success quota of only 29% in his one-on-ones. His overall performance, however, must be assessed taking into consideration the performances of other midfielders and team-mates in his zone of action. If Bender's actions are evaluated in more detail, his six losses of possession (5 offensive, 1 defensive) and his shortcomings in trying to prevent attackers from realizing their aims become evident (Fig. 3).

Important evidence is provided by the distribution of his one-on-ones in time, which shows an extreme load between the 20th and 45th minutes (Fig. 4). Eighteen one-on-ones in only 25 minutes is a far too heavy strain even for a player in optimum physical and mental shape. In comparison, Reuter and Wohlfahrt had fewer than 18 one-on-ones in the entire game; if Bender had played at this tempo for 90 minutes, he would have had to enter 65 one-on-one-situations. It is therefore reasonable to attribute Bender's deterioration in performance to fatigue. The resulting lapses in concentration may also serve as an explanation for his wrong position in the counter-attack leading to Belgrade's first goal, when Bender could not prevent Binic's run and set-up for Pancev's goal.

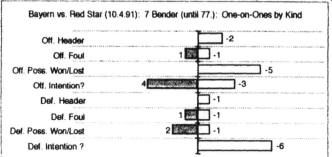

Fig. 3. *FC Bayern Munich vs. Red Star of Belgrade (Game 1 on 10.04.91): Action profile of one-on-one-situations for Bender.*

Immediately preceding that goal, Bender had to sprint several times at very short intervals. Bender carried out only four one-on-ones in the second half. In addition with Augenthaler's insufficient performance (he was often positioned too far in front of his own defence, thus being unable to interfere with the dangerous counter-attacks), the weakness on the left side had detrimental effects for Bayern's game plan.

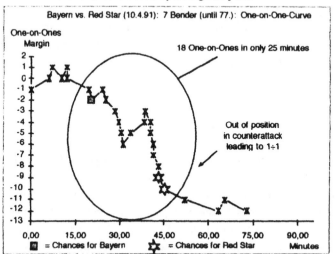

Fig. 4. *FC Bayern Munich vs. Red Star of Belgrade (Game 1 on 10.04.91): One-on-one-curve for Bender.*

The shortcomings of certain Bayern players were complemented by particularly strong performances by a number of Red Star players. Midfielder Prosinecki's performance, generally acknowledged as being outstanding in this match, may serve as an example.

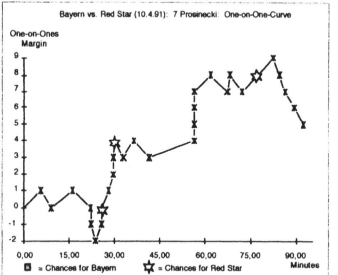

Fig. 5.   *FC Bayern Munich vs. Red Star of Belgrade (Game 1 on 10.04.91): One-on-one-curve for Prosinecki.*

Especially when Bayern increased the pressure towards Belgrade's goal, Prosinecki turned the game by a series of successful one-on-one-situations. In critical phases, he demanded the ball and relieved the pressure on his defence by long dribbles into the opponent's half of the field, thus often initiating dangerous counter-attacks at the same time (Fig. 5).

4   Conclusion

The fact shall not be questioned that the decisive goal for the Red Star team fell under "lucky" circumstances, and that Bayern could have left the field as winners if Wohlfahrt's shot had found its way into the goal instead of hitting the post. However, our analysis has provided evidence that Red Star proved to be the better team at least as far as one-on-one-situations are concerned, and also created more chances than Munich – particularly during the period when the score was 1:2 and both games were tied overall. In this crucial phase, the pre-eminent team leaders of Red Star – Belodedic, Prosinecki, Savicevic, Binic – proved that they wanted a decision (rather than extra-time) and were prepared to bring it about themselves. Several Bayern players – Augenthaler, Schwabl, Wohlfahrt and also Aumann – were not in optimum form, and their substandard performances could not be compensated for by the rest of the team.

Our study shows that a computer- and videobased analysis can support and enhance the trainer's impressions and evaluations, if the complex material is prepared in a clear and coherent way tailored to practical demands. Video and computers are continually growing closer together through technological advances and will soon be integrated devices, opening tremendous possibilities for complex match analysis in the near future. For this purpose, however, further discriminative investigation of the important performance factors is required, along with a system of categories and improved methods of analysis. The game of soccer is particularly complex and difficult to analyse – thus presenting us with a stimulating challenge to increase our efforts.

5   References

Bisanz, G. and Gerisch, G. (1988) Aspekte der Europameisterschaft '88 und Konsequenzen für das Konditionstraining, in **fußballtraining** 7/88, pp. 25-34.

Gerisch, G. and Reichelt, M. (1991) Erhebungstechniken und praktische Anwendung der computer- und videogestützten Spielanalyse im Fußball, in **Video und Computer im Leistungssport der Sportspiele** (eds K. Weber, E. Kollath and G.J. Schmidt). Sport und Buch Strauß, Cologne, pp. 145-161.

Harris, S. and Reilly, T. (1988) Space, teamwork and attacking success in soccer, in **Science and Football** (eds T. Reilly, A. Lees, K. Davids and W.J. Murphy). Spon, London, pp. 322-328.

Loy, R. (1989a) AC Mailand – Fußball der Zukunft, in **fußballtraining** 8/89, pp. 3-13.

Loy, R. (1989b) Wie fallen in der Bundesliga die Tore? 1. Teil, in **fußballtraining** 12/89, pp. 3-9. 2. Teil. In: **fußballtraining** 1/90, pp. 26-30.

Reichelt, M. (1990) **Der Zweikampf im Fußballspiel**. Unpublished thesis for the diploma. Deutsche Sporthochschule Cologne.

Reichelt, M. and Gerisch, G. (1991) Entstehung von Torchancen unter besonderer Berücksichtigung des Zweikampfverhaltens, in **Kongreßbericht des Internationalen Trainer-Kongresses des BdFL 1990**. Sport und Buch Strauß, Cologne, pp. 31-39.

Winkler, W. (1985) Fußball analysiert – Hamburger SV-Inter Mailand I, II, III, in **fußballtraining** 9&10/85, pp. 22-25; 11/85, pp. 25-30; 12/85, pp. 19-22.

QUANTIFICATION OF GAMES - PRELIMINARY KINEMATIC INVESTIGATIONS IN SOCCER

W.S. ERDMANN
Academy of Physical Education, Gdansk, Poland

1 Introduction

Analysis of a sport game can be performed either qualitatively or quantitatively. Since the first way is often imprecise, subjective and ambiguous, the use of the latter way is proposed. It should be based on mechanical quantities (temporal, kinematic, static, dynamic) when concerned with a technical or tactical approach. The analysis can cover the following characteristics - kinds of player behaviour, goalkeeper's reaction and movement, kinematics of outfield players (forward, midfield and defending formations or players involved in the action) in relation to the pitch, to the goal, to other players, and to the ball. This can be done with the help of lines of displacement, isochrons, mean line and point of position and their kinematics.

Analysis of soccer matches for many years has been based on 'observation sheets' filled in during the match. Modern ways of match analysis were developed in the early 1980's. Erdmann (1987) described a method of match analysis with a stationary TV camera having the whole pitch in the view-finder. Until now it has been utilized in analysis of European handball games (Erdmann and Czerwinski, 1989; Czerwinski, 1990).

2 Methods

For the analysis of soccer kinematics a match of the Polish Third division was televised in the 1990-91 season. The teams analysed were Comindex Damnica (A) and Baltyk Gdynia (B).

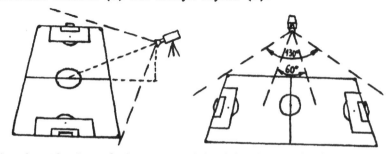

Fig. 1. Placing of the camera (A) with wide-angle lens (B).

For kinematic investigations a videogrammetry method was used. For analysis of the players' movement on the pitch a stationary TV camera with wide-angle (130°) lens (half fish-eye) was placed at an elevated level on the floodlights' mast, so the whole pitch was televised (Fig. 1). For a displacement analysis side-lines of the soccer pitch played a role in the reference system. The match was played back on a video tape player frame by frame (frequency 50 Hz). A transparent foil was put on a monitor's screen and pitch lines with a grid of 1 x 1 m were drawn on the foil. The irregular shape of the grid was known from the previous investigations (Erdmann and Czerwinski, 1989) where a 5 cm wide white tape was put on the pitch before the match. The tape was televised in a position of every 1 m as longitudinal and transverse to the pitch. Next, on separate foils a displacement line and a position of the player (striker, left-wing) in the time intervals of 1 s were drawn for the first 5 min of the match. The foil with the grid and the foil with the player's displacement were matched together (Fig. 2) and the player's position for every second was written down. Then, his kinematic quantities were calculated - displacement, velocity, and acceleration.

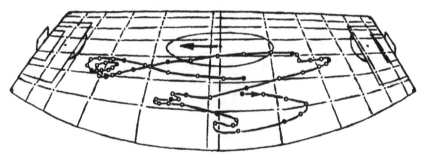

Fig. 2. A grid of lines matched with a displacement of a player.

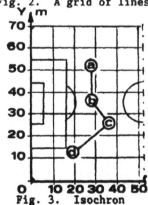

Fig. 3. Isochron

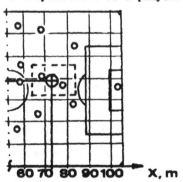

Fig. 4. Team point of position

For the analysis of kinematic quantities of the striking formation, isochrons, i.e. lines connecting positions of players at the same time, were used (Fig. 3).

For describing a position of a whole soccer team on the pitch, a mean value and its standard deviation of every team member's position (team point of position) were used. The time interval adopted here was 5 s. An example of team point of position is presented in Fig. 4.

For analysis of a goalkeeper's movement during penalty kick executions, the TV station's recordings of the Soccer World Championships 1990 in Italy were used. The time interval for these analyses was 0.01 s.

3 Results and Discussion

3.1 One player
During the first 5 min of the match a forward player ran 741 m with a mean velocity of 2.5 m/s. His maximal velocity was 7.8 m/s. During this period of time he was only twice near (less than 5 m) the side-line of the pitch. He also only twice crossed the 40 m line from the opposing team's goal. His nearest position from that goal was 25 m. He never crossed the longitudinal centre line. The whole distance covered by this player as well as the consecutive points of position for every second are presented in Fig. 5.

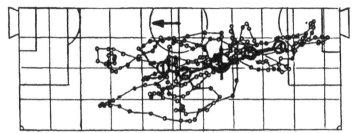

Fig. 5. A distance covered by left-wing striker in 5 min.

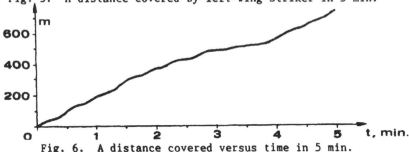

Fig. 6. A distance covered versus time in 5 min.

The distance covered versus time is shown in Fig. 6. Fig. 7A presents an example of instantaneous (with 1 s intervals) velocity, while Fig. 7B presents instantaneous acceleration of that forward player. Attention should be paid to the large changes in time of velocity and acceleration.

3.2 Group of players
Fig. 8A presents by means of isochrons an action of striking formation which appeared after the ball's take-over, while Fig. 8B presents a displacement of the mean point of position of the striking

formation. The highest velocity of this whole formation was 5.5 m/s.

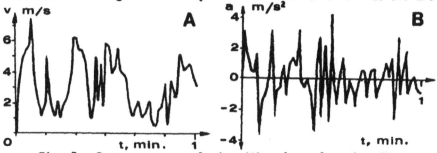

Fig. 7. Instantaneous velocity (A) and acceleration (B).

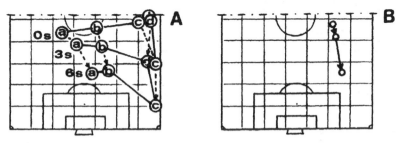

Fig. 8. Displacement of strikers with isochrons (A) and of their mean point of position (B).

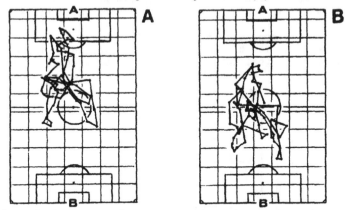

Fig. 9. Displacement of the team point of position of the team A and B in 5 min.

3.3 Team

The mean point of position of the whole team A moved 404 m during 5 min of the match, while for team B it moved 426 m (Fig. 9A and B). One can see that team A attacked twice on the wings, while team B attacked twice through the centre of the pitch. As can be seen in Fig. 10, the shapes of the team's simplified displacements (means for

every minute) are very similar. Also presented are the mean
positions of the teams during 5 min of the match. It can be stated
quantitatively how much one team was defensive (38 m from its own
goal for team A) and how much was offensive (51 m from its own goal
for team B).

There were also similar mean velocities, 1.3 m/s for team A and
1.4 m/s for team B, counted for t = 5 s. The maximal velocities were
3.5 and 4.2 m/s, respectively. The score for the first 5 min of the
match was 1:0 for team B.

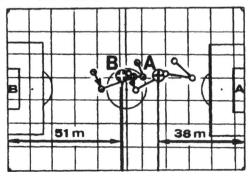

Fig. 10.   Mean positions for every minute and for five minutes for
the teams A and B.

3.4 Goalkeeper and ball during a penalty kick
In all ten penalty kicks analysed, the goalkeeper's foot moved before
the penalty kick was executed. The mean time of pre-execution for
the goalkeeper's movement was 0.20 s. This was about a half of the
ball's mean flight time to the goal after the kick (0.42 s)(Fig.
11). The biggest mean velocity of the ball's movement between the
penalty point and the goal was 36.3 m/s (131 km/h).

In 70% of the shots the ball moved closer to the left side of the
goal (looking from the goal toward the pitch). On average it went
through the goal about 1 m from the post and about 1 m from the
ground.

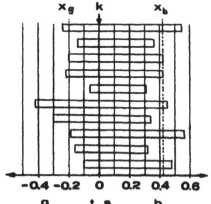

Fig. 11. The goalkeeper's foot movement (g) prior to the kicker's
contact with a ball (k) and ball flight (b).

178

4 References

Czerwinski, J. (1990) The characterization of a play in the team
    handball. Academy of Physical Education, Gdansk.
Erdmann, V.S. (1987) Assumption of investigations of players'
    movement in sport games by optical method. Technical Report
    1987-6, Dept. of Biomechanics, Academy of Physical Education,
    Gdansk.
Erdmann, V.S. and Czervinski, J. (1989) A method of investigation a
    movement of the team handball players in the whole field. VII
    International Symposium of Biomechanics in Sports,
    Melbourne-Footscray, July 3-7, 1989.

FIGURES DO NOT CEASE TO EXIST BECAUSE THEY ARE NOT COUNTED

NEIL LANHAM
'Ivy Todd', Helions Bumpstead, Nr. Haverhill, Suffolk, CB9 7AT

1 Introduction

'Soccer is dominated by chance' was the conclusion of Reep and Benjamin (1968). Furthermore, for all teams everywhere at every level, however they play, there are the same patterns of chance that occur and recur over a series of games, and these were classified 'near constants' (Benjamin et al., 1971). Whilst not exact, they are near enough for this description.

It is the aim of this paper to show that there is a 'near constant' figure, with a variation of 10% either way, for the number of possessions required on average, at every level of the modern professional game, to score a goal, i.e. this is the number of times that possession is lost and won back, on average, before a goal is scored. What is more important, the number of possessions less than this that a successful team takes for its goal on average over a season, or series of games, the same number more it will make its opposition take to score its average goal against them.

2 Method

Over the last ten years, ten English League teams, by whom the writer of this paper has been professionally employed, have been recorded and analysed (see Table 1). This has been done by a shorthand code that records every move within every possession, for both the home and away teams. This has been analysed through a Database computer system.

From the average number of possessions per match and the average number of goals scored per match, per team, the average number of possessions taken per goal for each team can be ascertained over a series of games and, likewise, the average number of possessions taken against that team. The average of all the 1988 European Cup Final and the 1990 World Cup Final games are included in the sample of 479 games. Whilst these matches were played more slowly, as shown by the number of possessions taken per match, the number of possessions taken per goal remains 'near constant' in spite of this.

The Spearman Rank Correlation Coefficient is -0.11, but this is not significantly different from zero.

180

Table 1. Football matches fully recorded and analysed 1981-1991 in the English Barclays Leagues

Team	Div	Final Pos'n	No. games	Average No. of goals recorded/ full match For/Against	Average No. of poss'ns recorded/ full match For/Against	Average No. of poss'ns therefore per goal scored For/Against	Average of the poss'ns For and Against per goal
A	I	6	47	1.43/1.17	253 / 255	176.9/217.9	195.28
B	I		24	1.48/1.10	253 / 256	170.9/232.5	197.00
C	I		10	1.90/1.10	269 / 270	141.6/245.4	179.57
D	I		22	1.00/1.72	233 / 237	233.0/137.8	173.10
E	II	2	50	1.84/1.04	256 / 256	139.1/246.2	177.76
F	II		30	1.73/1.30	265 / 266	153.2/204.6	175.21
G	II		24	1.79/1.42	268 / 268	149.7/188.7	166.90
H	II	2	55	1.60/1.20	257 / 259	160.6/215.8	184.15
I	III	1	60	1.62/0.95	262 / 265	161.7/279.9	204.00
J	III		12	1.66/1.23	264 / 264	159.0/214.6	182.66
K	III	2	55	2.00/1.22	275 / 275	137.5/225.4	170.80
L	IV	4	23	1.74/1.13	258 / 258	148.3/228.3	179.81
European Cup Final 1988			15	1.134	191.93		169.25
World Cup Final 1990			52	1.048	175.5		167.44
Sample of games			479		Average all 479 games		181.62

Formula for averaging possessions 'For' and 'Against' per goal where x and y are the average number of possessions for the teams, 'For' and 'Against'.

$$\frac{x \times y}{x + y}$$

3 Results and discussion

It will be seen that the average number of all lost possessions taken between all teams in total is 181.62 possessions that have been lost and won back before a goal is scored. The samples show that similarly the number of possessions below that that any team has taken, the same 'near constant' number more it has forced its opposition to take for its average goal. Thus, where the opposition has scored fewer goals per match, the home team has scored more.

Table 2.   English Barclays League Tables   1987-91

	Total goals	Average goals per team	Average goals/ match/ team	Est. poss'ns per goal	Average poss'ns therefore per match
Season 1987/88					
Division I	1049	49.95	1.248	180	224.64
" II	1389	60.39	1.372	180	246.96
" III	1485	61.87	1.345	180	242.10
" IV	1404	58.50	1.272	180	228.96
Season 1988/89					
Division I	972	48.60	1.279	180	230.22
" II	1466	61.08	1.328	180	239.04
" III	1495	62.29	1.354	180	243.72
" IV	1495	62.29	1.354	180	243.72
Season 1989/90					
Division I	986	49.30	1.290	180	232.20
" II	1524	63.50	1.380	180	248.40
" III	1414	58.90	1.280	180	230.40
" IV	1426	59.40	1.290	180	232.20
Season 1990/91					
Division I	1047	52.35	1.381	180	248.58
" II	1481	61.70	1.341	180	241.38
" III	1381	57.54	1.250	180	225.00
" IV	1415	58.95	1.281	180	230.58
European League Tables 1989-91					
Season 1989/90					
England	986	49.30	1.290	180	232.20
Germany	789	43.83	1.280	180	230.40
France	863	43.15	1.135	180	204.30
Holland	842	46.77	1.346	180	242.28
Spain	921	46.05	1.211	180	217.98
Italy	693	38.50	1.132	180	203.76
Belgium	809	49.94	1.468	180	264.24
Season 1990/91 as at 12th May, 1991					
England	1047	52.35	1.381	180	248.58
Germany	735	40.83	1.408	180	253.44
France	773	36.65	1.018	180	183.24
Holland	683	37.94	1.308	180	235.44
Spain	717	35.85	1.086	180	195.48
Italy	640	35.55	1.146	180	206.28
Belgium	728	40.44	1.304	180	234.72

An analysis of the English League Tables over the past four years is shown in Table 2. For each goal scored, a rounded figure of 180 possessions per goal is assumed. This shows the number of possessions per game, which would indicate an assumed number of possessions of around 240 per match. The number of possessions per match in the English Leagues tends to vary from 220 to 270 possessions, and approx-imately 240 on average would appear to be a reasonable assumption to be correct.

Table 3. Barclays League Division I as at 12.5.91 (1 match to play)

20 teams scored 1,047 goals over 38 matches. This averages 52.35
goals per team = 1.377 goals 'For' and 'Against' on average per match.

If we take an estimated average of 240 possessions per game we find:-

	Total goals		Average goals per match		Possessions taken per goal			
	For	Ag.	For	Ag.	For	Ag.	Diff.	Average
Arsenal	74	18	1.947	0.473	123	507	+384	197.97
Liverpool	77	40	2.026	1.052	118	228	+110	155.51
Crystal Palace	50	41	1.315	1.078	182	223	+ 41	200.42
Leeds United	65	47	1.710	1.236	140	194	+ 54	162.63
Manchester City	64	53	1.729	1.432	138	167	+ 29	151.12
Manchester United	57	44	1.500	1.157	160	207	+ 47	180.49
Wimbledon	53	46	1.394	1.210	172	198	+ 26	184.08
Nottingham Forest	65	50	1.71	1.315	140	182	+ 42	158.26
Everton	50	46	1.315	1.210	182	198	+ 16	189.66
Chelsea	58	69	1.526	1.815	157	132	- 25	143.41
Tottenham	50	49	1.351	1.324	177	181	+ 4	178.97
Queens Park Rang.	44	53	1.157	1.394	207	172	- 35	187.88
Sheffield United	36	55	0.947	1.447	253	166	- 87	200.46
Southampton	58	69	1.526	1.815	157	132	- 25	143.41
Norwich	41	64	1.078	1.684	223	143	- 80	174.25
Coventry	42	49	1.105	1.289	217	186	- 31	200.30
Aston Villa	46	58	1.210	1.526	198	157	- 41	175.13
Luton	42	61	1.105	1.605	217	150	- 67	177.38
Sunderland	38	60	1.000	1.578	240	152	- 88	186.12
Derby City	37	75	0.973	1.973	246	122	-124	163.10
	1047	1047						175.53

The figure of approximately 1.33 goals, more or less, occurs constantly,
at each level for each season. This is undoubtedly part of the laws of
chance that control the game.

European tables over the last two seasons may be examined for
countries known to play their game slowly, i.e. Spain and Italy.
Consequently, fewer goals are scored per match than in other countries
where the game is known to be played at a faster pace, i.e. England
and Germany.

Results for the English First Division for the 1990/91 season are
summarised in Table 3. If we assume an average 240 possessions per
game, which we know from experience to be more or less correct, we find
that the ball has changed hands on average 175.52 times before a goal
has been scored.

The least number of possessions per goal that a team has taken at
the top end of the table, the more it has consequently made its opposition take, and vice versa at the bottom, but the average is still
within our 'near constant' range. Where there are extreme figures outside of our reckoning, one might add that we do not know the performance

of those teams' Cup games as they are not necessarily included in the League Table, and could well affect the overall figures for the season. Occasionally, at the top end and the bottom end of small League Tables, one may find a warp in the figures because these teams could be of such a high, or low, standard that they can be considered to be almost out of the level of their League.

It is fair to assume that there are above 240 possessions per match. Some teams, who the writer has worked for, have tended to endeavour to play at a faster pace than the normal game, and the average number of possessions in their matches is generally higher than the average number of possessions for other teams in their League.

The least number of possessions that a team takes per goal is the simplest expression of what it has achieved on the field of play over the season, or over a given series of games.

Within this simplest expression there are similar probability rates (and very often 'near constant' ratios of success that apply to all teams) of every possession of the ball, or movement with it. It is the broadest summary of **the large picture of fooball performance** and is made up of rate per goal that can be applied as quantity per match for success in scoring the most goals on average per match. (Table 4)

'Facts do not cease to exist because they are ignored' according to Aldous Huxley in Proper Studies and, similarly, the laws of chance determining the lost possessions per goal apply to every team everywhere, and will not cease to exist because the possessions are not counted. If we treat football as purely an art form we deceive ourselves, for football is not a one versus one sport but 11 versus 11, in which the patterns of chance that these 11 versus 11 make under all conditions and rules of the game are manifold. The economics of these can be contrary to the delight taken from the self-expressive art form of the individual. The complete knowledge of how goals are brought is the understanding of the economics of all team possessions, and particularly their relationship to the many smaller, 'near constant' laws of chance that go to make the 'near constant' of the **'large picture'** of 182 average of lost possessions of goal. This because they occur for all teams, wherever and however they play, and are the same at every level.

If you have money in your pocket and have counted it, then you know how much there is, but if you have not and do not know the amount, that amount still remains the same. The principle is the same in soccer for all teams. Do you, the Coach, know what is the rate for your team per goal and the possibility of improvement, according to the 'near constant' laws of chance that control soccer and are the same for every team at every level.

The 'near constant' figures of performance remain the same, and the least number of possessions a team takes less than the 'near constant' of 182 possessions for its average goal, the same number **more** it will make the opposition take for their average goal against them. Whether you have measurement or not, these figures will not cease to exist because they are not counted.

Table 4. The broadest summary of the **large picture of football performance** made up of **rate** of possessions per goal as applied to **quantity** of possessions per match

	The **rate** of shots taken to score a goal	The **rate** of 'Reachers' (Attacking Third poss'ns) per shot	The **rate** of 'Reachers' taken to score a goal	The **rate** of all other poss. lost short of A/3 per goal	The **rate** of **all** poss'ns taken to score a goal	
Our Team	A x	B =	AB +	C =	?	
						182 = +/- av.
All Opposition	A x	B =	AB +	C =	?	
The difference			+	=	?	
			=========================			

Average

All 15 European Cup '88 Games	9.59 x	9.00 =	86.31 +	82.94 =	169.25	
All 52 World Cup '90 Games	10.62 x	8.27 =	87.87 +	79.62 =	167.44	

A 'Reacher' is a possession that reaches shooting distance (30 metres) of the opposition's goal.

Acknowledgement

I would like to acknowledge the help of Dr. D.A. East of Cambridge in the preparation of this paper.

References

Benjamin B. and Reep C. (1968) Skill and Chance in Association Football
J. Royal Stat. Soc. A., 131, 581-585
Benjamin B., Pollard R. and Reep C. (1971) Skill and chance in ball games
J. Royal Stat. Soc. A., 134, 623-629

A TASK ANALYSIS OF GAELIC FOOTBALL

L. DOGGART, S. KEANE, T. REILLY and J. STANHOPE
Centre for Sport and Exercise Sciences, Liverpool Polytechnic, Byrom Street, Liverpool, L3 3AF, England.

1 Introduction

Since its inception in 1884 Cumann Luthchleas Gael or the Gaelic Athletic Association (G.A.A.) has been responsible for the promotion and strengthening of the national identity, in a 32-county Ireland, through the preservation and promotion of Gaelic games and pastimes. National games such as hurling, Gaelic football, handball and rounders are organised and controlled by the G.A.A. The two major sports in Ireland are hurling and Gaelic football and this study is concerned with Gaelic football.

Gaelic football is a field game contested by two teams of fifteen players, in which a round ball may be caught and kicked from the ground or the hands. Passing is by means of the fist or hand, ie. by striking the ball while it is held stationary in the opposite hand. Also passing may be by means of the foot, along the ground or from the hands, ie. the ball is dropped from the hands onto the foot. Movement while carrying the ball is restricted to four steps, unless the player either hops the ball or does a 'solo' run. A solo run requires the player in possession of the ball to drop it from the hands, onto a foot and then gently tap the ball back into the hands. The player cannot hop the ball twice in succession, but is allowed to 'solo' in succession as often as necessary.

Tackling is performed in a number of ways. The shoulder charge, where the player in possession may be hit on the shoulder by the opponent's shoulder, is used in an effort to knock the ball from the player's grasp or knock him to the ground and thus gain possession. The ball may also be knocked from the player in possession by the use of the open hand, or it may be blocked, using the hands while the player in possession is attempting to pass or shoot. The player in possession may also be shadowed or shepherded at all times by his opponent in order to reduce his advantage.

A goal is scored by kicking the ball into the goal, ie. below the horizontal cross-bar and between two uprights, which is worth three points. Kicking the ball over the cross-bar scores one point.

Each of the 15 players is designated a position on the field, which in effect divides the pitch into sectors. The player is then responsible for winning the ball in that sector of the field. The team formation is 1 (goalkeeper), 3 (full-backs), 3 (half-backs), 2 (mid-field players), 3 (half-forwards) and 3 (full-forwards). Although each player is allocated a positional role, he is not restricted to any one area on the pitch. Some players may wander in search of the ball or to cover their markers. A player's positional sense is individual but it is influenced also by the team's playing pattern.

One of the attractions of Gaelic football is the speed with which the ball may be played from one end of the pitch to the other. A consequence of this is that scoring is frequent. The smooth flow of play is disrupted when the ball goes out of play (over the end-lines or the side-lines) or play is stopped due to a foul or an injury.

The rules of Gaelic football were amended in 1990 with a view to increasing actual playing time and enhancing its attractiveness. The rule changes related to side-line kicks which under the new rules are taken from the hand. For free-kicks the player fouled now has the option of kicking the ball from the hands to provide his team with an advantage. Players are also permitted to take frees resulting from technical offences from either their hands or from the ground (Cumann Luthchleas Gael, 1991). The aims of this study were to determine: 1) the time saved by the rule changes; 2) the specific aspects of play which contribute most towards the increase in playing time.

2 Method

All-Ireland (inter-county) semi-final and final championship matches in 1989 (Old Rules) and 1990 (New Rules) seasons were examined. Video analysis was performed by measuring the time of actual play and aggregate stoppage time. Durations of stoppages due to free-kicks, side-lines and goal kicks were measured. Flow of play was indicated by recording the number of times the ball crossed the 20 m line. The results for the old and new rules were examined using both parametric and non-parametric tests.

3 Results and Discussion

The results show a 2.0% increase in the actual playing time as a result of the rule changes. This figure is the result of a 69.1% reduction in the total amount of time spent taking side-lines and 21.7% reduction in the amount of time wasted by fouls. This means there is a 47.1% and 15.0% difference in the amount of time taken up by one side-line and one foul between the old and the new rules. Thus there has been a reduction from 23.1 to 22.1 s in the average duration of a single stoppage because of the rule changes. On the face of it this difference may not seem a lot; however, with an average of 105 stoppages per match this decrease did prove significant for both side-lines and frees (P<0.01). Frees occurred once every 91 s under the Old Rules compared to every 92 s under the New Rules. Corresponding figures for scores were one every 179 and 185 s; wides one every 217.5 and 208.5 s; sidelines one every 362.5 and 610.5 s and kick-outs one every 98 and 98 s for the Old Rules and the New Rules, respectively. There is an 85% difference in the time to take a free from the hand as opposed to off the ground.

This study also classified the reasons for other stoppages in play. With the change in rules it can be seen that 24.1% and 25.1% of total time was spent by stoppages due to fouls and kick-outs. There is a difference of 28% in the amount of time it takes to kick the ball out after a wide as opposed to after a score, the longer time occurring after a score.

Table 1. Mean playing time and stoppage time per game for Old Rules and New Rules conditions

| | Old Rules | | New Rules | |
	Frequency Mean	Duration (min)	Frequency Mean	Duration (min)
Total time		72.5		71.23
Actual playing time		31.82		32.45
Stoppage time		40.72		38.78
Stoppage Time:				
Frees; from the ground	48	18.62	36.5	14.58
out of the hands	0		15.5	2.66
total	48	18.62	52	17.15
Sidelines;	12	3.62	7	1.12
45's;	1.6	1.00	3	1.85
Kickouts; total	44.3	17.79	43.5	17.88
after wides	20	7.22	20.5	7.48
after scores	24.3	10.52	23	10.25

Table 2. Mean time taken by the various events

| | Old Rules | | New Rules | |
	Time (s)	Total Time (%)	Time (s)	Total Time (%)
Frees; from the ground	23.27	25.68	23.97	20.48
out of the hands	-	-	3.60	3.60
total	23.27	25.68	19.79	24.08
Side-lines;	18.08	4.99	9.57	1.57
45's;	37.50	1.38	37.00	2.60
Kickouts; total	24.02	24.46	24.67	25.11
after wides	21.65	9.95	21.90	10.51
after scores	25.98	14.51	27.13	14.60
% Actual playing time		43.89		45.56
% Stoppage time		56.16		54.44
Number of times ball				
crossed 21 m line		76		54

Frees from the ground under the Old Rules resulted in the side losing possession (or failing to gain clean possession) 12% more often than for frees taken from the hand under the New Rules. Thus the opportunity to take a free-kick immediately from the hand provided an advantage to the team in possession. Values obtained for side-lines were not significantly affected by the rule changes.

With possession playing a vital part in any football game, any means, be it by rule changes or skill alterations, to increase the retaining of possession must be a positive contribution not only to the team but also to the spectators' perception of the speed and flow of the game and to the elimination of negative tactics. The results for the number of times play crossed the 21 m line failed to provide evidence of a smoother flow of play with the New Rules. This may be an artefact of the small number of games available for analysis at the time the study was conducted.

The main finding was the saving in time provided by the introduction of the new rules. This saving, albeit small, was concentrated more on sidelines than free-kicks. Taking frees from the hand reduced the time wasted after foul play and provided an advantage to the team in possession. Further work is recommended to explore ways in which the incidence of fouls might be reduced or time lost at free-kicks might be further decreased.

4 References

Cumann Luthchleas Gael (1991) **Referee's Guide to the Playing Rules of Hurling and Football.** Central Council of the G.A.A., Dublin.

AN INVESTIGATION INTO THE VALIDITY OF THE USE OF CENTRALITY AS A CRITERION FOR STACKING STUDIES IN SOCCER

G. Nicholls, T.McMorris, A. White and C.Carr
West Sussex Institute of Higher Education, Chichester, England.

1 Introduction

Following a landmark study (Grusky 1963) into the stacking of black players into the least important positions in baseball, a number of studies have examined this phenomenon in various North American sports (see Curtis and Loy, 1978, for a comprehensive review). In these sports the least important positions were defined as the non-central positions (Grusky, 1963). Recent studies (Maguire, 1988; Melnick, 1988) have applied theories of centrality to soccer, when examining the possibility of stacking taking place in the English Football League.

The purpose of this study was to examine the validity of centrality as a criterion for determining the importance of various positions in soccer.

Unlike North American sports where positional roles are clearly defined, soccer is a fluid game (Hughes, 1980), with mobility as one of the principles of play (Wade, 1967). Both Maguire (1988) and Melnick (1988) were aware of this and both expressed some misgivings about using centrality as their criterion for stacking. The situation is further compounded by the fact that both used different definitions of central positions. Maguire (1988) based his centrality on the concept of a central spine - goalkeeper, centre backs, centre midfield, centre forward. Maguire (1988) supported this concept by referring to the "World Cup Technical Committee Report" (F.I.F.A., 1974). Melnick (1988), however, claimed that the central positions were occupied by those players playing in the centre of midfield. His rationale for this was based on one coaching text, Docherty (1978).

Recent coaching literature (Worthington, 1977; Hughes, 1980, 1990) does not support either concept of centrality. Equal importance is given to all positions and the emphasis in team organisation is on the ability to utilise strengths and hide weaknesses. In the words of Hughes (1980), " the sum of the whole should be greater than the sum of the individual parts." It is with this in mind that the present study set out to examine the validity of centrality as a criterion for stacking in soccer.

2 Methods

The relative importance of central and non-central positions was examined by means of a) match analysis, b) questionnaires sent to English Football League First and Second Division managers (managers in English soccer terminology are the equivalent of chief coaches in most other countries) and c) semi-structured interviews with selected managers. For this study the central positions were operationally defined as the central spine used by Maguire (1988). This was used rather than Melnick's central midfield players as it a) also included Melnick's (1988) central positions and b) provided a larger sample size for central players, thus making statistical analysis more viable. As well as examining the central versus non-central issue, a sociomatrix to measure the interaction between players, during a game, was also drawn up.

Following a pilot study it was decided that the factors to be covered in the match analysis should be a) efficiency (i.e. the number of successful passes made), b) number of possessions, c) passes made, d) passes received, e) shots on goal, f) tackles made, g) tackles received, h) interceptions made, and i) set pieces taken (throw ins, free kicks, corners).

The questionnaire required the managers to rank, in order of importance, the most important positions in the following formations 4-4-2, 4-3-3, 1-4-3-2. The questionnaire also provided opportunity for managers to add their own comments. The semi-structured interviews were designed to expand on the managers' questionnaire replies.

The sociomatrix was derived from Moreno's (1967) protocol, and highlighted passing interactions between team-mates. The questionnaires were sent to 42 English Football League managers. Four managers agreed to be interviewed. Six First Division teams were used for match analysis. The analysis was made from video recordings as this allowed the analyst to stop play in order to mark down the appropriate statistic, thus not missing any of the action.

3 Results

Of the 42 managers who were sent questionnaires, 26 replied. The questionnaire results failed to provide unequivocal support for the relative importance of central positions over non-central. Mann Whitney U tests demonstrated no significant differences ($P>0.05$) between central and non-central players for efficiency, possession, shots, tackles and passes. Central players did intercept more ($P<0.05$) while non-central players took more set pieces ($P<0.05$). Chi squared tests indicated that each team had individual players who were significantly ($P<0.05$) more involved than the rest of the team. Players thus identified were found in both central and non-central positions.

The sociomatrix also highlighted these individual players.Overall interaction tended to be among players who were positionally closest to one another.

4 Discussion

The managers consulted in the questionnaire and interviews were divided in their perception of the importance of central and non-central positions. Some managers supported Maguire's (1988) concept of a central spine while an equal amount felt that no positions were more important than any other. This finding, in itself, questions the use of centrality as a valid criterion for stacking studies, regardless of the results of the match analysis. Even if the match analysis were to show that central positions were more important than non-central positions, then the validity of centrality as a criterion for stacking would still be in question as many managers do not percieve these positions as being more important. The manager's perception of the importance of a player's role is a more important criterion than the simple spatial location.

The match analysis demonstrated the equal importance of central and non-central positions. This finding supports the claims of Worthington (1977) and Hughes(1980,1990). The greater number of set pieces taken by non-central players may be due to the fact that many wing players specialise in crossing the ball, hence their use at corners and free kicks. The greater number of interceptions by central players was probably due to the large amount of headed interceptions from crosses, by central defenders. Overall no position or group of players could claim to be more important than any other.

A finding in this study was that certain players proved to be more dominant than other members of the team regardless of position. It would have been reasonable to expect such players to occupy central positions especially central midfield as Docherty (1978) claimed, but this proved not to be the case. In one team the dominant player was the left back and in another the left winger.

These results question the validity of using centrality, in the simple form of spatial location, as used by Maguire (1988) and Melnick (1988) as criterion for stacking studies in soccer. It would appear that better criteria would be a) the manager's perception of who are the key players, and b) match analysis to determine who are the dominant players. Indeed the latter criterion was put forward by Grusky (1963) but appears to have been superceded by spatial location.

References

Curtis, J. and Loy, J. (1978) Race/ethnicity and relative centrality of playing position in team sports. **Exercise and Sport Science Review,** 6, 285 - 313.

Docherty, T. (1978) **The ABC of Soccer Sense; Strategy and Tactics Today**. ARCO Publishing,New York.

F.I.F.A. (1974) **World Cup technical committee report**. F.I.F.A., London.

Grusky, O. (1963) The effects of formal structure on managerial recruitment: a study of baseball organisation. **Sociometry**, 26, 345-353.

Hughes, C.F.C. (1980) **The F.A. Coaching Book of Soccer Tactics and Skills**. B.B.C., London.

Hughes, C.F.C. (1990) **The Winning Formula**. Collins, London.

Maguire, J.A. (1988) Race and positions assigned in English soccer: a preliminary analysis of ethnicity and sport in Britain. **Sociol.Sport J.**, 5, 257-269.

Melnick, M.J. (1988) Racial segregation by playing position in the English Football League. Some preliminary observations. **J.Sport and Social Issues**, 12, 122-130.

Moreno, G.P. (1967) **A Primer of Sociometry.** University of Toronto Press, Toronto.

Wade, A. (1967) **The F.A. Guide to Training and Coaching**. Heinemann, London.

Worthington, E. (1977) **Learning and Teaching Soccer Skills.** Melvin Power, North Hollywood, Ca.

PATTERN OF A SPORT TECHNIQUE IN FOOTBALL BASED ON THE SYMMETRY OF MOVEMENTS

W. STAROSTA and J. BERGIER
Institute of Sport in Warsaw, Department of Sports Kinesiology and
Academy of Physical Education in Gorzow Wlkp., Department of Sports
Theory; Academy of Physical Education in Warsaw, Department of
Football, Poland.

1 Introduction

In sport, just like in many manifestations of life, athletes are
examples for others. Their behaviour, dress, technique of movements
are copied. Specialized literature pays little attention to the
pattern of technique of elite athletes; instead stress is placed upon
standard technique. A significant question arising for the training
of soccer players is whether they can have patterns of technique.
The answer is yes, but only partly. High efficiency in play is
assured mainly by individual technique, i.e. that comprising physical
traits, motor and psychological features of the given athletes.
Nevertheless there are elements of technique which are beneficial for
everyone. These include the symmetry of movements. This is seen in
football in the identical effectiveness of both legs. This could be
a pattern. In practice, it has been so for years, but not all had
been aware of it. It was well known a long time ago that an elite
soccer player is able to shoot and pass a ball precisely using either
his left or his right leg, and is able to dodge an opponent on either
side. A lot was written about such players who were considered
worthy examples to copy.

Is that pattern easily attainable? Unfortunately, copying
requires technical versatility and this becomes available just to the
few most talented players. Those less able, manage to copy the
pattern just partially. This way, the extent and level of
'symmetrizing' exercise technique, equalizing the capabilities of
both legs, will at the same time test the player's coordination
abilities. Even attempts to copy the elite are just one of the ways
to develop movement coordination and improve technique. Football,
with recent emphasis on physical conditioning, has left little time
to this.

Our discussion of a technical pattern in shooting at goal is based
upon fragmentary observations (Bergier, 1989; Kowal and Zuchora,
1962; Starosta, 1988, 1990) and does not have a full theoretical
back-up. Such could be given by the many tests which are being
conducted with players of various ages, during prestigious
competitions and with large time spaces in between. The present
purpose was to determine: 1) Do technique patterns exist in football
and do these refer to symmetrical shooting at goal, i.e. using both
left and right leg? 2) Are juniors copying these examples? 3) Is
accuracy of shots at goal dependent on whether the left, the right or

the leading leg is used?

2 Methods

Data were collected on 476 soccer players, including 221 juniors
participating in high rank competitions, i.e. European Championship
and World Championship. Results of observations were recorded using
a special table and reviewed on a video recording.

3 Results

3.1 Technical pattern in seniors

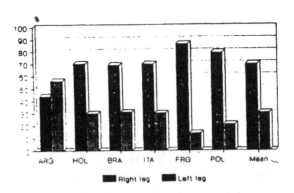

Fig.1. Shooting with the right and left leg of top
teams of the 1978 World Championship (n=64).

Observations made during the senior World Championship of 1978 were
used to seek a pattern for versatile technical preparation to
shoot at goal (Fig.1). The right leg had distinctly dominated
($\bar{x}$ = 69.8%), with this indicator varying between the teams from 69.1%
to 86.5%. The World Champions, Argentina, had different characteristics with domination of the left leg (56.2%) and highest symmetry
of shooting (r = 12.4%).

A detailed analysis of soccer players (Fig.2) of 6 leading teams
using both legs to shoot at goal showed a high movement symmetry
($\bar{x}$ = 45.6%). Players using both legs especially were in the
Argentinean (63.6%) and Dutch (60.0%) teams, with other teams varying
from 46.2% to 53.5%. West Germany was the exception, with no players
using both legs. These data point to high technical versatility of
world elite players in using the left and right leg to shoot at goal.
That didn't exclude the "leading" leg. Such technical preparation
could be considered as a desirable pattern, and one that has been
tested in practice with effectiveness and success.

3.2 Technical pattern in juniors
Further tests were made to explain the type of pattern seen in
juniors and whether this is similar to that of seniors. Answers were
sought during the Second International Junior Meeting "Syrena - 88"
organized in Poland, and during the Junior European Championship.

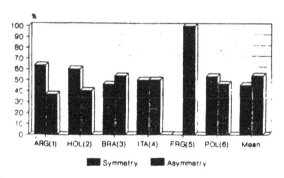

R-right, L-left
(1) - ranking
Symmetry(R and L leg) asymmetry(R or L)

Fig.2. Shooting with the R and L leg and both legs (symmetry) with
the players of top teams the 1978 World Championship (n=64).

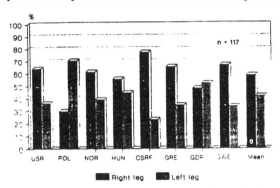

Fig.3. Shooting with the right and left leg of players
in the International Junior Meeting. "Syrena-88".

Analysis of shots on goal during the "Syrena - 88" Meeting (Fig.3)
showed domination of the right leg ($\bar{x}$) = 57.4%) at a low symmetry (r
= 17.2%). This differed between players of various teams from 48.0
to 77.1%. Domination of the left leg (70.3%) was reported in the
Polish team which finished in 2nd place in the competition. Averages
for shots of Junior European Championships (Fig.4) also showed a
domination of the right leg and slight functional asymmetry of lower
extremities (r = 14.8%). Detailed analysis of the results had shown
domination of the left leg in players of three teams (Czechoslovakia
- 1st, Poland - 3rd, Sweden - 6th).

The symmetry level of shots is given by a separate analysis of
results attained by the four finalists of the European Junior
Championships (Fig.5). Here, average results point to even higher
"fitness balance" of both legs, with domination of the right leg
reduced to 53.3%. However, such "balance" was spurious, because two
teams were dominated by right legged players (Yugoslavia, Portugal)
and two by left legged players (Czechoslovakia, Poland). Interesting
results were obtained for players using both legs in the best four

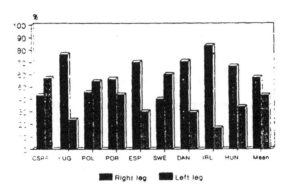

Fig.4. Shooting with the right and left leg of selected players in the 1990 Junior European Championship(n=104).

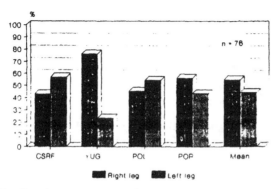

Fig.5. Shooting with the right and left leg of the best teams in the 1990 Junior European Championship.

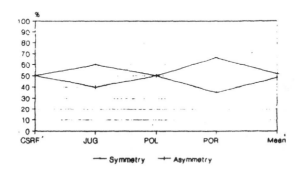

R-right, L-left , (1)-ranking
Symmetry (shots performed with R and L)
Asymmetry(shots performed with R or L)

Fig.6. Shooting with the R and L leg and both legged players of top teams in the 1990 Junior European Championship (n=52)

teams (Fig.6). Almost half of these players (48.3%) had symmetry in
shooting. In teams holding the first three places the number of
players using both legs was even higher, from 50% to 60%. These data
suggest that such technical versatility permits a solution of
tactical tasks during the game and facilitates success.

3.3 Comparison of technical patterns of juniors and seniors
The shooting technique used by senior and junior teams during the
recent period reflects the training system. Accuracy (Fig.7) shows

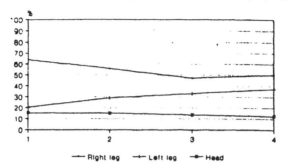

1-Polish 1st Division 1977/1978
2-World Champs 1978,3-Inter.Jun.Meeting
'Syrens-88'-1988, 4- Jun.E.Ch. 1990

Fig.7. Accurate shots at goal with the right and left leg of
        senior and junior level of the different competitions
        (n=476).

that symmetry of shooting at goal is taken more and more into account
during training. The differentiation in accuracy using right and
left leg in juniors was lower (13-14%) than in seniors (27-44%). This
was established by analyzing shots by the best shooters during the
three Championships (Fig.8). The domination of the right leg, over

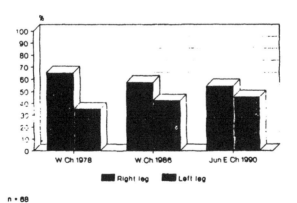

n = 68

Fig.8 Shooting with the right and left leg by the best senior and
      junior footballers - scorers in different Championships.

the last 12 years, had decreased from 30.2% during the 1978 World Championship to just 15.0% in 1986 and 9.0% during the 1990 European Junior Championships.

The growing number of players using both legs in junior teams was confirmed by comparing World Senior Championships with European Junior Championships (Figs. 9 and 10). Averages show that the number of players using both legs had increased by 3%, even though 5 senior teams were compared with 4 juniors teams. Note that the better the

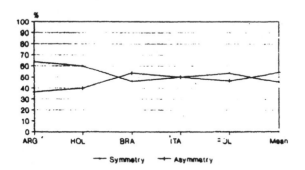

R-right, L-left ,
Symmetry (shots performed with R and L)
Asymmetry(shots performed with R or L)

Fig.9. Both-legged football players performing shots in Senior World Championship 1978 (n=31).

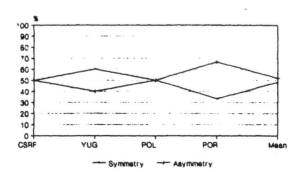

R-right, L-left , (1)-ranking
Symmetry (shots performed with R and L)
Asymmetry(shots performed with R or L)

Fig.10. Both-legged football players performing shots in the Junior European Championship 1990 (n=11).

result, the higher the number of players using both legs. This means that juniors are copying technical patterns set by the seniors. This is done even with some "surplus", i.e. there are more juniors using both legs than seniors. This tendency points to the value and efficiency of a pattern in practical training as well as to its effectiveness during the game.

4 Conclusions and recommendations

Analysis of shots on goal during the 1978 World Championships had pointed to an asymmetry in technical preparation of players, i.e. to a distinct domination of the right leg (69.8%) over the left leg (30.2%). A detailed analysis of these championships had shown that 45.6% players use both legs, i.e. have symmetrical technical abilities in shooting with the right and left legs. Elite juniors had lower (r = 6.6 - 11.9%) values than seniors (r = 12.4%) for the difference in the number of shots on goal made with the right and left legs. A comparison of results for seniors and juniors showed a distinct tendency for 'symmetrization' of the right and left leg shooting technique. Use of either leg for shooting at goal by seniors during the 1978 Championship was applied by some 50% of junior players. This could point to young players copying the technical pattern used by elite seniors.

An increase in the number of players using both legs could be forecasted for the next few years. The pattern is not new and has been observed previously. Pele provided one such individual pattern to copy; the 1950-1954 Hungarian team, in which "all players could shoot using the left or right leg from any place on the field" was another. But, no one pointed this out, and there was no serious theoretical backing. This pattern is a significant part of versatile technical preparation of soccer players and is perpetual, i.e. good for today and for the future. Therefore, it is worth popularizing among players, irrespective of their level. It is one of the universal patterns, the implementation of which leads to general and specialized improvement.

5 References

Bergier, J. (1989) Charakteristik der Schusstechnik der Juniorenmanschaften in Fussball. **International Symposiun "Motorik und Berwegungsforschung".** Abstract, Saarbrucken p.118.
Kowal, H. and Zuchora, K. (1962) Asymetria morfologiczna, dynamiczna i czynnosciowa u pilkarzay w wieku 14218 lat. **Kultura Fizyczna,** 11, 835-839.
Starosta, W. (1988) Symmetry and asymmetry in shooting demonstrated by elite soccer players, in **Science and Football** (eds T. Reilly, A. Lees, K. Davids and W.J. Murphy), E. and F.N. Spon, London, pp. 346-355.
Starosta, W. (1990) Symetria i asymetria ruchów w treningu sportowym. **Z zagadnien sportu.** Poradnik dla Trenera. Instytut Sportu, Warszawa, z.15.

PART SIX

Match Analysis: World Cup Soccer 1990

ANALYSIS OF THE GOALS IN THE 14th WORLD CUP

X. JINSHAN, C. XIAOKE, K. YAMANAKA & M. MATSUMOTO
Institute of Sports Sciences, University of Tsukuba, Japan.

1 Introduction

In a match, shooting at goal is perhaps regarded as the most
important feature of a game. In order to learn from the present
play of the highest-level teams, all 52 games of the 14th World
Cup were notated from video-tapes. An analysis of the 115 goals
was performed from a tactical view point(e.g. crosses, dribbling,
set-play, method of shooting). Some characteristics were noted as
a reference for demonstrating importance of soccer skills,
tactics and shooting abilities.

2 Method

The pitch was divided into eight areas according to the overlay
in Figure 1. Attacking methods considered included: crosses from
A-area, dribbling, crosses from B-area, central penetration, set-
plays, and exploiting opponents' mistakes. Each term recorded the
tactics, places and methods for the goals, whilst the final pass
played prior to the goal (an "assist") was used as a standard.
Goals from different types of volley were considered. The two-
sided statistical petcentage test (Hughes, 1971) was utilised
to compare the data of the 13th and the 14th World Cups.

3 Results

The tactics employed for the 115 goals are summarised in Table
1. Except for 4 goals scored in extra time, the remaining 111
goals were scored within the normal 90 minutes(Table 2). The
successful shooting techniques used are shown in Table 3. It
was found that the inside-of-the-foot accounted for 24.4%;
front, 18.3%; instep, 28.7%; outside, 1.7%; toe-kick, 0.8%; heading,
24.4%; sliding, 1.7%. Among the various shots, 8.7% of the total
goals were volleyed; these include volleys with a sharp turn
of the body. Finally, a comparison of the time at which goals
were scored during the 13th and 14th World Cup competitions
is given in Figure 2.

4 Discussion

Each team paid special attention to the width of its attack
to break the opposition's defence line. In this competition,
32 goals resulted from an attack down the wing(27.8%), most
of. which were completed by a cross; long crosses from B-area
obtained fewer goals than in the 13th World Cup(Liou, 1986).
Of course, if a team had used only the wings, this tactic would
have lost its effectiveness. In this competition, all the teams
used combination attacks in midfield(including various kinds

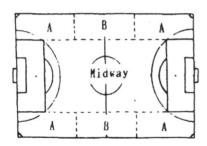

Figure 1. Pitch arrangement

A | B | A

Midway

A | B | A

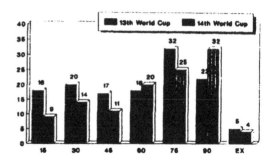

Fig. 2. Time analysis for goals

Table 1. Goals scored and attacking methods employed in the 13th and 14th World Cups.

Attacking methods	13th World Cup		14th World Cup		
Cross from B-area	19 goals	14.2%	5 goals	4.3%	p<0.05
Dribbling	16	12.1	13	11.3	NS
Cross from A area	30	22.7	32	27.8	NS
Central penetrate	28	21.2	21	18.3	NS
Set play	36	27.3	37	32.2	NS
Exploit.opp.miss	3	2.3	5	4.3	NS
Throw in assist	0	0	2	1.7	
Total	132		115		

Table 3. The shooting techniques used in the 13th & 14th W.Cups

Methods	13th W.Cup		14th W.Cup		
Inside	28,	21.2%	28,	24.4%	NS
Front	34,	25.7	21,	18.3	NS
Instep	42,	31.8	33,	28.7	NS
Outside	1,	0.8	2,	1.7	NS
Head	19,	14.3	28,	24.4	P<0.05
Slide	5,	3.8	2,	1.7	NS
Toe	3,	2.4	1,	0.8	NS
Total	132		115		

Table 2. A comparison of the goals scored in the 1st and the 2nd halves of the 13th & 14th W.Cups.

Time	13th W. Cup		14th W. Cup		
1st	56,	42.4%	34,	29.6%	P<0.05
2nd	71,	53.8	77,	66.9	P<0.05
Extra	5,	3.8	4,	3.5	NS
Total	132		115		

of 2 against 1 tactics), dribbling and crosses from B-area. The situation on the pitch is constantly changing, so the tactic chosen related to the proficiency and techniques of the team and tactical combinations of players; these factors are not independint. Goals scored from set-plays accounted for 26% of the total goals scored in the 12th World Cup, 27.3% in the 13th World Cup and 32.2%(37 goals, Jinshan, X.1986)in the 14th World Cup. There is an increasing tendency to take advantage of set-plays for creating scoring chances. Scoring from set-plays is mainly from free kicks near the penalty area, corner kicks ans penalty kicks. In the competition, except for 5 goals directly shot from the pivot instep kick and 13 goals from penalty kicks, 19 goals were executed from free kicks and corner kick assists. In terms of method, there were not only the simple, powerful, accurate "one puch-one shot", flexible "one pass-one shot" tactics; but also the "tactical-free-kick" was employed. All these helped to provide many scoring chances. Although most of the

time the ball is played on the ground,on occasions the ball is
in the air;this is dealt with by heading the ball,and is especially aparent for headers at goal.In this tournament 24.4% of
the 115 goals were scored by headers,underlining their importance,and the percentage of goals resulting from headers significantly increased (p<0.05).These occurred in 21 different
matches.Among these,in the game Czechoslovakia Vs Costa Rica,
with a final score of 4:1,4 of the 5 goals were scored by
headers.For every 15 min that the game progressed,the number
of goals scored increased gradually with time,(except for the
period between 30-45 min)with a peak located between 75-90 min.
This finding varies from the results reported by Jinshan(1986)
concerning the scoring in the 13th World Cup where scoring
peaked between 60-75 min in the second half.All other periods
resulted in a similar number of goals,expressing a balance in
the attack and the defence.In this competition some teams ov-
erweighted their defence,without positive attacking intentions,
wasted too much time in ineffective crosses,making many games
unattractive to watch.Table 2 indicates that the percentage of
goals scored in the first half was only 44.3% of those scored
in the second half(p<0.05),showing the caution employed in the
first half,and reflecting an imbalance in attack and defence.

5 Conclusion

The purpose of this study was to clarify the characteristics
of the goals scored in the 14th World Cup final.All 52 matches
were notated from video-tapes,an analysis of the 115 goals was
performed from the view point of technique and tactics;these
were then compared to the goals of the 13th World Cup final.
The tactics used,as a percent of the 115 goals were:crosses
from B-area,4.3%;dribbling and crosses,27.8%;central penetration,18.3%;set-play,32.2%.The successful shooting techniques
were:instep of the foot,28.7%;heading,24.4%;inside of the foot,
24.4%;front,18.3%.On comparing the 13th and 14th World Cups,
the percent of goals scored from crosses in the B-area and the
goals scored in the first half were found to decrease(p<0.05).
In contrast the percent scored in the second half and the percent resulting from headers significantly increased(p<0.05).

6 References

Hughes, G. (1971) Statistics: A Foundation for Analysis. Addison-
    Wesley Publishing Company, Reading, Massachusetts, pp.189-222.
Jinshan, X. (1986) The analysis of the techniques, tactics and the
    scoring situations of the 13th World Cup. Sandong Sports Science
    and Technique, April, 87-91.
Liou, L. (1986) The analysis of the scoring situations of the 13th
    World Cup. Chinese Sports Science and Technique, October, 10-14.

AN ANALYSIS OF PLAYING PATTERNS IN THE 1990 WORLD CUP FOR ASSOCIATION FOOTBALL

*Kunio Yamanaka, Mike Hughes & Michael Lott

Centre for Sport and Exercise Sciences, Liverpool Polytechnic, England.
* - Institute of Sports Science, University of Tsukuba, Japan.

1 Introduction

Early research utilising notation analysis concentrated on either movement and work rates (Reilly and Thomas, 1976; Withers et al., 1982) or simple analysis of event outcomes, such as the number of passes preceding a goal or the number of shots compared to the number of goals scored (Reep and Benjamin, 1968; Hughes, 1973). As the degree of sophistication of notation systems increased in the mid-eighties, the depth of analyses also increased, so much so that playing patterns and tactics in a number of sports have been traced and analysed (Hughes, 1988; Partridge and Franks, 1989a,b). The rapid technological advances in microcomputers have enhanced these computerised systems so that learning time for data entry has been minimised, and the inherent data handling ability of computers has enabled greater quantities of data to be processed.

Analysis of patterns of play completed on the 1986 World Cup for soccer, demonstrated the individual characteristics that sides develop (Hughes et al., 1988; Pollard et al., 1988). Other researchers attempted to define those patterns of play or tactics that could be associated with success (Bate, 1988; Harris and Reilly, 1988).

Because of the different ways in which soccer has developed throughout the world, the range of climates in which it is played and the varying temperaments associated with individual nations, there would appear to be styles of play unique to areas of the globe. It is hypothesised that nations representing South America, Europe and the British Isles exhibit different styles of play. Also, the nations within these groupings do not vary in the tactics played.

The first aims of the study were to take representative teams of these three groups and to compare the patterns of play of the three groups of teams using computerised notational analysis techniques.

A number of nations in the 1990 World Cup did not have the tradition and footballing pedigree of those from the British Isles, Europe or South America. Despite this lack of tradition and a small base of players from which to develop, the Cameroun team was successful within the competition. This study examined the playing patterns of the Cameroun team, and compared these patterns with those of the European, British Isles and South American teams.

2 Method

The software used for data collection and processing was a modified version of that developed by Hughes et al. (1988). It was rewritten to run on IBM compatible machines, and the output was extended and improved in format. The general data for each match were entered via the "QWERTY" keyboard, whilst the detailed data entry was completed using a Concept keyboard. The latter is a digitisation pad with 128 touch sensitive cells that can be programmed. By the use of an overlay placed over the keyboard, data entry is quick and simple. Twenty four action variables and outcomes encompassed all possible activity in the game; in addition the pitch was divided into 24 areas.

Twelve matches were selected for each group of teams. These matches were notated using the software and then merged and collated to produce mean patterns played by the three groups over twelve games. The twelve matches in each group were balanced, as much as was possible, for factors such as games won, games drawn, games lost, first round matches, knock-out matches, goals for and goals against.

Four matches played by Cameroun were notated and analysed. These data were then merged and collated to produce mean patterns played by the team over these four games. This profile was then compared with profiles of the patterns of play exhibited by teams from Europe (Germany, Italy and Holland), South America (Argentina, Uruguay and Brazil) and the British Isles (England, Eire and Scotland). These profiles were produced by notating twelve matches of the teams from each group. These twelve matches were balanced, as much as was possible, for factors such as games won, games drawn, games lost, first round matches, knock-out matches, goals for and goals against.

3 Results and discussion

The 24 action and outcome variables were reduced to only ten variables for which there were sufficient data for statistical testing. The pitch was also reduced to six strip areas across the pitch, signified by 'A' at the defensive end through to 'F' at the attacking end, by summing the frequencies in the relevant cells. A Chi-square analysis was applied to the sets of data and those areas that had significant differences are summarised in Tables 1 and 2.

From Table 1, it can be seen that the British Isles teams performed more headers ($P<0.001$) in areas A, D, E, and F, the sixth in front of their own goal and the whole of their opponents' half of the pitch. This suggests a superiority of the British Isles teams in winning headers, a dominant aspect of British club football.

Comparing the passes of the three groups across the 6 pitch divisions, the British Isles teams can be seen to have had significantly fewer passes ($P<0.001$) in areas C, D, and E, the midfield area, whilst the South American teams had fewer passes ($P<0.01$) in area A, their defensive sixth of the field. The European teams, however, had more passes ($P<0.001$) in areas C, D, and E. Significantly, all three groups played down the centre of the field in areas A, B, C and D whereas the European and South American teams played more centrally in area E and then towards the wings in area F. The British Isles teams' attacking play favoured the wings in both areas E and F. This pattern was identified by Hughes et al. (1988) to be similar to those displayed by successful teams in the 1986 World Cup finals. Since two of the teams from each group went on to reach the later stages of the tournament, this pattern could have been expected.

The British Isles teams had a very low ratio of shots to crosses (87:200), see Table 1, whereas the South American teams had a ratio of 128:157 implying a greater ability to make a good cross which results in a shot. The South Americans had fewer crosses ($P<0.05$) in areas D and E which suggested that they made a higher percentage of crosses from the final sixth of the field.

The British Isles teams had significantly more goal kicks ($P<0.001$) than did the other teams. This underlines one of the main tactical differences between the three groups with

Table 1. Comparison of variables that had significantly higher frequencies for the team listed in the first column. The letter in parentheses indicates the area of the pitch in which these difference occurred, (A) being the defending one sixth, (F) the attacking one sixth.

TEAMS	BRITISH	EUROPEAN	SOUTH AMERICAN
BRITISH ISLES		*** Goal kick *** Goal throw *** Goal catch *** Dribble(A) * Lost cont. (BCDEF) *** Headers (ACDEF) ** Shot block(F)	*** Goal kick * Goal save *** Goal catch * Dribble(A) * Run(F) ** Pass(A) * Lost cont. (CDEF) *** Headers (ADEF) *** Shot wide
EUROPEAN	** Dribble(A) * Run(BCDE) *** Pass(CDE) *** Shot(EF) * Crosses(F) * End of poss. (ABCDEF)		*** Goal throw *** Goal catch ** Dribble(EF * Run(CD) *** Pass(ABCDE ** Lost cont. (EF) ** Shot(EF) *** Headers(AF * Crosses (DEF)
SOUTH AMERICAN	** Foul(CD) ** Dribble(CD) *** Pass(CDE) * Run * Free kick(D) * Shot high(F) *** End of poss. (ABCDEF)	* Foul(D) *** End of poss. (BCDEF)	

Significance levels:-

'*' :- p<0.05 ; '**' :- p<0.01 ; '***' :- p<0.001

Table 2. Comparison of variables between Cameroun, European, Brit Isles and South American teams along 6 lateral pitch divisions.

6 pitch divisions ( )		A	B	C	D	E	F
Header	European	***	(..)	(...)			
	Brit.Isles		(...)	(...)	(...)	(...)	(...)
	S.American	**	(...)	(..)			
Pass	European	**	(...)	(...)	(...)	(...)	(...)
	Brit.Isles	***	***	***	***	***	(...)
	S.American	***	***	(..)	(...)	(...)	(...)
Crosses	European						(...)
	Brit.Isles					(.)	(...)
	S.American				**		(...)
Shot	European					(..)	(...)
	Brit.Isles					**	***
	S.American						***
Goal Kick	European	***					
	Brit.Isles	(...)					
	S.American	***					
Goal Throw	European	*					
	Brit.Isles	***					
	S.American	***					
Dribble	European	***				(...)	(...)
	Brit.Isles	***		*	***		
	S.American	***	(..)			(..)	
Run	European	*	(...)	(...)	(...)	(.)	
	Brit.Isles	(..)	***	**			(..)
	S.American	**	***	..			
End of Possession	European	***	***	*	***		***
	Brit.Isles	**	**	(...)	(...)	(...)	(...)
	S.American	(...)			***		
Foul	European	***			*	**	**
	Brit.Isles	***		*		(.)	
	S.American	***	(..)		(..)		(..)

( ): Direction of attack,
*, (.): P<0.05, **, (..): P<0.01, ***, (...): P<0.001,
*, **, ***: Cameroon had more actions than the other groups,
(., .., ...): Cameroon had less actions than the other groups.

the British Isles teams using the goal kick as a means of transporting the ball downfield, into the opponent's half of the field. Even though there is a risk of immediately losing possession, this tactic is used so that, by tight marking and good tackling, possession can be regained quickly with an overall gain being made. The basis for this is the recurring statistic that 60% of goals are scored as a result of possession regained in the attacking one third of the playing area (Hughes, 1973).

The British Isles teams had significantly fewer (P<0.05) runs in area C and dribbles in area D whereas the Europeans tended to run more (P<0.05) in areas C and D and dribbled more (P<0.01) in areas E and F. This indicates the different way of transporting the ball into the opponents half of the field used by the European teams.

There was a significantly greater number of end of possessions in areas C, D and F for the teams from the British Isles, which is the result the tactics involving goal kicks and long forward passes. This tactic naturally has a greater probability of an end of possession ensuing.

From line 1 in Table 2, it can be seen that Cameroun performed less headers than the British Isles teams in all pitch divisions, except for headers in front of their own goal (P<0.001). The Cameroun players headed the ball significantly less (P<0.01-0.001) in their own half of the pitch, save again for the last one sixth in front of their own goal. The unusually high distribution of headers by Cameroun players in the defensive area of the pitch would seem to be due to the defensive nature of the Cameroun game, resulting in all the variables having high frequencies in this area for this team. The high number of headers by the British Isles teams is a significant factor in the definition of the patterns of their game. Sending long balls towards the opponent's goal is a simple tactic favoured by all the British teams to a greater or lesser extent. This necessarily results in a large number of headed balls.

Line 2 (Table 2) compares the passing distributions of the three groups to Cameroun and shows clearly that Cameroun had significantly more passes than the teams from the British Isles (P<0.001) except for immediately in front of their opponents' goal. The European teams passed more than Cameroun in every area of the pitch (P<0.001) except for the defensive sixth in front of their own goal (P<0.01), whilst the South Americans had more passes than Cameroun (P<0.001), except for the defensive one third of the pitch (P<0.001).

This distribution emphasises again the defensive nature of the Cameroun game. In addition two other patterns of Cameroun's play emerge; the passing pattern is skewed to favour the right wing, a bias which an individual team often exhibits but which would not be expected to be present in group data processed from a number of teams. In addition the distribution for the British Isles' and the European teams in pitch divisions exhibit a greater distribution of play out to both wings - a pattern Hughes et al. (1988) identified for successful teams. Two of the three teams in each of these groups reached the later stages of the tournament, and so their data could be expected to manifest this property. The passing patterns of the Cameroun players showed that they did not play wide in this area of the pitch and so would not have been classed as a successful side on this criterion.

Although they crossed the ball significantly less (P<0.001) than all the three groups (see line 3 in Table 2), Cameroun players still managed to have significantly more shots than the teams from the British Isles and South America (P<0.001). This is probably one of the keys to the team's success in this tournament; the more a team shoots, the more goals the team scores (Hughes, 1973; Franks, 1989).

The goalkeeper of the Cameroun team was used almost as much as those of the British Isles, but the distribution of kicking and throwing was significantly different (P<0.001). Although the kicking and throwing frequencies of the Cameroun goalkeeper were significantly higher (P<0.001) than those of South American goalkeepers, reflecting again the defensive game of Cameroun, the pattern was similar - slightly more kicks than throws. The European goalkeepers were used less than that of Cameroun, in addition the pattern was different, with there being more throws by the European goalkeepers than kicks. Nevertheless the Cameroun goalkeeper threw the ball significantly more (P<0.05) than the European goalkeepers. The kicking frequencies differed in favour of the Cameroun goalkeeper (P<0.001).

Additionally Cameroun players dribbled with the ball less than both the European and the South American teams in the attacking one third of the pitch (see line 5 in Table 2), but more than all the groups in the defensive one sixth in front of goal (P<0.001).

The distribution of the end of possessions (line 9 of Table 2) shows a close similarity in play between Cameroun and the teams from South America. The differences between Cameroun and the other two groups indicate the disparate tactics employed by these groups, the long ball game of the teams from the British Isles and the possession tactics of the European teams.

The overall patterns employed by the teams from the British Isles differed considerably from those of Cameroun, apart from the use of the goalkeeper, and even then the distribution of kicking to throwing was very different. Although there were significant differences in most of the areas for the variables, when comparing Cameroun to the two other groups, the main reason for this would seem to be the defensive tactics employed by Cameroun. There were similarities to the South American game in the distribution of passing, the relative number of goal-throws to goal-kicks, the low number of headers in the attacking half of the pitch, the overall number of runs with the ball and dribbles, the distribution of the ends of possession and the number of crosses.

The Cameroun team played a passing game that favoured the right wing but failed to exploit either of the wings enough in the final third of the pitch. Although the Cameroun players employed highly defensive tactics, playing a great deal in their own defensive one third, and despite the fewer crosses than the other groups, they had more shots per game than South American and British Isles teams.

4 Conclusions

It is clear that the overall patterns of the British Isles teams differ from the other groups examined in the way they build up their attack from defence, using the goal kick and long forward passes. They also showed a dominance in the air. European teams tended to build up the play using short passes, runs, and dribbles, reducing the risk of losing possession. The South American teams had a high ratio of shots to crosses with a higher percentage of crosses coming from the final sixth of the field.

It was also concluded that Cameroun exhibited similarities to the game patterns played by the teams of South America, more so than the other two groups, from the British Isles and Europe. The main differences were attributed to a more defensive emphasis to their game.

5 References

Bate, R. (1988) Football chance: tactics and strategy, in **Science and Football,** (eds T.Reilly, A.Lees, K.Davids & W.Murphy), E. and F. Spon, London, pp. 293-301.

Franks, I.M. (1989) Analysis of association football. **Soccer Journal**, Coaching Association of Canada: pp.35-43.

Harris, S. & Reilly,T. (1988) Space, teamwork and attacking success in soccer, in **Science and Football** (eds T.Reilly, A.Lees, K.Davids & W.Murphy), E. and F. Spon, London, pp. 322-328.

Hughes, C. (1973) **Football Tactics and Teamwork.** Wakefield, E.P. Publishing Co. Ltd.

Hughes, M.D., Robertson, K. & Nicholson, A. (1988) An analysis of 1984 World Cup of association football, in **Science and Football,** (eds T.Reilly, A.Lees, K.Davids & W.Murphy), E. and F. Spon, London, pp.363-368.

Partridge, D. & Franks, I.M. (1989a) A detailed analysis of crossing opportunities from the 1986 World Cup. (Part I) **Soccer Journal,** May-June, 47-50.

Partridge, D. & Franks, I.M. (1989b) A detailed analysis of crossing opportunities from the 1986 World Cup. (Part II) **Soccer Journal,** June-July, 45-48.

Pollard, R., Reep, C. & Hartley, S. (1988) The quantitative comparison of playing styles in soccer, in **Science and Football,** (eds T.Reilly, A.Lees, K.Davids & W.Murphy), E. and F. Spon, London, pp. 309-315.

Reep, C. & Benjamin, B. (1968) Skill and chance in association football. **J. Royal Stat. Soc.,** Series A,131, 581-585.

Reilly, T. and Thomas, V. (1976) A motion analysis of work-rate in diferent positional roles in professional football match-play. **J. Human Movement Stud.,**2, 87-97.

Withers R.T., Maricic, Z., Wasilewski, S. & Kelly, L. (1982) Match analyses of Australian professional soccer players. **J. Human Movement Stud.,** 8, 158-176.

A STATISTICAL EVALUATION OF OFFENSIVE ACTIONS IN SOCCER AT WORLD CUP LEVEL IN ITALY 1990

P.H. LUHTANEN
Research Institute for Olympic Sports, Jyväskylä, Finland

1 Introduction

In soccer games, the players, coaches and spectators will get positive experiences when the attacking play is successful. This means a lot of attacking attempts, scoring chances and goals. Positive attacking play will in the future be a key point for attractive football. This may explain why the majority of match analysis and tactics employed in soccer has been related to attacking play (Franks & Goodman, 1986; Harris & Reilly, 1988; Ali, 1988; Chervenjakov, 1988; Winkler, 1988). In general, the team dominating will win the game but not always. Many exceptions were found in the 1990 World Cup in Italy.

The purpose of this study was to compare the number of offensive actions and the efficiency of the offensive actions between teams in respect to their final ranking using a method which could be applied easily and manually in match conditions.

2 Methods

A special sheet depicting the playing field was constructed in order to observe the offensive actions in the attacking third of the ground. The observation method was applied both in match conditions, live TV broadcasting and video recording. The offensive actions observed were defined as follows:

i) The action was registered when the ball was controlled by the attacking team in the attacking third of the field.

ii) The ball was lost when the opponent took the ball in the attacking third or when the attacking team ran with the ball to the middle third and lost the ball there.

iii) The offensive action was not lost when the attacking team won in the attacking third, a free kick, corner, throw-in or penalty kick.

iv) When the attack included in the attacking third a centre, header or shot and goal, these offensive actions were recorded.

v) When the attacking team scored a goal after a standard situation, such as a shot or header and goal, these were recorded.

The specific symbols were used for all observed actions. The summary of offensive actions was calculated in each match for a single team. In the matches with extra time, the number of offensive actions was standardized according to the normal duration of the match. The penalty kick after the extended time was not included in this analysis.

Three kinds of efficiencies of offensive actions were calculated in percentages.

i) The efficiency of attacks not lost out of the total number of observed offensive actions.

ii) The efficiency of scoring trials out of the number of attacks not lost.

iii) The efficiency of goals scored out of the number of scoring trials (shots and headers).

The analysis included in total forty-seven matches.

The reliability of the different analysis methods was evaluated with conventional correlation analysis. The correlation coefficients were higher than 0.88 in all observed variables both between the video and live observation, and between the observation in match condition and video observation. Playback was used in all video observations.

The statistical differences in respect to the final ranking were tested using one-way analysis of variance (Table 2).

3 Results

The number, average, minimum and maximum values of each observed variable are shown in Table 1. Significant differences were found in respect of the final ranking order in the number of total offensive actions, the number of attacks, where the ball was not lost, the number of centres, scoring trials shots and goals (Table 2).

Table 1. **Total number and average, (± S.D.) minimum and maximum values of observations for one team.**

Variable	Number	Average	Minimum	Maximum
Centres	1627	17.3 ± 7.4	3	38
Shots	972	10.3 ± 4.6	1	23
Headers	263	2.8 ± 2.3	0	17
Free kicks	580	6.2 ± 3.1	0	18
Corners	425	4.5 ± 3.0	0	14
Throw-ins	561	6.0 ± 4.7	0	40
Penalties	16	0.2 ± 0.4	0	2
Losses	1995	21.2 ± 8.5	4	45
Goals	105	1.1 ± 1.1	0	5
Total	6365	67.7 ± 21.1	30	117

Non-significant differences were found in the number of the free kicks, corners, penalty kicks and throw-ins.

Table 2. The number of total offensive actions (1), the number of attacks, where the ball was not lost (2), the number of centres (3), scoring trials (4), shots (5) and goals (6)

Ranking	1	2	3	4	5	6
1 FRG	87±6	60±5	23±3	22±3	17±1	2.3±0.6
2 ARG	53±5	33±4	9±2	9±2	7±2	0.7±0.3
3 ITA	77±4	53±3	19±2	15±2	11±1	1.4±0.2
4 ENG	63±6	42±4	16±2	11±1	8±1	1.3±0.4
5- 8	61±3	44±3	17±1	12±1	9±1	1.3±0.3
9-16	64±4	45±3	17±1	12±1	10±1	1.0±0.2
17-24	60±5	41±3	16±2	11±1	9±1	0.7±0.2
MEAN	64±2	45±1	17±1	13±1	10±1	1.1±0.1
F=	3.536	3.443	2.421	5.717	5.467	2.359
P=	0.004	0.004	0.029	0.001	0.001	0.036

The efficiency of attacks, where the attack was not lost, where a scoring attempt was achieved and where a goal was scored can be seen in Figure 1. The mean values for these efficiencies were 69 %, 28 % and 9 %, respectively. The differences between teams according to the ranking order were not statistically significant in any variables. The teams in the positions 9-16 and 17-24 typically had a low number of offensive actions in total but successful offensive actions and frequently, high efficiency in

The highest percentages for (1) the efficiency of attacks not lost out of the total number of the observed offensive actions, (2) the efficiency of scoring trials out of the number of attacks not lost and (3) the efficiency of goals scored from the number of scoring attempts (shots and headers) was 76% (Costa Rica), 36% (U.S.A.) and 23% (Belgium), respectively.

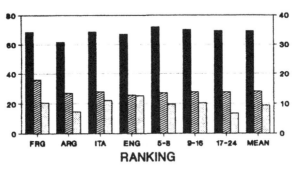

Fig. 1. Efficiencies in the offensive actions where the ball was not lost, where a scoring attempt was achieved and where a goal was scored. The numbers in the right vertical axis refer to the goals scored.

4 Discussion

According to this study, Germany was the strongest team in the World Cup. Germany had the highest number of attacking trials, the lowest number of lost attacks and the highest number of scoring trials both with shots and headers. However, Argentina had less attacking trials than the teams on average for positions 17-24. The situation was also the same in the number of attacking trials, where the ball was not lost and in scoring trials.

The efficiency of scoring goals by the German team was 10.3%. The highest efficiencies for scoring goals among the eight best teams were found in the English team (12.6%), Italy (11.1%), and Yugoslavia (15.2%). Among the eight best teams in percentage of the attacking attempts not lost, Czechoslovakia, Cameroun and Ireland were all more efficient than Germany. In efficiency of creating scoring attempts the best teams were Cameroun and Germany.

Germany used the middle and attacking third of the pitch more than all other teams for long runs with the ball. Their team played wide and deep long passes well. In building offensive actions in their patterns of play they were also successful in overlapping, long runs by the defenders, "scissors" and combinations of wall passes and double wall passes.

The strength of Argentina in attacking play was in the high individual skills and free combination play without any fixed patterns. The real efforts for scoring were performed by Maradona and Caniggia who were very effective in the few attacks they had.

The final ranking correlated positively with the statistics of Germany, Italy and Czechoslovakia. Argentina's placing was clearly not reflective. Also the position of the real surprise team Cameroun, was slightly non-representative.

Analysing teams in respect of the continental point of view, these statistics revealed that European teams mastered the total number of offensive actions, balls not lost in the attacking attempts and scoring trials better. The only variable where South American teams had higher numbers was standard situations. In general, South America ranked second in the statistical list. On average teams from Africa, Asia and North and Central America were equal in all variables. One exception was found in the number of scoring attempts, where on average Africa was the best.

It can be concluded that in a long tournament like the World Cup in Italy the successful teams, except Argentina, mastered the games in terms of numbers, in the attacking third, creating more scoring chances with shots than teams with a lower ranking. The standard situations did not play very important roles in respect of the whole tournament. Likewise the efficiencies in percentages did not indicate the teams' successful offensive manoeuvres, creating chances to score and scoring goals. The success of Argentina was based on the strong defence, excellent goalkeeper, good interplay between Maradona and Caniggia and perhaps fortune.

Acknowledgement: The author would like to thank Mr. Stephen Clarke for his assistance in this research.

5 References

Ali, A. H. (1988) A statistical analysis of tactical
movement patterns in soccer, in **Science and
Football** (eds T. Reilly, A. Lees, K. Davids, and
W.J. Murphy), E. & F. N. Spon, London, pp. 302-308.
Chervenjakov, M. (1988) Assessment of the playing
effectiveness of soccer players, in **Science and
Football** (eds T. Reilly, A. Lees, K. Davids, and
W.J. Murphy), E. & F. N. Spon, London, pp. 288-292.
Franks, I.M and Goodman, D. (1986) A systematic approach to
analysing sport performance. J. Sports Sci., 4,
49-59.
Harris, S. and Reilly, T. (1988) Space, teamwork and
attacking success in soccer, in **Science and
Football** (eds T. Reilly, A. Lees, K. Davids, and
W.J. Murphy), E. & F. N. Spon, London, pp. 322-328.
Winkler, W (1988) A new approach to the video analysis of
tactical aspects of soccer, in **Science and Football**
(eds T. Reilly, A. Lees, K. Davids, and W.J.
Murphy), E. & F. N. Spon, London, pp. 58-79.

A COMPUTER ASSISTED ANALYSIS OF TECHNICAL PERFORMANCE - A COMPARISON OF THE 1990 WORLD CUP AND INTERCOLLEGIATE SOCCER

D. PARTRIDGE, R.E. MOSHER, & I.M. FRANKS
School of Physical Education, University of British Columbia,
Vancouver, Canada.

1 Introduction

Quantitative analysis of the game of soccer has been conducted by many researchers (Reep & Benjamin, 1968; Hughes et al., 1988; Pollard et al., 1988; Partridge & Franks, 1989). In order to conduct such analyses numerous computer systems have been developed. These computer systems have been used to collect, store, and analyze large amounts of data from an extensive number of games (Franks et al., 1983; Hughes, 1988). Much of the research in soccer, however, has been conducted on games played at the elite professional level. As yet few data have been collected on other levels of soccer performance (e.g. collegiate, youth etc.), and little is known, therefore, about the generalizability of previous research to these other levels of play.

At the Center for Sport Analysis at the University of British Columbia a computer assisted analysis system was designed to undertake a comprehensive technical analysis of the 1990 FIFA World Cup Finals. Data about the technical performance of a team were gathered from all 52 games played in the 1990 World Cup. The same system was then used to analyze 7 elite level University games from the 1990 World Collegiate soccer championship in Las Cruces, New Mexico. Participating in this tournament were the National Collegiate soccer champions from the United States, Canada, Mexico, Brazil and Germany.

The purpose of this paper is twofold. Firstly, it is to describe and explain the computer assisted analysis system that was used to collect the data from these games. Secondly, it is to compare the results from the two levels of playing performance, namely the 1990 FIFA World Cup Finals and the 1990 World Collegiate soccer championships.

2 Methods

The 1990 Analysis System

To collect data on each teams performance during the 1990 World Cup a data capture routine was written for an IBM compatible microcomputer. The data were entered into this program by an analyst using a touchpad. This touchpad (a modified digitization tablet) was specifically adapted to meet the needs of the computer program. The data were entered in "real time" and the analysis component of the program allowed for results to be accessed immediately, both at half and full time. Analysis was completed on all 52 games of the 1990 World Cup which were broadcast live by T.S.N. (Canadian Sports Television Network).

Prior to the start of the 1990 World Cup an analyst underwent a 25 hour training process using the data entry program. Following this training program, data were collected on scenes of pre-recorded games so that the reliability and validity of the system could be measured. The methodology involved the analyst and an independent observer inspecting the incidence and position of each event from these pre-recorded games. This procedure was continued during the initial stages of data collection for the World Cup Finals, with the data from each game taking approximately three hours to verify. As the analyst became proficient in collecting the data it was found that not all events needed to be verified, and although data from every game was re-examined, the accuracy of recording was such that only major events of the game action needed verification (e.g., positions of shots, crosses, opportunities to shoot or cross, possession changes and so on). The data capture routine also allowed the analyst to depress an "error" key. This key was entered whenever the analyst felt a possible mistake had been made in collecting the data. After a data collection session was complete careful checks were made of instances when this key had been entered and any necessary corrections to the data were made.

The inclusion of one other key should also be noted. An "advert" key allowed the analyst to record when television advertisements interrupted the broadcasting of a game. This was important to the running of the "analysis" component of the computer program. For example, a passing sequence started before an advertisement would be discontinued during the advertisement and upon returning to the game a new possession would have been registered by the program.

Entering the data

As the analyst observed the play, he entered events using the touchpad presented in Figure 1. In order to collect data on all the events which took place during a game the touchpad was divided into two areas. The first area, on the right hand side of the touchpad, consisted of a series of "event keys" (e.g., Cross opportunity, Free Kick (Direct), Throw-in, Shot on, Backpass). The analyst used the right hand to depress these event keys as they occurred during a game. The second area, on the middle and lower left side of the touchpad, consisted of an outline of a soccer field. As the ball was moved around the field, the analyst used the left hand to mirror this ball movement on the field outlined on the touchpad. For example, each time a pass was completed a new position was depressed on the touchpad field which corresponded to that position on the game field. Also, if a player ran or dribbled with the ball the analyst would mirror this action by moving his finger across the touchpad, only releasing the finger from the touchpad when the player released the ball. Tracing the path of play in this manner allowed the computer program to automatically record the field position where each of the game events took place. Data were collected and stored in the computer as a sequential history of events and positions. The time of each event occurrence was also recorded.

Some problems were encountered in collecting the data. "Close in" camera shots, and the insertion of instant replay and advertisements resulted in small pieces of action being missed and ultimately lost. Reliability checks made at the end of each game, however, did produce as complete and accurate an account of each game as was possible, given that the data were collected from television coverage.

Figure 1.

Powerpad
(Modified Digitization Tablet)

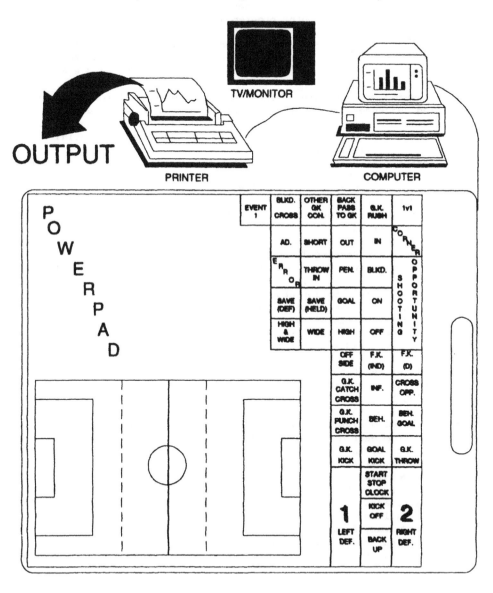

TV/MONITOR

OUTPUT

PRINTER   COMPUTER

Description of the data collected

Data were collected on a number of performance factors. The following information was collected and stored by the computer program:

i) **Administration** - this information was particular to each game and consisted of the teams, round of competition (first, second, quarter, semi-final, and final), venue, and playing conditions at that venue. It was entered prior to the start of any data collection.

ii) **Events** - data were gathered on certain "events" which took place during a game. Each time one of these events occurred the analyst entered it with the computer program automatically recording the position on the field that the event took place. Listed in Table 1 are definitions of each event that was recorded. Operational definitions were designed for both crossing and shooting opportunities (for a detailed definition of a "crossing opportunity" see Partridge and Franks, 1989a, p. 49).

iii) **Passing** - the nature of the program allowed for information about passing sequences to be gathered. Information about where each passing sequence began and finished, and the length of each of these passing sequences (i.e., the number of successfully completed sequential passes) was collected for analysis.

iv) **Position of Possession Loss** - each time a team gained possession of the ball the event key "Possession Team Right (or Left)" was depressed depending upon which end of the field that team was defending. This was followed by the recording of the position on the touchpad field where possession was regained. The computer stored the data and the analysis program converted the raw totals of where these possession changes occurred, into percentages for each team for each third of the field.

v) **Successful Attacking Third Entries** - the outline of the soccer field on the touchpad was divided into thirds of the field (attack, middle, defending). Consequently, the data capture program allowed for the collection of information about where (position on the field,) and how (run or pass) a team successfully entered its own attacking third of the field (a successful passing entry into the attacking third was defined as one in which a team passed the ball into its own attacking third of the field and then made the next contact with the ball).

Analysis of the Data

The analysis component of the computer program offered two methods of examining the data. The "Detailed Analysis" provided immediate results on a number of the events from a game. The "Summary Analysis" extended the detailed analysis and produced a more comprehensive package of results from each game. It also compiled summaries of a teams performance by half (first, second), and across rounds (first, second, quarter, semi-final, and final).

The **"Detailed Analysis"** program was menu driven and provided the results for a number of performance factors. Firstly, a specific data file was loaded. After loading this file the computer returned to the menu and allowed a choice of results to be viewed.

The **"Summary Analysis"** included all of the results available from the Detailed Analysis plus other summary information about a team's performance. One important feature of the summary analysis was the way in which it categorized the results for each team's performance during

224

Table 1. List of possible event keys that could be entered via the touchpad during a game

---

1. LEFT DEFENCE - possession to team defending left hand goal.
2. RIGHT DEFENCE - possession to team defending right hand goal.
3. KICK OFF
4. START/STOP CLOCK
5. DIRECT FREE KICK
6. INDIRECT FREE KICK
7. OFFSIDE
8. GOALKEEPER THROW - goalkeeper throws/passes ball out of pen. area.
9. GOAL KICK
10. GOALKEEPER KICK - ball is punted by goalkeeper.
11. BEHIND GOAL - ball is crossed behind opponents goal = goal kick.
12.* BEHIND - ball is crossed "Behind" of defenders.
13. GOALKEEPER PUNCHES CROSS - cross taken which goalkeeper punches.
14. CROSS OPPORTUNITY - opportunity to cross that is not taken.
15.* INFRONT - the ball is crossed "Infront of the defenders.
16. GOALKEEPER CATCHES CROSS - cross taken which goalkeeper catches.
17. SHOOTING OPPORTUNITY - opportunity to shoot that is not taken
18. OFF - shot is taken and is off target.
19. HIGH - shot high.
20. WIDE - shot wide.
21. HIGH & WIDE - shot high and wide.
22. ON - shot taken and is on target.
23. GOAL - shot taken and goal scored.
24. SAVE (HELD) - shot taken on target - saved and held by goalkeeper.
25. SAVE (DEFLECTED) - as 24 but shot is deflected by goalkeeper.
26. BLOCKED - shot is blocked.
27. PENALTY KICK
28. THROW-IN
29. ERROR KEY - used when error was made in entering the data.
30. CORNER
31. IN - inswinging corner.
32. OUT - outswinging corner.
33. SHORT - corner played short.
34. AD - advertisement key. Used when ads. or instant replay
    interrupted data collection.
35. GOALKEEPER RUSH - goalkeeper rushes from pen. area to clear ball.
36. BACKPASS - defending team passes ball back to its goalkeeper.
37. OTHER GK. CONTACT - e.g., collects errant pass by attacking team.
38. BLOCKED CROSS - cross is attempted but blocked.

---

* (For a definition of "Cross Behind" and "Cross Infront" see
  Partridge and Franks, Soccer Journal, May-June 1989a, p. 49).

the World Cup. Firstly it presented the results for each team either by round, by half or all results combined for that team. Secondly, it allowed the possibility of combining the results of all teams together, either by half, by round or all games together. At the same time, while the Summary Analysis could aggregate the results of one team, it did the same with results of a team's opponents over the games they played, therefore allowing comparisons to be made between a team and its opponents.

The **Summary Analysis** also provided results about a teams performance in passing the ball. The following totals were computed:

   i) The number of sequences in which 0,1,2,3,4,5,6,7,8,9 or 10+ consecutive passes were successfully completed.
   ii) The position on the field that each of these pass length sequences began and ended.
0 iii) The number of passes successful within each third of the field.

Statistical Testing

The above system was used to collect data on both the 1990 FIFA World Cup Finals and the 1990 World Collegiate soccer championships. Specific game related data for these two playing levels of soccer were compared using a Hotelling T^2 test. In order to account for the possible inflation of statistical significance due to the large differences in sample size between the World Cup (n=52) and Collegiate (n=7) data, six random sub samples of 7 or 8 games were drawn from the World Cup data. As no significant differences were found between the sub-samples, only the results of a comparison between data from Collegiate games and all World Cup games together, are reported in this paper.

3   Results

Descriptive summary totals for Collegiate and World Cup teams are presented in Table 2. Table 3 contains results of the statistical comparison between the two playing levels on selected events recorded during a game and Table 4 presents the statistical comparison of Collegiate and World Cup teams in terms of their passing performance.

Results in Table 2 indicate that Collegiate teams created approximately the same number of shooting opportunities per team per game (15.8), as World Cup teams (14.8). The shot to goal ratio is also very similar between Collegiate (11.9 : 1) and World Cup teams (11.5 : 1). With regard to crossing, World Cup teams created more opportunities to cross (19.3) than did Collegiate teams (14.4). Collegiate teams, however, averaged a similar number of <u>successful</u> (crosses that were first contacted by an attacker in the penalty area) crosses (2.9) per game when compared to World Cup teams (3.1). In addition the ratio of crosses taken to those successful was almost identical for the two levels of play.

Table 3 shows no significant differences between Collegiate and World Cup teams in the skill of shooting. Crossing performance was significantly different (p <0.01), however, although the category of crosses played "Behind" defenders accounted for most of the difference. Significant differences were also found in regard to possession loss (p <0.0001). Collegiate teams lost a significantly higher mean percentage (46.11%) of their possessions in the middle third of the field (p <0.05), than World Cup teams (40.53%).

Results from the analysis of passing performance (Table 4) show World Cup teams successfully completed significantly more passes (347.3 : 230.3) in a game and had less changes of possession (180.1 : 240.6)

Table 2. Descriptive summary totals for Collegiate and World Cup teams

	COLLEGE Total (AvTG)*		WORLD CUP Total (AvTG)*	
Total Shot Opps. Created	221	(15.8)	1535	(14.8)
Total Taken	179	(12.8)	1256	(12.1)
Goals	15	(1.07)	109	(1.04)
Total Crossing Opps.	201	(14.4)	2003	(19.3)
Crosses Taken (CT)	157	(11.2)	1600	(15.4)
Successful Crosses (SC)	33	(2.9)	321	(3.1)
Goals from crosses	8	(0.57)	33	(0.31)
Shot \ Goal Ratio	11.9 : 1		11.5 : 1	
CT \ SC Ratio	4.8 : 1		4.98 : 1	

* (AvTG) = Average per team per game.

Table 3. Results of statistical tests on selected events
         from computer assisted analysis

	COLLEGE Mean* (S.D.)	WORLD CUP Mean (S.D.)	HOTELLINGS T^2	t	p
SHOOTING			1.33	(df=116)	NS
On Target	4.71 (3.89)	4.41 (2.90)		0.29	NS
Off Target	5.79 (3.81)	5.15 (3.09)		0.70	NS
Blocked	2.36 (1.34)	2.50 (2.03)		-0.79	NS
Not Taken	2.43 (1.60)	2.69 (2.28)		-0.42	NS
CROSSING			16.45	---	<0.01
Infront	4.79 (2.97)	4.83 (2.76)		-0.05	NS
Behind	4.14 (2.41)	8.33 (4.58)		-3.35	<0.01
Behind Goal	0.58 (0.76)	0.73 (0.80)		-0.70	NS
Blocked	1.71 (1.73)	1.63 (1.76)		0.16	NS
POSSESSION LOSS (%)			13.43	---	<0.001
Att. 1/3	41.30 (9.15)	47.36 (11.09)		-1.89	NS
Mid. 1/3	46.11 (5.37)	40.53 (8.40)		2.47	<0.05
Def. 1/3	12.71 (4.70)	12.11 (5.41)		0.36	NS

* Mean per team per game

Table 4. Results from statistical tests on computer assisted analysis
of passing performance

	COLLEGE	WORLD CUP	HOTELLINGS		
	Mean[*] (S.D)	Mean (S.D)	T^2	t	p
Sequential Passes			161.40	(df=116)	<0.001
0	125.86 (15.75)	71.10 (16.25)		11.88	<0.001
1	60.10 (11.20)	35.40 (9.86)		8.62	<0.001
2	22.86 (8.0)	22.68 (5.71)		0.10	NS
3	16.50 (7.17)	15.0 (4.18)		1.14	NS
4	8.50 (2.38)	11.30 (3.44)		-2.94	<0.01
5	3.36 (2.41)	7.47 (3.06)		-4.94	<0.001
6	1.71 (2.20)	6.18 (2.69)		-4.89	<0.001
7	1.16 (1.66)	3.04 (2.07)		-3.24	<0.01
8	.40 (.57)	2.42 (2.07)		-3.99	<0.001
9	.29 (.46)	1.44 (1.56)		-3.30	<0.01
10	.07 (.27)	4.02 (3.24)		-4.59	<0.001
Possessions in a Game	240.64 (24.97)	180.12 (23.46)		8.99	<0.001
Completed Passes	230.29 (43.87)	347.32 (74.41)		-5.89	<0.001

* Mean per team per game

Collegiate teams (p <0.001). World Cup teams also completed more
passing movements that included a high number of sequential passes
(4,5,6,7,8,9,10+). Conversely, Collegiate teams had a higher number of
possessions where either 0 (Zero) or 1 pass was completed. These
results indicate several difference between Collegiate and World Cup
teams in passing.

4 Discussion

The purpose of this paper was to compare the results of a computer
assisted analysis of two levels of soccer performance, namely the 1990
FIFA World Cup Finals and the 1990 World Collegiate soccer
championships. A statistical comparison of the results from this
analysis revealed significant differences between the two levels in
several facets of playing performance. Significant differences were
found in the categories of "Crossing", "Possession Loss", "Passing",
"Total Possessions in a Game," and "Completed Passes". No significant
differences were found with regard to "Shooting".
    The significant differences between Collegiate and World Cup data in
the categories of "Possession Loss", "Passing", "Completed Passes" and

"Possessions in a Game", suggest that Collegiate games can be characterized by passing movements which include a low number (0,1,2, or 3 passes) of sequential passes, hence a large number of changes of possession with much of this action taking place in the middle third of the field.

In the category of "Possession Loss" the mean percentage of possessions lost in the defending third of the field remains similar between the two levels of play. The average for the percentage of possessions lost in the middle and attacking thirds of the field appear to differ with collegiate teams losing a higher mean percentage of their possessions in the middle third (46% for Collegiate teams compared to 41% for World Cup). This figure appears to be offset, however, by figures for the mean percentage of lost possessions in the attacking third. World Cup teams had a higher mean percentage of lost possessions in the attacking third of the field (47%) than did Collegiate teams (41%). While the difference in mean percentage for the middle third was found to be significant, the difference in the attacking third was **not**. The lack of significance between the two levels in terms of possessions can be accounted for, however, by the large standard deviation amongst results for World Cup teams in this category. That is, there was a large variation amongst the results of World Cup teams in mean percentage of possessions lost in the attacking third of the field.

In trying to speculate as to why significant differences occurred in the categories of "Possession Loss", "Passing", "Completed Passes" and "Possessions in a Game", a possible answer could lie in the fact that after a change in possession, Collegiate teams **did not** drop back deep into their half in order to begin defending. Instead, by trying to win the ball back much more quickly play became congested in the middle third of the field. Consequently, it was difficult for teams to complete a large number of sequential passes each time they gained possession of the ball particularly if they tried to "play through" this middle third of the field. In addition, individual players in Collegiate soccer are less technically skillful in passing and receiving the ball under pressure, which again results in more frequent changes of possession. Collegiate teams did not execute large numbers of passing sequences which included a high number of sequential passes each time they had the ball.

When examining the category of "Crossing", significant differences according to multivariate Hotellings T^2 were found between Collegiate and World Cup teams. Within this category, however, the factor of crosses played "behind" defenders is mainly responsible for differentiating between Collegiate and World Cup teams. While World Cup teams created more crossing opportunities (19.3) per game than Collegiate teams (14.4), significant differences in crossing between the two levels existed primarily due to World Cup teams delivering more crosses that went "behind" defenders (8.33), than did Collegiate teams (4.14).

Crosses have been an important source of strikes on goal and goals scored in the previous two World Cups (1986 = 38 goals, 1990 = 33 goals) and the same can be seen in Collegiate soccer. In the 7 Collegiate games analyzed there were 31 strikes on goal and 8 goals as a result of crosses. These 8 goals accounted for over 50% (8 of 15) of the total goals scored in the games that were analyzed.

The importance of crosses delivered "behind" defenders was shown by Partridge and Franks (1989a, 1989b). They found in the 1986 World Cup that of 38 goals scored from crosses 37 evolved from crosses played "behind" defenders. In the Collegiate games there were 31 strikes on goal from crosses, 10 of which were played "behind" defenders. Of these 10 strikes on goal 4 goals were scored. In Collegiate games, therefore, crosses played behind defenders for a strike on goal were more likely to produce goals (4 of 10) than crosses played infront of defenders which produced a strike on goal (4 of 21).

Given these findings on crossing, shooting, possession loss and passing, one can begin to speculate as to what the priorities of performance are to which Collegiate teams should attend during the practice and playing of the game of soccer. **Firstly**, Collegiate teams may be able to create more shooting and particularly crossing opportunities during a game and ultimately score more goals, if they were to use specific tactics that resulted in a higher percentage of their possessions reaching their own attacking third of the field. That is, attempting to make passing movements that include a high number of sequential passes and which move the ball from their own defending third and through the middle third before entering the attacking third, may not be effective in Collegiate soccer due to the compact and congested nature of play. Given the nature of Collegiate soccer as evidenced by results from this study, Collegiate coaches who present the play of World Cup teams as a model of performance, focusing primarily on passing movements which include a high number of consecutive passes, may in fact be utilizing an inappropriate model of performance. **Secondly**, Collegiate teams should attempt to create more opportunities to cross and then deliver these crosses into the space which is "behind" defenders but in-front of the goalkeeper. Coupled with this is a need to have other players attempt to contact these crosses in the penalty area. Practices need to be designed to help players understand and improve their specific roles in exploiting crossing opportunities.

World Cup teams might increase the effectiveness of each of the possessions they have during a game. This could be achieved by using more "pressurizing" techniques to regain possession of the ball in their own attacking and middle thirds of the field. The tactic employed by most teams playing in the 1990 World Cup, of "dropping back" to set a defensive line on or around the half way line on losing possession, is certainly not utilizing such "pressurizing" techniques, or reducing the number of attacking third entries made by an opponent. Logically it is these attacking third entries that result in the creation of crossing and shooting opportunities.

There purpose of this paper was twofold. Firstly, to describe and explain the computer assisted analysis system that was used to collect the data. Secondly, to compare the results from two levels of playing performance, namely the 1990 FIFA World Cup Finals and the 1990 World Collegiate Soccer championships. It would appear, that the results from this comparison have several implications for soccer coaches, particularly at the Collegiate level. The most important of these is that significant differences exist between the two playing levels in several aspects of technical performance, most notably in the areas of passing and possession loss. It can be concluded, therefore, that Collegiate coaches need to be very selective when presenting the play of World Cup teams as an appropriate model of performance for the play of their own team.

Acknowledgements

The research reported in this paper was funded by grants from the Coaching Association of Canada, the Canadian Soccer Association, and the Social Sciences and Humanities Research Council of Canada.

5 References

Franks, I.M., Goodman, D. & Miller, G. (1983). Analysis of performance: Qualitative or quantitative. Science Periodical on Research and Technology in Sport. GY-1.

Franks, I.M. & Goodman, D. (1986). Computer-assisted technical analysis of sport. Coaching Review, May/June, 58-64.

Hughes, M. (1988). Computerized notation analysis in field games. Ergonomics, 31, 1585-1592.

Hughes, M.D., Robertson, K. & Nicholson, A. (1988). An analysis of the 1986 World Cup of Association Football, in Science and Football (eds T. Reilly, A. Lees, K. Davids & W. Murphy), London: E. & F.N. Spon, pp 363-368.

Partridge, D., & Franks, I.M. (1989a). A detailed analysis of crossing opportunities from the 1986 World Cup - part 1. Soccer Journal, May-June, 47-50.

Partridge, D., & Franks, I.M. (1989b). A detailed analysis of crossing opportunities from the 1986 World Cup - part 2. Soccer Journal, July-August, 45-48.

Pollard, R., Reep, C., & Hartley, S. (1988). The quantitative comparison of playing styles in soccer, in Science and Football (eds T. Reilly, A. Lees, K. Davids & W. Murphy), London: E. & F.N. Spon, pp 363-368.

Reep, C., & Benjamin, B. (1968). Skill and chance in Association Football. J. Royal Stat. Soc., Series A, 131, 581-585.

COMPUTER ANALYSIS OF THE EFFECTIVENESS OF COLLECTIVE TECHNICAL AND
TACTICAL MOVES OF FOOTBALLERS IN THE MATCHES OF 1988 OLYMPICS AND
1990 WORLD CUP

A. BISHOVETS, G. GADJIEV and M. GODIK
Russian Sports Committee, Central Institute of Physical Culture,
Moscow, Russia

1 Introduction

Overall analysis of the game of football during competitive
situations includes the following parameters:
  (1) individual technical and tactical moves (ITTM);
  (2) collective technical and tactical moves (CTTM);
  (3) volume and intensity of players' moves during play (VIPM);
  (4) changes in biological parameters (HR, HLa, $\dot{V}O_2$max, and so on)
  during matches.
Studies have been conducted on each of these directions, and the
results presented at the First Congress "Science and Football"
(Reilly et al., 1988) as well as being published elsewhere (e.g.
Winkler, 1991). By the end of 1970s when the fundamental principles
of CTTM were established, analysis was started in the Soviet Union
(Gadjiev and Bazilevich, 1981; Gadjiev et al., 1982; Godik, 1988).
Results of the quantitative analyses indicated the scope of such
studies for theory and practical aspects of football and demonstrated
that the results of these studies could be utilized for the better
understanding of the rules of the game. Results offered the
possibility to construct models for team play and to plan the
training programmes effectively.
    Quantitative estimation of CTTM indicated a lot of variations. In
order to establish the statistical reliability of the results, a
large size of sample was needed. Preliminary results showed that
CTTM structure comprised a number of factors. Therefore the
importance of these factors on match results was to be established.
    The aim of the present study was to analyze the structure of the
moves of footballers and the effectivness of CTTM during matches in
the 1990 World Cup. Realization of these objectives would enable us
to identify which of the various CTTM factors positively affects the
results of the game. Results might be used for training programmes
and modelling of CTTM for training sessions.

2 Methods

Details of the measurements and definition of terms had been given by
Gadjiev (1984). During the 1990 World Cup the variables registered
were: number of attacks (including the centre and side attacks),
zones in which these attacks were started and completed (total 4
zones), number of units of play in each attack (0-3, 4-6 and more

than 6), numbers of shots in an attempt to score), places from where these shots were taken, number of critical situations created by the footballers using CTTM and so on. A total of 32 moves was registered during 52 matches of the World Cup. The values were used for the calculation of the coefficients of effectiveness of the offensive and defensive moves, central and side attacks, success of the shots at goal, width of attack, effectiveness of offensive moves and so on.

Initial matrices were compiled based upon the observations, and were processed by RIVAL 386SX PC by Arche Technology, Inc. The first matrix consisted of the data of the winning teams, the second of the losers, and the third was a combination of both. Correlation and factor analyses were conducted.

3 Results

The average values and relative differences of the parameters of winners and losers are given in Figure 1. It is evident that losers did not differ much on the main parameter of the game (number of attacks in which the ball was propelled to the 4th zone) as compared to winners (50.1±17.8 and 55.4±16.2 attacks). Both groups did not differ much on the effectiveness of the defensive moves: the difference was only 6% less in the case of losers compared to the winners.

The differences were found on the following parameters:- in the effectiveness of attacks (test 4) and, particularly, in attacks through the centre (test 15), effectiveness of shots (test 6), coefficient of effectiveness of the moves (test 8), effectiveness of attacks which were the result of a combination of 1-3 passes (test 22). The winners were effective in attacks when the move started in the 1st zone (test 26), and from the 2nd zone after getting the ball from the opponents (test 28). The winners were more effective than losers while making use of critical situations which they could create frequently (4.85±2.2 vs 1.96±1.6).

For the evaluation of moves during play, the authors had been using a standard battery of tests over several years. In this case the use of factor analysis is appropriate, by means of which the most important factors could be grouped and identified. In our opinion, each of these factors represents one of the substantial moments of the game. A part of the factor analysis is given in Table 1.

Statistical analysis showed that the most important factor among the various criteria of the effectiveness of CTTM was the attacking moves, number of critical moments and the shots from within the penalty area.

The important determinant of attacking moves was the loss of the ball in the first three zones of the pitch. This applied especially after the first pass.

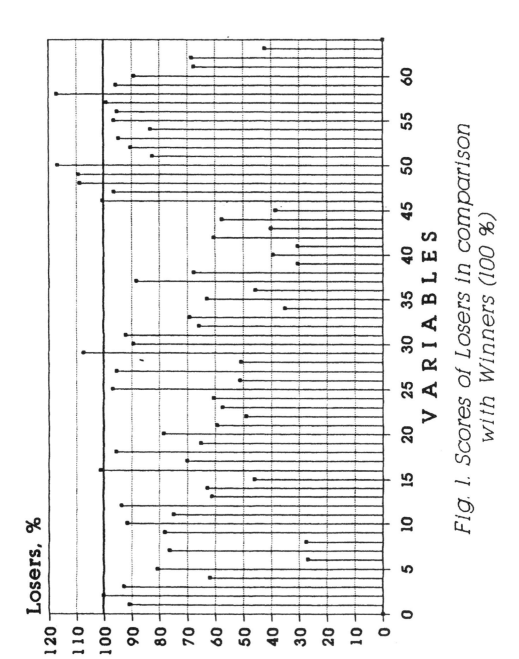

Fig. 1. Scores of Losers in comparison with Winners (100 %)

Table 1. Factor matrix for various variables of effectiveness of CTTM (winners, n=27)

| Variables | Factors | | | | Commun |
	I	II	III	IV	ality
1. Effectiveness of defensive moves	.345	.785	-.344	.308	.934
2. Effectiveness of offensive moves	.945	.279	.136	.016	.975
3. Coeff. of effectivness of game	.599	.689	-.146	.048	.973
4. Number of critical moments	.864	.211	.259	-.085	.902
5. Number of successful attacks	.005	.089	.063	.577	.332
6. Number of goals scored	.409	-.065	.782	.102	.639
7. Number of goals missed	.000	-.143	.691	.032	.442
8. Total score	.884	.269	-.020	-.024	.860
9. Shots taken from penalty area	.847	.069	.202	.172	.778
Factor scores, %	65.8	23.1	7.5	2.7	

4 Discussion

The results of the analysis between the number of CTTM variables and its factors showed the high relationship between offensive and defensive moves for the winners. The factor structure of CTTM of such teams consisted of a lower number of factors than the losers. It was due to more effective collective moves of the winners. This was the result of a more consistent and reliable understanding between players, irrespective of the various destructive factors.

The increase in the number of factors in the losers was because they were less consistent and unreliable in team-play. This applied especially when shifting from defensive to offensive moves or vice versa.

All these factors were taken into account while preparing the USSR team for competitions. The training exercises depended upon the fundamental principles of CTTM described above. For example, special attention was paid to mastery and proficiency of the individual exercises modelled for the final stages of attacking moves and a better understanding for team-play. In our opinion the number and effectiveness of such exercises form the foundation of the training in the preparation of footballers.

5 References

Gadjiev, G.M. (1981) Structure of competitive moves as a base for complex control and planning for preparation of top class footballers. Ph.D. thesis, Moscow, (in Russian)

Gadjiev, G.M. and Bazilevich, O.P. (1981) Modelling of competitive moves of the teams based upon the quantitative parameters of collective moves during play. Football. Fizkultura i Sport, Moscow, pp. 34-38. (in Russian)

Gadjiev, G.M., Godik, M.A. and Zonin, G.S. (1982) Control of competitive moves for the top class footballers. Methodological recommendation. Fizkultura i Sport, Moscow, (in Russian)

Godik, M.A. (1988) Sports Metrology. Textbook for the Institutes of Physical Education. Fizkultura i Sport, Moscow.

Reilly, T., Lees, A., Davids, K. and Murphy, W.J. (1988) Science and Football, E. and F.N. Spon, London.

Winkler, W. (1991) Match analysis and improvement of performance in soccer with the aid of computer controlled dual-video-systems (CCDVS). Science and Football, 4, 6–10.

PART SEVEN

Physiological Aspects of Soccer Skills

ADVANCE CUE UTILIZATION IN SOCCER

A.M. WILLIAMS and L.BURWITZ
Division of Sport Science, Crewe and Alsager College, Cheshire ST7 2HL, England.

1 Introduction

The importance of the penalty kick in deciding the outcome of a soccer match has been much debated. During the 1990 World Cup finals 4 of the 16 final stage matches were decided by the outcome of a penalty kick. As more games are being decided by a single goal (Hughes, 1990), or by the intervention of a penalty shoot-out, the ability of the goalkeeper in these situations is increasingly important.

Recently, it has been suggested that goalkeepers in penalty situations should react to the ball based on the initial portion of ball flight (Hughes, 1990). However, temporal limitations in terms of ball speed (Keller et al., 1978) and the goalkeeper's response time (Morris and Burwitz, 1989) would prevent the goalkeeper from saving a reasonably struck penalty. An alternative approach would be to anticipate ball direction by careful analysis of advance (pre-impact) cues from the penalty taker's technique (eg. angle of run-up and body orientation in addressing the ball).

The ability of experienced sports performers to utilise advance visual cues is well documented within the research literature (Abernethy, 1987). However, very little work has to date been carried out in soccer. The following experiments were designed to examine the ability of soccer goalkeepers to utilise advance visual cues in the context of a penalty kick.

2 Experiment 1

2.1 Objective

The objective of experiment 1 was to examine the effect of playing experience on anticipatory performance during a penalty kick. Further, the investigation was designed to identify whether there were any specific input cues which allow players to anticipate ball direction.

2.2 Methodology

A filmed occlusion paradigm was used where the perceptual display available to a goalkeeper during a penalty kick was selectively manipulated by varying the duration of the kick that was visible.

The test film included 40 penalty kick situations taken by right-footed players. The camera was placed in the goalkeeper's normal penalty position and each filmed trial included the penalty taker's preparatory stance, run-up and kicking technique up to the point of occlusion. Four restricted viewing conditions were used 120 ms before foot-ball impact, 40 ms before impact, at impact and 40 ms after foot-ball contact.

Two groups of experienced (n=30), and inexperienced soccer players (n = 30) viewed the penalty kicks on a video projection screen. The experienced group had played an average of 396 competitive soccer games (SD ± 99.22), whereas, the inexperienced group had played an average of 56.46 competitive matches (SD ± 36.64). The subjects were required to make perceptual judgements, in terms of a pen and paper response, regarding which corner of the goal the ball was directed to. Response accuracy was the dependent variable measured.

Subjects also completed a questionnaire following the session of testing. This was used to obtain information regarding the importance of various areas of the penalty taker's technique in anticipating ball direction.

2.3 Results and Discussion
Analysis of experimental results in terms of percentage accuracy (Table 1) showed differences in performance between the two groups and across each temporal occlusion condition.

Table 1. Mean percentage of correct responses for experienced and inexperienced goalkeepers in each of four conditions (SD ±).

	Condition 1 120 ms prior impact	Condition 2 40 ms prior impact	Condition 3 at foot impact	Condition 4 40 ms after impact
Experienced Players	51.00 (± 15.13)	62.66 (± 12.89)	82.66 (± 9.55)	83.33 (± 7.88)
Inexperienced Players	39.33 (± 14.22)	54.00 (± 15.18)	78.00 (± 12.20)	85.33 (± 5.62)

Statistical analysis of the above scores, using a two way analysis of variance with repeated measures, showed significant differences both between groups and across conditions ($p < 0.01$). Further post-hoc Newman Keuls analysis revealed that the superior performance of the experienced group was significant ($p < 0.01$) only under the shortest durations (pre-impact conditions 1 and 2).

These results, expressed graphically in Figure 1, showed that experience plays a major role in the ability of goalkeepers to make use of advance visual cues in anticipating ball direction. Differences between experienced and inexperienced players were more apparent at earlier occlusion periods, with experienced players being able to make better use of earlier potential sources of information.

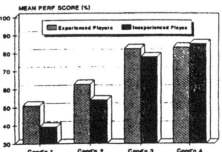

Figure 1. Mean percentage correct responses for both groups across conditions.

In addition Chi square analysis showed that both groups scored significantly better than 'chance' (p< 0.01) across all conditions. It therefore appeared that it was possible to anticipate the direction of a penalty kick from the preparatory movements of the penalty taker.

The questionnaire responses revealed that information was obtained in anticipating the appropriate side from the angle of run-up, arc of leg on approach to the ball and the angle of kicking foot and hip prior to ball contact. The hip position at impact was regarded as being the most important of these information sources. If the right hip was in an "open" or angled position relative to the goalkeeper, the ball went to the kicker's right. If the hip was "square on" to the subject, the ball went to the kicker's left. Similarly, the lean of the trunk was deemed to be most important in anticipating the correct height of the ball. A ball that went high was characterised by a leaning back of the trunk on ball impact; while the trunk tended to lean forward, with the head and shoulders over the ball, when the kick was kept low.

Further breakdown of the results (Table 2) showed that the majority of errors (61.8%) were associated with incorrect height judgements. In contrast very powerful differential cues seemed to be available in distinguishing the correct side where only 25.71% of errors occurred. Analysis of error rates for incorrect height decisions shows that there was a marked improvement in height judgement only after initial ball trajectory had been viewed (condition 4). For example, in condition 1 71.23% of errors were of an incorrect height nature, compared to, only 40.62% of errors in condition 4. In contrast the error rate for incorrect side was relatively low even under the earliest occlusion condition (condition 1).

Table 2. Variations in error type, as a proportion of total error made, across all four conditions for both groups combined.

Response Category	Condition 1	Condition 2	Condition 3	Condition 4
Incorrect Height	71.23%	67.00%	68.35%	40.62%
Incorrect Side	17.36%	26.91%	25.64%	32.91%
Height & Side Incorrect	11.41%	6.09%	6.51%	26.47%

On the basis of the results a suitable penalty saving strategy was suggested. Goalkeepers should attempt to anticipate the direction of a penalty kick prior to foot-ball contact. Information regarding correct side should be extracted from the run-up, kicking leg and specifically the hip position prior to impact. Adjustment of position according to shot height should occur initially on the basis of trunk position prior to foot-ball impact, but firstly on the basis of the initial portion of ball flight just prior to breaking ground contact in the diving phase.

3 Experiment 2

3.1 Objective
The objective of this second experiment was to determine whether a beginner's anticipatory performance could be improved by a video based coaching programme.

3.2 Method
Ten novice players were selected from experiment 1 to participate in approximately 90 minutes of visual simulation training using video film. Relevant anticipatory cues, drawn from the questionnaire study administered in experiment 1, were highlighted using video film of six different penalty takers. The training film included a total of forty-eight different penalty kicks.

3.3 Results and Discussion
Statistical comparison of pre-and post-training performance scores, using a two way analysis of variance and Newman Keuls procedure, showed significant improvements for the experimental group as opposed to a control group (p< 0.01). Analysis of Figure 2, showed that the improvement in performance was due to an improvement across all response categories. It appeared, therefore, that the film based training programme improved anticipation performance. Given that this type of training rarely occurs in practice this was considered to be of practical significance.

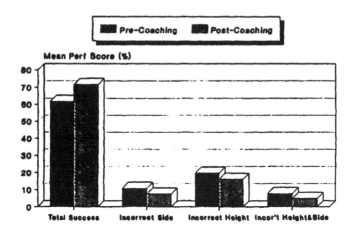

Figure 2. Distribution of response alternative pre and post coaching treatment.

4 Conclusion

The results of this study showed that experienced goalkeepers can successfully make use of pre-impact cues to anticipate ball direction. The results also demonstrated that this ability can be enhanced through effective video based coaching. The data would therefore support the adoption of an anticipation based penalty saving strategy.

References

Abernethy, B (1978) Anticipation in sport: A review. **Phys. Educ. Rev.** 10, 5 -16.

Hughes, C (1990) **The Winning Formula: The Football Association Soccer Tactics and Skills.** William Collins Sons & Co Ltd. London.

Keller, D; Hennermann, M.C; and Algeria, J (1979) Fussball: Der Elfmeter. **Leistungsport** 5, 394 - 398.

Morris, A and Burwitz, L (1989) Anticipation and movement strategies in elite soccer goalkeepers at penalty kicks. **J. Sports Sci.**, 7, 79-80.

TESTING THE ABILITY OF ANTICIPATION-COINCIDENCE OF SOCCER PLAYERS

WERNER KUHN
Free University of Berlin, Germany

1 Introduction

Passing into open space and placing the ball accurately and timely for a moving team mate are important skills in soccer (Williams, 1973; McMorris and Copeman, 1991). This ability of anticipation-coincidence can be defined as the timing of an own response to coincide with a response triggered by an outside source. Since testing this skill under field conditions is difficult to achieve, a strict laboratory situation was chosen at the beginning (Henry and Grose, 1968; Abernethy, 1987). In our study two movements - the movement of a team mate and of a ball (which was controlled by a ball-possessing player) - had to be anticipated and coordinated. Anticipation of direction was not required. Most of the studies carried out so far, have chosen a typical one-on-one situation with the opposing player and/or the object (e.g. the racquet, the ball) moving towards the subject. A new aspect was brought into this investigation in so far as the subject had to coordinate the speed of his own pass with the movement of a player who was running away from him.

Thus, the purpose of this study was to develop a test for anticipation-coincidence that differentiated between soccer players of different levels.

2 Methodology

An overview of the experimental set-up is shown in Figure 1. The speed of the pass recipient was simulated with a Bassin anticipation timer of 2.88 m in length. After a fixed fore-period warning signal, a red light travelled on a runway from left to right with an adjustable, yet constant velocity. The ball was placed on the microswitch of a self-constructed wooden platform. When contact with the ball was established, the timer was set in motion. The clock was stopped when the ball touched the contact mat prepared as vertical target area. The subject had to "time" the pass to coincide with the arrival of the light at the target point on the runway. This test was carried out from two perspectives: Perspective A (frontal) corresponded to a diagonal passing situation, perspective B (lateral) to a forward passing situation. In order to increase the difficulty of the task, the second part of the runway was covered up in half of the trials. Thus, four conditions resulted: frontal-full view, frontal-half view, lateral-

244

full view, lateral-half view.

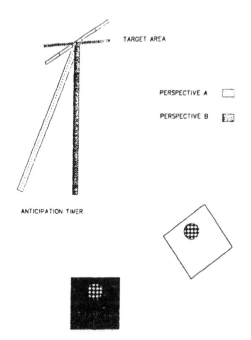

Fig. 1. Overview of the experimental set-up.

Two lengths of presentation (2.88 and 1.44 metres) and two perspectives (frontal and lateral) were used as independent variables. The two runway light speeds (1.79 and 2.68 m/s) were administered alternately over the 10 trials. A composite score was computed. Accuracy of passing ($\bar{x}$, SD) and timing error (constant error, absolute error and variability error) were used as dependent variables. An overview of the design is given in Table 1. Two groups of subjects performed three test situations twice one week apart (test-retest):

i) A test for passing accuracy (single task condition)
The accuracy of passing (score: 3-2-1-0 from the inside to the outside of the target) was registered only from the frontal perspective.

ii) A test for anticipation (single task condition)
The subject had to press a foot button to make it coincide with the arrival of the red light at the target point. The timing error was registered under all four conditions: frontal-full view, frontal-half view, lateral-full view, lateral-half view.

iii) A test for anticipation-coincidence (dual task condition)
Both tests were combined. Passing accuracy and timing

error were registered under all four conditions.

Table 1. Design structure for Test-Retest

GROUP	SINGLE TASK CONDITION					DUAL TASK CONDITION				
	passing accuracy	timing error				passing accuracy	timing error			
		f-f	f-h	l-f	l-h		f-f	f-h	l-f	l-h
experienced (n = 13)										
inexperienced (n = 11)										

Key: f-f: frontal-full view
     f-h: frontal-half view
     l-f: lateral-full view
     l-h: lateral-half view

The temporal progression of this test situation is illustrated in Figure 2. After a warning signal the light sequence was started two seconds later. The subject had to program the speed of the ball on the basis of the speed of the light sequence. Simultaneously or successively he had to program the accuracy of the pass. After a certain latency the movement started with the preparatory phase. Contact with the ball took place according to the speed of the ball about 0.80 or 1.14 s after the start of the light sequence. After a flight time of about 0.40-0.50 s the ball hit the contact mat. Precision of the pass and timing error were registered.

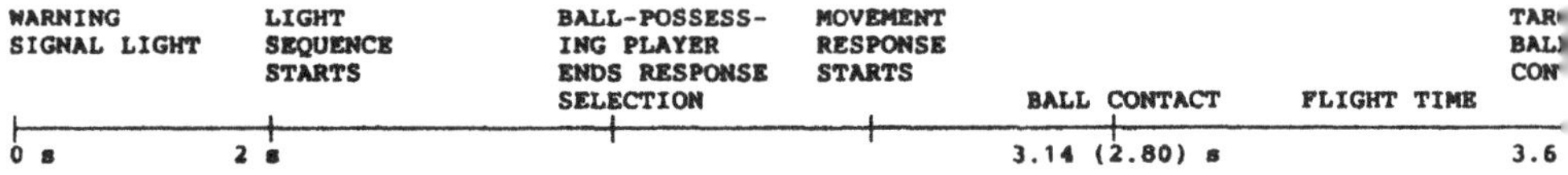

WARNING SIGNAL LIGHT	LIGHT SEQUENCE STARTS	BALL-POSSESS- ING PLAYER ENDS RESPONSE SELECTION	MOVEMENT RESPONSE STARTS			TAR BALL CON
0 s	2 s			BALL CONTACT 3.14 (2.80) s	FLIGHT TIME	3.6

Fig. 2. Temporal progression of the anticipation-coincidence test

All subjects were physical education students. The experienced group had played soccer in a club on an average for 14.15 (SD = 1.60) years and consisted of amateur players of different levels from the Berlin area. The inexperienced group was enrolled in a compulsory basic soccer course. The original number of 14 subjects in both groups dropped to 13 respectively 11 at the retest condition due to illness or injury.

The following questions were asked:

1. What are the coefficients of objectivity and

reliability?
2. What are the differences between experienced and
   inexperienced players with regard to accuracy of
   passing and the timing error?

Data were treated with ANOVAs (group, perspective,
length of presentation, single-dual task, test-retest) with
repeated measurements.

3 Results

3.1 Coefficients of objectivity and reliability

The coefficients of objectivity are presented in Table 2
for both groups (in parentheses: inexperienced group). They
were computed for passing accuracy only since all other
scores were measured electronically. The coefficients are
considered to be high for both groups. The coefficients of
reliability reflect the common fluctuations of precision-
tests (Table 3). There were no pronounced differences
between the two groups (in parentheses: inexperienced
group) and coefficients were not higher under single task
condition than under dual task condition. The majority of
coefficients are not suitable for individual diagnosis.

Table 2. Coefficients of objectivity for passing accuracy
         (in parentheses: inexperienced group)

Single task:	r = 0.98 (0.99)
Dual task:	
frontal-full view	r = 0.99 (1.00)
frontal-half view	r = 0.98 (0.99)
lateral-full view	r = 1.00 (0.99)
lateral-half view	r = 0.99 (1.00)

Table 3. Coefficients of reliability for passing accuracy
         and timing error (in parentheses: inexperienced
         group)

Accuracy of passing	
single task condition	r = 0.81 (0.68)
dual task condition	r = 0.56-0.79 (0.53-0.74)
Timing error	
single task condition	r = 0.66-0.82 (0.73-0.92)
dual task condition	r = 0.53-0.76 (0.55-0.79)

3.2 Differences between experienced and inexperienced players

3.2.1 Test for passing accuracy (single task condition)

Analysis is restricted to the group effect which is important for test validation. A two-way ANOVA (factor: group, test-retest) with repeated measurements revealed significant F-ratios for the group factor for both dependent variables ($\bar{x}$, SD): $F_{1,22}$ = 10.03 and 8.37, P $\leq$ 0.01. The experienced group scored a significantly higher number of points and had less dispersion of scores in the pass precision-test than the inexperienced group.

3.2.2 Test for anticipation (single task condition)

Significant F-ratios for the group factor for the CE and Abs E ($F_{1,22}$ = 9.85, P $\leq$ 0.01; 4.60, P $\leq$ 0.05) were obtained only for the condition lateral-full view. In a few cases there was a tendency in favour of the experienced group.

3.2.3 Test for anticipation-coincidence

With respect to passing accuracy there were significant F-ratios for the group factor for both dependent variables ($\bar{x}$, SD) except for the standard deviation under the condition lateral-half view (Table 4). With regard to the timing error significant F-ratios for the group factor were obtained only for the CE (lateral-half view), the Abs E and Var E (lateral-full view and lateral-half view). In contrast to passing accuracy the timing error did not differentiate between both groups under all four conditions. Virtually this held true only for the lateral perspective. If one considers all three error measurements, significant group differences exist only for the condition lateral-half view.

<u>Table 4</u>. F-ratios (df: 1,22) for the two dependent variables ($\bar{x}$, SD) for the group factor under dual task conditions for passing accuracy and timing error

CONDITIONS	PASSING ACCURACY		TIMING ERROR		
	$\bar{x}$	SD	CE	Abs E	Var E
frontal-full view	13.61**	7.84*	0.00	2.41	0.87
frontal-half view	11.40**	11.97**	0.05	1.32	2.73
lateral-full view	4.73*	7.74*	1.32	5.99*	13.99**
lateral-half view	4.84*	2.48	5.20*	10.12**	12.16**

** = p < 0.01
* = p < 0.05

4 Discussion

The study was conducted in a strict laboratory context entailing a number of limitations. First, the anticipation-coincidence situation in a real game was reduced in its complexity (e.g. short pass over 4.70 m; no anticipation of running direction of pass recipient; no progressive, fast speed of the light sequence). Second, both "pass recipient" and pass initiator could act without direct/indirect pressure from the opposition and without the physical and psychological loads of a real game situation. As the laboratory situation favours the inexperienced group, it can be assumed that the superiority of the experienced players is even higher under the complex conditions of a game. Under the conditions of this study it is concluded that two of the four situations (lateral-full view, lateral-half view) of the anticipation-coincidence test are valid (if one uses as criterion of validity the expert-novice paradigm), highly objective and sufficiently reliable (with regard to group comparisons).

In the near future it is intended to leave the strict laboratory context and move into a more controlled field situation. In order to improve ecological validity, the running speed will no longer be simulated by the Bassin anticipation timer but by several live subjects moving with an ultra sound speed device. With this experimental set-up, the question of whether the test differentiates between experienced players of different skill levels will also be examined. Further, a training phase before actual testing will be implemented with the goal of enhancing coefficients of reliability.

5 References

Abernethy, B. (1987) Anticipation in sport: A review. **Phys. Educ. Rev.**, 1, 5-16.

Henry, F.M. and Grose, J.E. (1968) Coincidence timing apparatus. **Res. Quart.**, 794-797.

Lafayette Instrument Company (without year) **Instructions for the Bassin anticipation timer # 50575.** Lafayette, IN.

McMorris, T. and Copeman, R. (1991) **Anticipation of soccer goalkeepers facing penalty kicks.** Paper presented at the 2nd World Congress 'Science and Football', 22.-25.5.1991 Veldhoven, Netherlands.

Williams, L.R.T. (1973) Anticipation and timing in motor skills. **New Zealand J. Health, Phys. Educ. Recr.**, 49-51.

ANTICIPATION OF SOCCER GOALKEEPERS FACING PENALTY KICKS

T. McMorris, R.Copeman, D. Corcoran, G.Saunders, and S. Potter.
West Sussex Institute of Higher Education, Chichester, West Sussex,
England.

1 Introduction

The purpose of this study was to examine the ability of soccer
goalkeepers to anticipate the direction of a penalty kick. Kuhn (1988) has
shown that for a goalkeeper to save a penalty struck at more than
20.83 m/s he must initiate his movement before or as the striker makes
contact. Only if the ball is struck at less than this speed can the
goalkeeper wait until after contact before moving. As the goalkeeper does
not know what the ball velocity will be, it is important that he begins his
movement, at the latest, at contact. If this is the case then the goalkeeper
must use some form of perceptual anticipation in order to determine the
direction of the flight of the ball.

Morris and Burwitz (1989) found that soccer goalkeepers anticipate
ball flight while Salmela and Fiorito (1979) made similar findings for ice
hockey goaltenders. Recent studies have shown that pre-contact cues are
used in a number of sports (see Abernethy, 1987, for a comprehensive
review). Most of these studies have examined expert-novice differences in
anticipation; the present study accepts that such differences occur and,
therefore, concentrates on the changes in accuracy of anticipation between
temporal stages for experienced goalkeepers.

2 Method

Ten experienced collegiate goalkeeper's watched a video recording
of penalties being taken, from the goalkeeper's perspective. A temporal
occlusion paradigm was used, with the video being stopped two frames
before contact (-2), at contact (0), and two frames after contact (+2). Eight
shots were shown for each condition and order of presentation was
randomised. The subject marked, with a cross, on a scaled map of the goal,
where he anticipated that the ball would cross the goal line. Radial,
horizontal and vertical error were recorded. Post-hoc interviews were
carried out in order to determine what, if any, pre and at contact cues
were utilised.

3 Results

Mean radial error for each occlusion period differed (see table 1). A one-way ANOVA (with repeated measure) showed that the difference was significant (P<0.01). Tukey post-hoc tests revealed that the only significant differences were between +2 and the other conditions, with +2 being more accurate.

Table 1 Mean error (mm)

Occlusion	-2	0	+2
Mean Radial Error	74.72	69.98	48.72
Mean Vertical Error	56.56	42.21	33.92
Mean Horizontal Error	48.55	30.09	31.13

A two way ANOVA (with two repeated measures) showed no significant (P>0.05) differences between horizontal and vertical errors. There was, however, a main effect for occlusion (P<0.01) and an interaction effect (P<0.05). Tukey post-hoc tests revealed that vertical error was significantly different for all conditions while for horizontal error -2 differed significantly from the other conditions.

During post-hoc interviews the goalkeepers claimed to have used the point of foot-ball contact, angle of the player's trunk and angle of run up as the main pre-contact and contact cues.

4 Discussion

As expected, for radial error, the +2 condition resulted in significantly fewer errors than the other two conditions. More importantly however, the results show that there was no significant difference between the -2 and 0 occlusion stages. This result suggests that the goalkeeper could initiate his movement before contact as waiting until contact would provide no more significant information. If this is the case then initiating a movement before contact would allow a goalkeeper more time to execute the movement; this, however, is an infringement of the rules of play. Nevertheless, the decision could still be made prior to contact and the movement initiated at contact, thus not infringeing the rules. This would be faster than waiting to process the 'at contact' cues.

Observation of the results pertaining to horizontal and vertical error suggest, however, that the above is an oversimplification. Although no overall significant difference was found for horizontal and vertical error, observation of Table 1 and the fact that a significant interaction effect was found suggest that these findings are the result of the similarities in mean error for the +2 condition. In the other situations the vertical position was more difficult to anticipate than the horizontal.

The +2 condition obviously provides the most information but the goalkeeper can only wait until this moment before initiating a movement if the ball is travelling at less than 75 km/h (Kuhn, 1988). If the goalkeeper knows that the penalty taker is someone who strikes the ball at below this speed, what Kuhn (1988) described as slow to medium paced, then he can wait and collect more information. If, however, the goalkeeper is in any doubt or he knows that the pace will be fast (over 20.83 m/s) then he must initiate his movement at contact, at the latest.

According to the data presented here the goalkeeper would gain no advantage, as far as horizontal position is concerned, by waiting until after contact, as the 0 and +2 conditions do not differ significantly. The +2 condition does, however, supply extra valuable information concerning the height of the ball. This information could possibly be used to refine the movement during its execution. Abernethy and Russell (1984) suggested that cricket batsmen initiate a "ball park" or generalised motor programme early in the batting sequence and refine it in the later stages. It is possible that goalkeepers can, and do, do this.

A ball struck at 20.83 m/s takes 600 ms to reach the goal (Kuhn, 1988); therefore the movement made by the goalkeeper could be closed loop in nature and alterations made after initiation. Whether or not such alterations or refinements could be made when the ball is travelling very fast, say 27.77 m/s, which takes 400 ms to reach the goal, is debatable. Stubbs (1976) claimed that 500 ms is the lower limit in which feedback can be utilised. This figure would take into account the reaction to initial stimulus (at contact), the reaction to the second stimulus (+2), the psychological refractory period and movement time. If this is indeed true then the goalkeeper would not be able to alter his movement quickly enough to save a 27.77 m/s penalty kick.

Stubb's (1976) stance follows information processing theory models (e.g. Welford, 1968; Adams, 1971), which suggest that the goalkeeper could only alter his position following a sequence whereby information was received by the sensory cortex via the visuoreceptors. This information would then be processed by the central nervous system (CNS), a decision made and the appropriate motor programme selected and organised by the CNS. This information would then be passed to the limbs by the peripheral nervous system (PNS). This process takes one reaction time, somewhere between 170 and 200 ms, depending on the individual and arousal levels. Movement time i.e. time to execute the movement also needs to be taken into account.

This approach is not without its critics, however, and action systems theorists (Turvey, 1977; Reed, 1982) provide a holistic approach in which perception and action are combined. According to an action systems approach it is possible that refinements could be handled by lower regions of the CNS and PNS thus shortening the total response time. Nevertheless in practical terms the implications for the goalkeeper do not change. He must initiate his response at contact and try to utilise subsequent information to refine his movement.

Although it is recommended that the goalkeeper wait until contact before initiating his movement, this does not mean that the pre-contact information is irrelevant. On the contrary, pre-contact cues can help the goalkeeper narrow down the possible ball flight. Narrowing down the possible areas to which the shot will be directed will reduce the reaction time as it reduces the number of possible responses. Therefore observation of such pre-contact cues as angle of run up and trunk position may help the goalkeeper respond more quickly. Indeed future research should focus on eye mark recorder and spatial occlusion studies in order to determine exactly which cues provide the most information.

5 References

Abernethy, B. (1987) Anticipation in sport : a review. **Phys.Educ.Rev.**, 10, 5-16.

Abernethy, B. and Russell, D.G. (1984) Advance cue utilisation by skilled cricket batsmen. **Austr.J.Sci.Med.Sport,** 16, 2-10.

Adams, J.A. (1971) A closed-loop theory of motor learning. **J.Motor Behav.**, 3, 111-149.

Kuhn, W. (1988) Penalty kick strategies for shooters and goalkeepers, in **Science and Football,** (eds T.Reilly, A. Lees, K.Davids and W.J.Murphy), E. and F.N.Spon,   London. pp.489-492.

Morris, A. and Burwitz, L. (1989) Anticipation and movement strategies in elite soccer goalkeepers at penalty kicks. Paper presented at the British Association of Sports Science Annual Conference, Exeter, September.

Reed, E.S. (1982) An outline of a theory of action systems. **J.Motor Behav.**, 14, 98-134.

Salmela, J.H. and Fiorito, P. (1979) Visual cues in ice hockey goaltending. **Canad.J.Appl.Sports Sci.,** 4, 56-59.

Stubb, D.P. (1976) What the eye tells the hand. **J.Motor Behav.**, 8, 43-58.

Turvey, M.T. (1977) Preliminaries to a theory of action with refernece to vision, in **Perceiving, Acting and Knowing,** (eds R.Shaw and J.Bansford),. Erlbaum, Hillsdale, N.J. pp. 211-265.

Welford,A.T.(1968) **Fundamentals of Skill.** Methuen, London.

CHANGING THE KICKING ACCURACY OF SOCCER PLAYERS DEPENDING ON THE TYPE, VALUE AND AIMS OF TRAINING AND COMPETITIVE LOADS

M. GODIK, I. FALES and I. BLASHAK
Central Institute of Physical Culture, Moscow, Russia.
Institute of Physical Culture, Lvov, Ukraine.

1 Introduction

Attacking actions in soccer imply the collective creation of goal situations and their individual completion. Shots at goals from an advantageous position can either improve or negate team work. That is why high demands are made for accuracy in shooting and much attention is paid to the methods of estimation and predition of its structure. The accuracy of motor actions is considered as one of the most important components of a motor skill (Godik, 1988; Mechdi, 1984; Popov, 1986; Zatsiorsky and Smirnov, 1976).

Motor actions are very specific in different kinds of sports and their accuracy depends on various factors. Although there is no general theory of accuracy of motor actions, investigations of this problem have been carried out nevertheless.

Investigations in sports games have been aimed at determining the accuracy of kicks and passes as well as finding out the factors upon which accuracy depends (Babudjan, 1978; Gadjiev et al., 1982; Godik and Skomorokhov, 1981; Smirnov, 1975; Sherstakov, 1984). Analysis of results of different authors' investigations shows that:

(i) there are considerable contradictions in the methods of measuring accuracy;
(ii) there are some differences in views regarding the influence of the speed of movements, mass and inertial characteristics of players, their age and sex, the standard of physical fitness, fatigue when performing motor activities.

It is thought that elaboration of effective methods to improve accuracy of shots at goal in soccer is possible when the following questions have been answered:

(i) What is accuracy and how it can be measured?
(ii) What factors does it depend on?
(iii) What are the most effective exercises for its improvement?

To solve these problems an experiment was carried out. The aim was to determine the level and structure of accuracy of footballers' kicks and how accuracy is affected by different training loads. In particular the aims were:

(1) to define the level and structure of the accuracy of shots at

goals by soccer players;

(2) to determine the dependence of the shooting accuracy on the run-up speed;

(3) to find out the relationship between fatigue, caused by different types of training sessions, and shooting accuracy.

2 Methods

The method of examining accuracy was based on the relation of the number of shots placed on target at the goal posts to the total number of shots at goal. These shots were registered in games at the World Cup 1990 and the International Junior Tournament devoted to the memory of V.N. Granatkin as well as at training sessions.

Three positions were taken into account when recording shots at the training sessions: i) from the 16 m mark, place-kick; ii) from the same mark, a kick with the ball on a standing base from a run-up; iii) from the same mark, kicking a ball rolling in the opposite direction with a run-up.

Besides, juniors undertook a special test where a soccer player had to shoot with a run-up on to a stationary ball from 16 m distance to the target measuring 240x240 cm, marked on the goal net.

The conditions of performing a run-up were standard for all players tested. By means of a photoelectronic optical system the speed of the run-up in 1 m segments, placed 2 m before the ball, was measured.

This test consisted of two series of kicks done before and after training. In the first one the player took 10 kicks towards a target after a run-up at a customary speed; in the second, the same kicks were taken but after a run-up at maximum speed. These two series of kicks were done before training and two after it. For each of the series the accuracy of the kicks, the speed of the run-up and the heart rate were recorded.

The following criteria were used to estimate the target accuracy:

1) the value of systematic error (SE) that numerically is equal to the value of deviation of the ball's hits from the geometrical centre of the target;

2) the value of random error (RE), numerically equal to the diversity of results of some attempts relative to the mean value.

Besides, the absolute (AE) and complex (E) constituents of accuracy were estimated.

The physiological load of the test was determined by the heart rate and the total heart beats using short range radio telemetry (Sporttester PE-3000). The influence of three types of loads on the accuracy of kicks was measured at the training sessions.

The first type was characterized by using the non-specific aerobic exercises during warm-ups (the heart rate was 130-150 beats/min); the training session consisted of technical and tactical combinations of the same quality and the duration of the training sessions was 80-90 min.

In the second type, both when warming-up and in the main part, specific aerobic-anaerobic (150-170 beats/min) and anaerobic (180-190 beats/min) exercises were used; the duration of training sessions was

45-60 min.

In the third type, games (11 or 10 a-side) were employed. These also included small-sided drills as well, such as exercises aimed at "retaining" the ball (squares 4x2, 4x4, 3x5 and so on).

Among the players tested were 14 footballers aged 14-15 from the junior team "Karpaty" (Lvov), the winner of the Ukrainian championship. They included 4 backs, 6 half-backs and 4 forwards. The course of these players' studies lasted from 2 to 10 years (5.6±2.1), the height of the players ranged from 150 to 185 cm (167±10.5), the body mass - 40-75 (60±18.1) kg.

3 Results

There were no noticeable differences between the total number of kicks hit at goals of rivals by the soccer players of different teams whether winners, losers or those who played in a draw. The players of teams that lost matches or played a draw proved to be more accurate (if accuracy is estimated by the number of kicks at the goal). This accuracy had no positive influence on the results of the game as the kicks were done from positions well known to the goalkeeper.

The case with accuracy is different if the kicks were done from the penalty area. It is worth remembering that they were performed under severe competitive conditions, and here the accuracy of the winners' kicks was statistically higher than that of the losers.

It should be noted that in competitive criteria of accuracy, juniors differed little from highly qualified footballers. The only difference between the World Cup participants and qualified juniors was in the total number of kicks and the number of shots at goal. Here the winners' values were much higher; besides, almost all the differences between the three groups of teams were statistically significant.

The accuracy of shots in the training sessions proved to be not very high. When calculating the coefficient of efficiency as the ratio of kicks with which the ball hit the goal, to the total number of kicks, the highest value was 0.83. In those cases when the kicks were performed under more strenuous conditions (dribbling, feinting, juggling and so on) the value of this coefficient decreased to 0.42 - 0.60.

Thus we may conclude that the poor accuracy during training may be one of the reasons for accuracy not being very high in competition.

Figure 1a shows the accuracy of kicks performed at the customary and maximum speed (evaluation - the value of systematic error SE along the vertical axis). It also shows that the accuracy of kicks after a run-up at customary speed is much higher than that after a run- up at maximum speed (2.94±0.27) and 3.70±0.33 m/s respectively; the differences are statistically significant at P < 0.05.

In Figure 1b are the indices of accuracy calculated on the basis of another criterion - the horizontal constituent SE. The level of accuracy here is almost the same as in the previously mentioned case, with one exception - rather noticeable asymmetry. The value of systematic error indicates that the majority of the kicked balls hit the horizontal line much higher, coming across the centre of the target. This is explained by the fact that the vertical accuracy is positively related to the closeness of the centre of the support foot

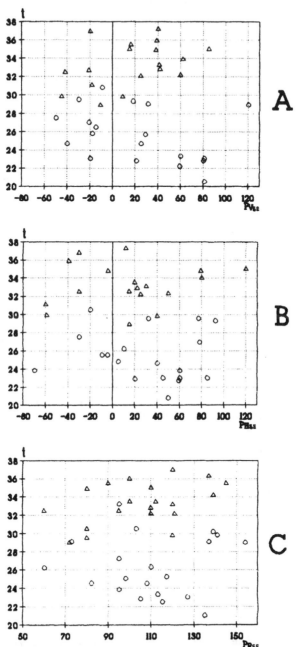

ig.1. Relationship between the speed of run-up and accuracy of
hots at a target (A - vertical constituent of SE, B - horizontal
onstituent of SE, C - radial constituent of SE; △ - run-up at
ustomary speed, O - run-up at maximum speed).

257

to projection of the ball onto the longitudinal axis of that foot.

Figure 1c shows a graphical description of dependency between the speed of the run-up and the radial constituent of the accuracy of getting the ball onto the target. It is noteworthy that if the kick is performed at the speed customary for the player, then it is more accurate for players with the higher customary speed. This dependency changes when kicking the ball at the maximum speed. In this case those with the lower maximum speed are the more accurate. All the results of the tests conducted show that there is an optimal speed for the run-up, at which speed the accuracy of getting the ball onto the target is greatest.

It is known from soccer experience that accuracy of kicking gets worse under fatigue. To prove it a special test was carried out, during which junior footballers hit a target before and after training sessions. The comparative data showed how the accuracy of kicking changed after the run-up with the customary speed under the influence of the different training sessions.

If footballers did both specific and non-specific aerobic exercises (HR < 150 beats/min), then the accuracy increases. In this case the increase in accuracy was noticeable in all criteria without exception. Accuracy in kicking under the influence of anaerobic load (HR = 180-190 beats/min) deteriorated on all the criteria.

The influence of game exercises (the third type of load) on the accuracy of kicks after the run-up at the customary speed is manifold. For example, if the horizontal constituent of systematic error increases, then the vertical and radial constituents decrease.

When characterizing the influence of the first type of load, it is necessary to point out that there is a tendency to keep or to improve the indices of accuracy. A decrease in indices of the vertical and radial constituents from 31 and 120 cm respectively to 16 and 102 cm occurred without any change in errors. Thus, the aerobic load resulted in some improvement of kicking accuracy performed at the maximum speed.

The same situation is noted in the second type of load. For example, increase in the horizontal constituent of the systematic error from 42 to 58 cm occurred in parallel with a worsening of the analogous indices of the random error from 87 to 89 cm. At the same time the absolute horizontal constituent of accuracy improved from 91 to 83 cm.

The influence of the third type of load on kicking accuracy performed at the maximum speed is also manifold. When the horizontal constituent of the systematic error decreased from 51 to 34 cm, the absolute value fell from 72 to 66 cm, and the complex - from 98 to 87 cm, the possibilities of random error increased.

4 Conclusions

The experiment allowed us to conclude:

1) in competitive games at the highest level (World Cups in soccer) the players perform shots at the opponent's goal up to 28 kicks. The number of shots at goal by the winners (15.93±6.65) was statistically greater than that of the losers (10.10±4.87);

2) in the games of the junior national teams from different countries the differences in these indices of accuracy are less noticeable. Junior winners are more accurate when shooting from the penalty area (3.83 ± 2.04 against 2.0 ± 1.79);

3) indices of kicking accuracy were set at the training sessions conducted by the soccer players from the national teams of different countries. They were considerably higher in the same indices in competitive games, but the conditions of shooting at goal during training mostly do not correspond to the conditions used for this purpose in games;

4) there is a relation between the speed of the run-up and the accuracy of kicking. If the kick is performed at the customary speed of a footballer, the more accurate is the player whose customary speed is the higher. This dependence proves to be different when kicks are performed at a maximum speed. In this case the players whose maximum speed is the lower are the more accurate. There is an optimal speed of run-up for getting the ball onto the target;

5) the accuracy of kicks at goal changes with fatigue caused by the training load. When training is mainly aerobic (HR < 130-150 beats/min) kicking accuracy is maintained at the customary speed, and when the speed is maximal the accuracy increases. Moreover, the anaerobic loading (HR = 180-190 beats/min) results in a decrease in accuracy when performing kicks at the customary speed.

5 References

Babudjan, S.G. (1978) Investigation of ways for perfecting accuracy of kicking actions of football players in special tasks. Ph.D. Dissertation, Moscow (in Russian).

Gadjiev, G.M., Godik, M.A. and Zonin, T.C. (1982) A control of competitive activity of the highly qualified football players. **Methodical Instructions.** USSR Sports Committee, Moscow (in Russian).

Godik, M. and Skomorokhov, E.B. (1981) Factor structure of special fitness of football players. **Theory and Practice of Physical Culture.**, 7, 14-15 (in Russian).

Godik, M. (1988) **Sports Metrology.** Fizkultura i Sport, Moscow (in Russian).

Mechdi, D.S. (1984) The accuracy of motor actions performed at maximal speed by the football players. Ph.D. Dissertation. Moscow (in Russian).

Zatsiorsky, V.M. and Smirnov, G.A. (1976) Factors influencing kicking accuracy of footballers. **Theory and Practice of Physical Culture**, 5, 19 (in Russian).

Popov, A.V. (1986) Types of shot movements in football and bio-mechanical criteria of their classification. **Theory and Practice of Physical Culture**, 4, 9-10 (in Russian).

Smirnov, G.A. (1975) Investigation of factors influencing the accuracy of footballers' kicks and some ways of its teaching. Ph.D. Dissertation, Moscow (in Russian).

Shestakov, M.P. (1984) Individualization of technical and tactical training of highly qualified football players with respect to their morpho-functional peculiarities. Ph.D. Dissertation Moscow, (in Russian).

THE EFFECT OF PHYSIOLOGICAL STRESS ON COGNITIVE PERFORMANCE IN A SIMULATION OF SOCCER

J. MARRIOTT, T. REILLY and A. MILES
Centre for Sport and Exercise Sciences, Liverpool Polytechnic,
Liverpool, England

1 Introduction

Studies of cognitive function in the sports of basketball (Allard et al., 1980), hockey (Starkes and Deakin, 1984) and rugby (Nakagawa, 1982) have shown that experts perform at a higher cognitive standard than do less experienced participants in their particular discipline. This is due mainly to superior methods of information processing. It is not clear what effect the exercise intensity and duration have on cognitive function during performance in games. This study is concerned with mental performance in a soccer context where little research has been undertaken. Of particular interest was the study of mental fatigue in a soccer-specific simulation. The aim was to examine cognitive function in skilful and low-skilled soccer players during sustained exercise modelled on the exercise intensity and duration of soccer match-play.

2 Method

Sixteen male undergraduates acted as subjects, with eight subjects forming the skilful group (members of Liverpool Polytechnic 1st XI). Another eight subjects formed the low-skill group, comprising athletes from non-team sports or team sports not cognitively similar to soccer as defined by Allard and Burnett (1985).

The study utilised three sessions in the research protocol. Session 1 was an extended incremental exercise test to volitional exhaustion which was undertaken in order to find the relation between speed and heart rate (HR). This allowed each subject's speed to be predicted for session 2 to induce a HR of 157 beats/min. This was the mean value found for soccer players during actual matches (Reilly, 1986). Heart rate was recorded using short range radio telemetry (Sports Tester PE3000).

Session 2 consisted of a 90 min treadmill run at the predicted speed, designated the "fatigue" session. The 90 min was divided into two periods of 45 min, separated by a 15 min break. At 0, 45 and 90 min of exercise a cognitive function test was administered and percentage error recorded. Throughout the 90 min HR was recorded, $\dot{V}O_2$ measured (Sensorimedics, Salford) and rating of perceived exertion (RPE) monitored according to Borg (1962). Session 3 was a 90 min laboratory visit, where the cognitive function test was undertaken at the same three times within the 90 min period but in a rested state.

The cognitive function test consisted of 45 slides depicting situations encountered in soccer. Each slide had a question regarding a decision to be made from five possible responses (Fig.1). Each was shown for approximately 20 s as determined by a timer on the projector. Questions and responses were played to the subjects via an audio tape in harmony with the timer. Full validation and reliability studies were undertaken with the help of qualified Football Association coaches.

- · Which is the best pass A1 can make to A2?
- · 1)Pass 1 to A2 left
- · 2)Pass 2 to A2 right
- · 3)Neither - lofted ball over D2's head
- · 4)Alternative not shown
- · 5)Do not know

Fig.1. Example of decision requested in cognitive function test

3 Results

The anthropometric characteristics obtained from session 1 are shown in Table 1. The subjects in the two groups were matched for age, height, body mass and $\dot{V}O_2$max (P>0.05).

Table 1. Subject data : values are means ±SD

Skilful soccer players (n=8)	Age 22.50(±3.12) years
	Height 1.75(±0.06) m
	Body mass 79.6(±9.8) kg
	$\dot{V}O_2$max 51.3(±2.9) ml/kg/min
Low-skill soccer players (n=8):	Age 20.88(±0.99) years
	Height 1.78(±0.05) m
	Body mass 74.4(±8.30) kg
	$\dot{V}O_2$max 54.7(±2.6) ml/kg/min

Mean HR during session 2 was 153 (±7) beats/ min for the skilful group and 151 (±6) beats/ min for the low-skill group. These were within ±6% of the values found for outfield players during actual matches by Reilly (1986).

Heart rate values of 80.1 (±6.2) and 76.4 (±4.5) % HRmax respectively were recorded during session 2, with a distinct cardiovascular drift (rise in HR, presumed fall in SV) throughout session 2 exhibited by both groups. Skilful players worked harder in terms of % $\dot{V}O_2$max, 63.0 (±5.3) to 59.7 (±5.1)%.

Both skilful and low-skill players found the second 45 min harder in terms of RPE (P<0.01). This confirmed that the predicted speed for each subject was sufficient to induce a trend towards subjective fatigue.

Sustained exercise, leading to increased subjective effort associated with fatigue, had no consistent effect upon the cognitive function of skilful and low-skill players (P>0.05) (Table 2). The trend in both experimental conditions, significant (P<0.05) in the non-fatigued condition, was for the skilful players to make less errors than the low-skilled.

Table 2. Analysis of cognitive function scores - percentage errors. Values are means (±SD) over the complete session.

	Non-Fatigue Session	Fatigue Session	Probability
Skilful (n=8)	42.22 (±6.06)	43.33 (±10.22)	NS (P>0.05)
Low skill (n=8)	51.40 (±8.84)	47.77 (±7.60)	"
Skilful vs Low-skill	-	-	"

Both subject groups experienced a positive effect (decrease in error) from 0 to 45 min, the low-skill subjects' decrease being significant (P<0.05). This facilitation remained in the skilful players, whereas the low-skill players underwent a negative effect (increase in error) after 90 min (Table 3).

Table 3. Analysis of effect of sustained exercise on cognitive function scores - percentage error. Values are means (±SD)

	0 min	45 min	90 min
Skilful (n=8)	49.16 (±10.65)	40.00 (±17.82)	41.67 (±13.21)
Low-skill (n=8)	52.50 (±8.31)	39.16 (±10.95)	* 51.86 (±19.76

*Significantly different from the other two time points

4 Discussion

The predicted speed enabled the subjects to exercise at relative exercise intensities that were close to heart rate values found in real soccer match-play (Reilly, 1986; Smodlaka, 1978; Ekblom, 1986). However, the % $\dot{V}O_2$max values were lower than those estimated for real game studies which have ranged from 70% (Reilly, 1986) to 80% (Ekblom, 1986). This could have been due to the more continuous exercise in the present study, the treadmill being unable to truly simulate the intermittent nature of soccer or allow the execution of game skills
Observations suggest that decision making in a soccer context is unaffected by the exercise intensity corresponding to match-play. Therefore, mental fatigue effects that were experienced and reflected in the perception of greater effort may be attributed to peripheral rather than central mechanisms.
The trend in both experimental conditions was for the skilful

263

players to make fewer errors. This is in agreement with findings of Allard et al. (1980) in basketball and Starkes and Deakin (1984) in hockey which suggest superior methods of processing task specific information among the highly skilled players.

The low-skill players firstly exhibited a facilitation and then a decrement in mental performance over 90 min. This reflects the mental benefits of "warming up" in this level of player. Exercise appeared to facilitate, although non-significantly, cognitive function in the skilful players, with little evidence of "fatigue" after 90 min. This suggests an ability to offset the effects of exercise-induced subjective fatigue on decision making.

The results of both subject groups can be linked to the relationship between exercise and arousal (Reilly and Smith, 1984) and its subsequent effect on attentional focus. The positive effect was attributed to arousal being at its optimum and attentional focus eliminating cues irrelevant to the task. The "fatigue" effect was attributed to failing to maintain arousal at this optimum, causing some task relevant cues to be excluded.

In summary, exercise intensity corresponding to match-play was found to have no consistent effect upon cognitive function in a simulated soccer context. It is recommended that further work should examine possible effects of exercise intensities corresponding to soccer play on decision making using dynamic displays of soccer-specific situations.

5 References

Allard, F. and Burnett, N. (1985) Skill in sport. **Canad. J. Psychol.**, 39, 294-312.

Allard, F., Graham, S. and Paarsalv, M.E. (1980) Perception in sport: Volleyball. J. **Sport Psychol.**, 2, 14-21.

Borg, G. (1962) Physical Performance and Perceived Exertion. Gleerups, Lund.

Ekblom, B. (1986) Applied physiology of soccer. **Sports Med.**, 3, 50-60.

Nakagawa, A. (1982) A field experiment on recognition of game situations in ball games. The case of static situations in rugby football. **Jap. J. Phys. Ed.**, 27, 17-26.

Reilly, T. (1986) Fundamental studies in soccer, in **Sportsuissenschraft Und Sportpraxis** (ed by R. Andresen), Verlag Ingrid Czwalina, Hamburg, pp. 114-121.

Reilly, T. and Smith, D. (1984) Influence of metabolic loading on a cognitive task, in **Contemporary Ergonomics 1984** (ed by E.D. Megaw) Taylor and Francis, London, pp. 104-109.

Smodlaka, V.N. (1978) Cardiovascular aspects of soccer. **Physician Sportsmed.**, 6, 66-70.

Starkes, J.L. and Deakin, J. (1984) Perception in sport: a cognitive approach to skilled performance, in **Cognitive Sport Psychology** (eds W.F. Straub and J.M. Williams), Sport Science Association, New York, pp. 115-178.

THE INFLUENCE OF DIFFERENT EXERCISE TESTS ON MOVEMENT COORDINATION LEVEL IN ADVANCED SOCCER PLAYERS

W. STAROSTA, Z. ADACH, J. ADACH, M. BAJDZINSKI, I. DEBCZYNSKA, H. KOS, M. RADZINSKA
Institute of Sport in Warsaw, Academy of Physical Education in Gorzow WLKP. Department of Sports Theory and Department of Physiology Poland.

1 Introduction

According to Farfel (1960) all sports disciplines may be divided into three groups depending on the levels of movement coordination. The most difficult disciplines require accurate and rapid movements under changing conditions. Football is one of these. Significant research attention has been given to the technical difficulty of this discipline and even more to development of physical fitness (Reilly and Thomas, 1977: Talaga, 1983, Reilly et al., 1988). However, little attention has been paid to the interdependence of efficiency and co-ordination or the effect of fatigue on the co-ordination level of soccer players. This is surprising, as the accuracy of movements during the whole match can decide the winner. The present study was undertaken to fill the existing gap. The purpose was to determine the changes taking place in co-ordination of players under variable physical loads.

2 Methods

Seventeen Third Division players were tested during the preparation period. Mean age was 21.5 years, and duration of career 8.8 years. The following tests were used: i) the Wingate anaerobic test on a bicycle ergometer (Bar-Or, 1983); ii) maximum oxygen consumption during a cycle ergometer test with increasing load until voluntary exhaustion; iii) ability to differentiate muscle strength of the lower extremity was determined using a tensiometric dynamometer with an electronic counter. First, maximum strength of the extremity was determined, and later the ability to differentiate the force corresponding to 50% of maximum capacity was taught, with immediate feedback on the extent of error made. Finally, the player tested had to reproduce the test five times as memorized. The discrepancies from this value were recorded in kg and were denoted as errors in differentiating force. Similar information was obtained for the other leg. To eliminate other information, except for kinesthetic data, the eyes were blindfolded; iv) Starosta's (1978) movement co-ordination test; v) to test the ability to differentiate motion amplitude, a prototype kinesthesiometer connected to a potentiometric goniometer was used to record the angle changes on flexion. The goniometer was fixed to the knee joint of the right, and next the

left leg.   Tests were made based on the method of Schulte and Puni
(Starosta and Aniol-Strzyzewska 1990; Starosta et al., 1990.).   This
resembled the method used in differentiating muscle force.
   Force and amplitude differentiation were statistically tested for
10 measurements (5 for each leg): averages and standard deviations
were calculated and correlation coefficients computed.   It was
acknowledged that collective consideration of the results could
"flatten" the overall tendency.   Tests were preceded by an interview
on functional asymmetry and combined with self-evaluation of results
achieved before and after the effort.

Table 1.   Physical capacity of soccer players (n = 17)

No.	Soccer player	Body mass (kg)	Height (cm)	Total work L 30/kg (kJ/kg)	Power Pmax/kg (w/kg)	$\dot{V}O_2$max (ml/kg/min)
1	R.S.	70.0	185	274	11.32	56
2	J.K.	68.0	176	263	10.92	60
3	M.S.	77.5	180	289	12.65	64
4	P.G.	69.0	172	272	11.30	64
5	W.P.	70.0	170	272	11.70	56
6	J.L.	86.0	180	259	10.71	57
7	D.C.	78.0	179	245	9.09	52
8	M.Z.	63.0	169	266	11.36	58
9	C.B.	65.0	172	245	11.48	60
10	P.N.	65.0	172	243	9.78	49
11	M.K.	81.0	183	261	11.54	54
12	M.N.	74.5	178	268	11.13	60
13	K.K.	75.5	175	245	10.22	48
14	R.B.	69.0	183	250	10.21	59
15	T.J.	75.5	185	247	11.27	54
16	P.B.	66.0	176	289	12.28	68
17	K.Cn.	65.0	181	249	9.82	64
	$\bar{x}$	71.6	177.4	261	10.9	57.8

3 Results

3.1
The fitness levels (Table 1) showed that the players tested had a
high maximal oxygen uptake ($\bar{x}$ = 57.8 ml/kg/min) and a moderate
anaerobic output.   A statistically significant correlation
(r = 0.531; P < 0.01) existed between the aerobic and anaerobic
power. ·

3.2
The influence of load upon selected coordination indicators is
illustrated in Figure 1.   The smallest differences under load were
reported for Starosta's test.   After the first loading the results
deteriorated slightly, and improved in the next attempt - but had not
reached the initial values.   More distinct post-effort changes were
observed in differentiating muscle force.   Here, the first and second
test had led to slight improvement in results.   The ability to

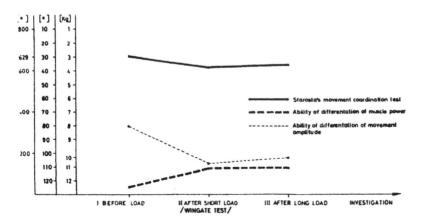

Fig.1. The influence of different exercise tests in movement
      co-ordination in soccer players: n = 17.

differentiate amplitude of motion turned out to be an extremely
senstitive indicator of co-ordination. Results deteriorated greatly
after the first test and little change was observed after the second
one. In summary, of the two co-ordination indicators tested, the
first loading led to a deterioration, and in one case to improvement.
The second loading always improved the result, but this was still
away from the initial figures. Though a statistically significant
dependence between the fitness measures and selected co-ordination
indicators was not reported, a distinct tendency existed. The
non-significant result could have been caused by a low level of
co-ordination and advancement of the players (3rd Division), unified
training cycles restricting individual means and methods, treatment
of the soccer team as a uniform group, the specific nature of soccer
as a game in which every player has a narrow specialization. Thus,
seeking a common tendency for all the players may be erroneous. More
such results are sought for elite players, even though each of them
is a distinct individual. Therefore, an analysis characterizing
individual results of each player is required.
    Results of such an analysis pointed to the high differentiation
between co-ordination level of players (Fig. 2). Individual
differences in results exceeded 300°. Here, the line for the first
effort was at a level distinctly higher than for post-effort results.
A similar, though less distinctive tendency for individual results is
reported in the differentiation of muscle force (Fig. 3). There,
results show great individual differences with large errors from 1 to
47 kg. Analysis shows that after the effort the results of many
players had improved as compared with the initial ones.

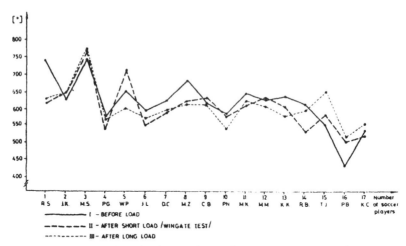

Fig. 2. Changes of individual results of Starosta's co-ordination
tests after different exercise test in soccer players: n = 17

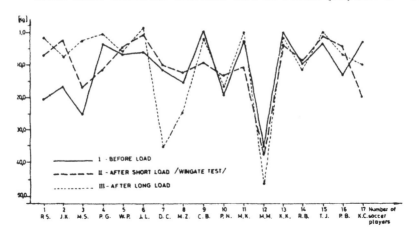

Fig. 3. Changes of individual results of ability to
differentiation of muscle power after different
exercise test in soccer players: n = 17.

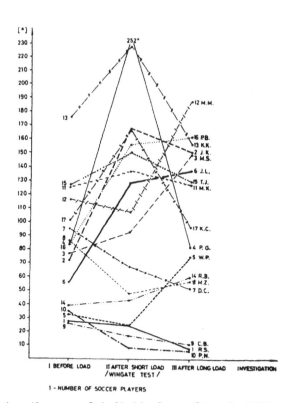

Fig. 4.　Changes of individual results of ability to
differentiation of movement amplitude in soccer
players: n = 17.

This is seen especially in the averages. An even higher spread of
results (Fig. 4) was observed in the ability to differentiate
amplitude of motion. The spread was over 250°. Almost an identical
number of improvements (7) as deteriorations (9) was recorded.
Similar results were reported in post-effort changes after high
loads. Finally, the changes taking place under the effort,
differentiated between two groups. Those improving and those
lowering their results are shown in Fig. 5. The co-ordination test
after the first loading showed a deterioration in 58% of the players
tested, increasing to 71% after the next test. Similar results were
obtained in differentiating amplitude of movement: a deterioration
was noted in 66% after test one and in 55% after test two. An
opposite tendency characterized differentiation of muscle force.
Here, a decisive majority (65%) had improved results after both the
first and the second tests. This could reflect a favourable
influence of effort upon the ability to differentiate muscle force
and confirms the necessity of an intensive warm-up period to improve
accuracy of movements. However, the use of this phenomenon in
practice has to account for individual features. This is shown by
results of over one-third of the players, in which both types of
effort had a detrimental effect.

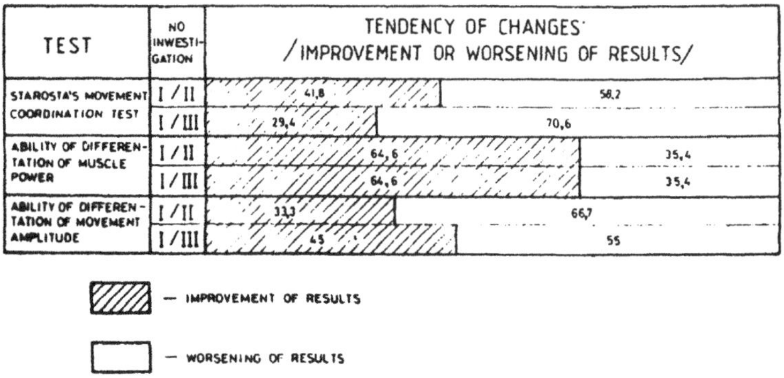

TEST	NO INWESTI-GATION	TENDENCY OF CHANGES /IMPROVEMENT OR WORSENING OF RESULTS/	
STAROSTA'S MOVEMENT COORDINATION TEST	I / II	41,8	58,2
	I / III	29,4	70,6
ABILITY OF DIFFEREN-TATION OF MUSCLE POWER	I / II	64,6	35,4
	I / III	64,6	35,4
ABILITY OF DIFFEREN-TATION OF MOVEMENT AMPLITUDE	I / II	33,3	66,7
	I / III	45	55

▨ — IMPROVEMENT OF RESULTS

☐ — WORSENING OF RESULTS

Fig. 5. Changes of results in movement co-ordination after
after physical exercise in soccer players(%): n = 17.

4 Conclusions

A general analysis of the results did not point to a significant link
between the level of power output and co-ordination ability of soccer
players. Neither did aerobic or anaerobic output significantly
affect the co-ordination indicators tested. This could have been
conditioned by an insufficient number of players tested, relatively
low co-ordination level and sports advancement, unified training
programmes, narrow specialization of each player, treatment of a
soccer team as a uniform group, inadequate testing methods and so on.
   The players had attained highest levels in two co-ordination
indicators before the effort. This was quite low compared with
athletes in other sport disciplines.
   Irrespective of the type of effort, an improvement in results was
reported only in the ability to differentiate muscle strength. This
points to the necessity to use an intensive warm-up period to better
utilize this ability during movements, taking into account the output
capacity of the player.
   Analysis of the influence of physical effort upon individual
co-ordination indices requires an individual approach, i.e. depending
on the type of function which is fulfilled by the player in the team.

5 References

Bar-Or, O. (1983) Paediatric sports medicine for the practitioner.
   in, Physiologic Principles of Clinical Applications. Springer
   Verlag, New York.
Farfel, V. (1960) Fizjologija Sporta. Fizkultura i Sport, Moskva.
Reilly, T. and Thomas, V. (1977) Effects of a programme of pre-season
   training on the fitness of soccer players. J. Sport Med. Phys.
   Fit., 17, 401-412.
Reilly, T., Lees, A., Davids, K. and Murphy, W.J. (1988) Science and
   Football. E. and F.N. Spon, London.
Starosta, W. (1978) Nowy sposob pomiaru i oceny koordynacji ruchowej.
   Monografie nr 96, AWF Poznan pp. 365-371.

Starosta, W. and Aniol-Strzyzewska, K. (1990) Die Veranderungen der
Fahigkeit zur kinasthetischen Differenzierung der
Bewegungsamplitude unter dem Einfluss dem Trainingsbelastungen bei
der Kanusportler, in Bewegungskoordination im Sport (ed W.
Starosta), Intern. Gesselschaft fur Sportmotorik. Gorzov Wlkp.
Warszava, pp.188-195.

Starosta, W., Kos, H. and Sadowski, J. (1990) Die Fahigkeit der
Muskelkraftdifferenzierung in Folge des kinasthetischen
Empfindungen (Fuhlens)der Fortgeschrittenen Wettkampfer, in
Bewegungskoordination im Sport (ed W. Starosta). Intern.
Gesselschaft fur Sportmotorik. Warszava-Gorzow Wlkp. pp. 211-217.

Talaga, J. (1983) Valori musurabili dell attivita del giocatore di
calcio a loro importanza per la practica, in Teaching Team Sports.
Intern. Congress. CONI-Scuola dello Sport, Rome pp. 363-371

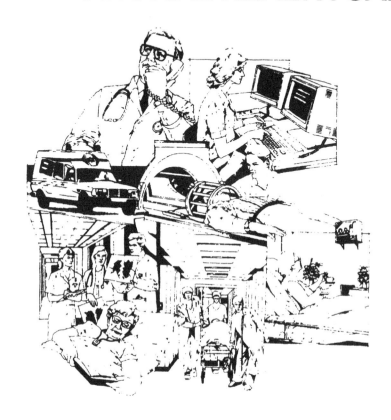

PART EIGHT

Paediatric Science and Football

DO YOUNG SOCCER PLAYERS NEED SPECIFIC PHYSICAL TRAINING?

Flemming Lindquist & Jens Bangsbo
August Krogh Institute, University of Copenhagen, Denmark.

1 Introduction

The importance of physical training for young athletes in order to ensure an optimal physical level as grown up athletes is still under debate. Studies on the effect of physical training with children are complicated by the fact that growth and maturation also influence the physical capacity (see Krahenbuhl et al., 1985). Physiological data such as maximal ventilation, oxygen uptake and heart rate, have been collected from children participating in sport activities (Daniels et al., 1978; Vaccaro and Clake, 1978; Mayers and Gutin, 1979), and this have also been the case in soccer (Caru et al., 1970; Berg et al., 1985; Bell, 1988). In the latter studies measurements have been obtained under laboratory conditions with continuous exercise protocols. However, it appears that intermittent field test results have higher validity for physical performance in soccer (Bangsbo and Lindquist, 1992). To throw further light on the need for physical training at a young age the intermittent exercise performance of youth soccer players in different age groups was evaluated.

2 Methods

The subjects were 112 youth soccer players (mean age: 13.7; range: 10.5-17.4 years), 10 young elite players (18.3; 18-19 years) and 75 adult elite players (24.3; 20-31 years), who participated voluntarily after receiving verbal information.

The youth group consisted of 5 goalkeepers, 36 defenders, 26 strikers and 45 midfield players. All players were members of soccer clubs in Copenhagen and participated in the best local league within their age group. The young elite and the adult elite players were playing in the Danish National League. All players took part in soccer training at least three times per week. For the players younger than 15 years no specific physical training was carried out, which means that no training was performed with the main purpose of improving the physical capacity. The physical characteristics of the youth players are given

Table 1. Physical characteristics of the youth players. Means ± SE are given

Age (years)	11	12	13	14	15	16	17
Body Mass (kg)	35.5 ±0.9	40.1 ±2.4	44.1 ±1.5	51.0 ±1.4	61.6 ±2.9	64.8 ±1.4	61.8 ±2.3
Height (cm)	144.4 ±1.3	150.5 ±2.1	154.2 ±1.5	163.7 ±1.4	173.0 ±2.2	174.7 ±1.6	172.6 ±2.8
n	15	15	14	29	12	20	7

in Table 1.

All players performed a soccer specific interval field test. The course for this test is shown in Fig. 1. The test was set up in a penalty area and each lap was 160 m. The activity alternated between high and low intensity exercise for 15 and 10 s, respectively, which was controlled by signals from a taperecorder. The total running time was 16.5 min. Thus, total durations of high and low intensity exercise were 10 and 6.5 min, respectively. During the high intensity periods the players followed the outlined course with different locomotion forms (side-stepping, backwards and forward running). The low intensity periods consisted of 10 s jogging to the centre and back to the stop-position. The test result was the distance covered during the 10 min of high intensity exercise. All tests were carried out during the competitive season.

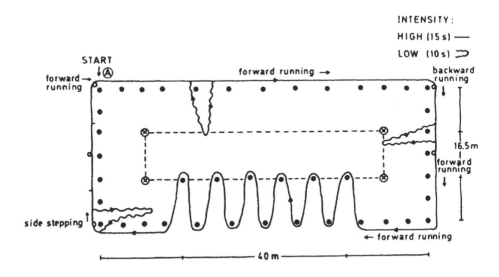

Fig. 1. The course of the intermittent field test.

During the test heart rate (HR) was recorded on 72 of the youth players and 23 of the adult elite players by a telemetric recorder (Sportstester, PE-3000). The maximal HR was determined at the end of a test where the players were running for 5 min at a moderate intensity and subsequent performed 400 m running with increasing intensity, ending with a sprint.

For 22 of the 112 youth players the test was repeated eight months after the first test. These players were divided into two age groups with 11 players in each. One group consisted of players from 11.2 to 14.0 years, another group of players from 14.1 to 16.2 years. The training during this period did not include any specific physical training for the younger group.

In addition, two groups of young elite players (15.8, 15.3-16.2 (n=5) and 18.4; 18.1-19.0 (n=7) years) and 50 adult elite players (25.1; 21-31 years) carried out a maximal test on a motor driven treadmill in order to determine the maximal oxygen uptake (VO_2max). The initial treadmill speed was 16 km/h for the youngest group and 18 km/h for the other groups. The speed was increased progressively with 2 km/h every 2 min until the subject was exhausted. Expiratory gas was collected in Douglas bags and the volume was measured with a Tissot spirometer. Oxygen (O_2) and carbon dioxide (CO_2) concentrations were determined with paramagnetic O_2 (Servomex) and infrared CO_2 (Beckman LB-II) analysers, respectively.

3 Results

The mean HR for the youth players and the adults during the field test was respectively 11 and 9 beats/min below their maximal HR (Fig. 2).

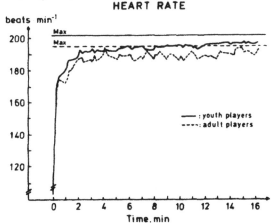

Fig. 2. Mean HR during the intermittent field test for youth (—) and adult (---) players.

Table 2. Running distance during the intermittent field test.

Age (years)	(n)	Test distance (m) Mean±SD	Range
11	(15)	1596±28	1397 - 1836
12	(15)	1660±25	1480 - 1825
13	(14)	1705±44	1315 - 1979
14	(29)	1802±18	1606 - 2014
15	(12)	1783±37	1563 - 1908
16	(20)	1872±15	1705 - 2002
17	(7)	1881±15	1817 - 1926
18 - 19	(10)	1955±28	1836 - 2014
20 - 31	(75)	1967±32	1717 - 2077

The running distances of the different groups are shown in Table 2.

For the youth players a relationship (r=0.65; P<0.05) between age and test distance was established. Players of age 12, 14 and 16 years had a longer (P<0.05) running distance in the test than players of age 11, 13 and 15 years, respectively. The difference in running distance between the 11 and 14 years old players was larger (P<0.05) than the difference between the 14 and 17 years old players. The performance of the 18-19 years old players was similar to that of the grown-up elite players (Fig. 3).

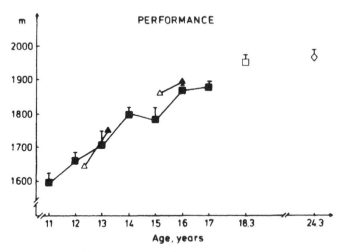

Fig. 3. Running distance during the intermittent field test for youth players (■), young elite players (□) and adult elite players (◇). Furthermore, values are given for two groups of youth players tested before (△) and after (▲) 8 months of ordinary soccer training. Means ±SE are given.

When re-tested after 8 months the group under 14 years had a better (P<0.05) performance (1738 m) than in the first test (1643 m). In contrast, the increase for players above 14 years was not significant (Fig. 3).

No difference in VO_2-max between the two young groups and the adults was observed (59.5, 61.3 and 61.2 ml/kg/min for the 15.8, 18.4 years old and adult players, respectively).

4 Discussion

The major finding in the present study was a larger difference in intermittent exercise performance between players of age 11 and 14 years, compared with the difference between players of 14 and 17 years, indicating that the physical development was more pronounced for the young players. This was supported by data from the players, who were re-tested. During the 8 months between the two tests, the players younger than 14 years had a greater improvement than players above 14 years. It should be noted that these differences occur even though physical training was not undertaken by the young players. Thus, it appears that changes in physical performance during early puberty are related to growth rather than to physical training. Consequently, in early puberty physical training seems to be of little significance. These findings are in agreement with Kobayashi et al. (1978), who reported that the maximal aerobic power for trained boys was not different from active boys until one year before reaching peak height velocity. It could be argued that physical training for young players is important for reaching a sufficient physical level as grown-up players. However, in the present study maximal aerobic power and the intermittent exercise performance for the 18.4 years old players were similar to the adult elite players. Thus, it appears that youth soccer players can obtain a physical performance level as high as adult players by ordinary soccer training in the young ages.

The running distance in the intermittent test was related to increasing age (r=0.65). However, a large range of performance within each group was observed. It was probably due to a large variation in maturation within each age group, which has been shown to influence performance (Tanner, 1980). The players HR during the field test indicates that the test is demanding for the aerobic energy system, and it has also been demonstrated that a significant anaerobic energy production occurs (Bangsbo and Lindquist, 1992). The reduced performance of the younger players can be attributed to these players' lower maximum oxygen uptake, endurance performance and anaerobic exercise performance, which have been observed in several studies (Åstrand, 1952; Caru et al., 1970, Eriksson et al., 1971; Van Den Eynde et al., 1989).

In conclusion, the present data suggest that specific physical training should have very low priority in soccer training until late puberty. The time could be better devoted to other types of training, e.g. technical aspects.

5 References

Åstrand, P. O. (1952) Experimental studies of physical working capacity in relation to sex and age. **Munksgaard**, Copenhagen.

Bangsbo, J. and Lindquist, F. (1992) Comparison of various exercise tests with actual physical soccer capacity. **Int. J. Sports Med.**, in press.

Bell, W. (1988) Physiological characteristics of 12-year-old soccer players, in **"Science and football" (eds. T. Reilly, A. Lees, K. Davids and W.J. Murphy)**, E. & F.N. Spon, London, pp. 175-180.

Berg, K.E. LaVoie, J.C. and Latin, R.W. (1985) Physiological training effects of playing youth soccer. **Med. Sci. Sports Exerc.**, 17, 656-660.

Caru, B. Le Coultre, L., Aghemo, P. and Limas, F.P. (1970) Maximal aerobic and anaerobic muscular power in football players. **J. Sports Med.Phys.Fit.**, 10, 100-103.

Daniels, J. Oldridge, N., Nagle, F. and White, B. (1978) Differences and changes in VO_2 among young runners 10 to 18 years of age. **Med. Sci.Sports**, 10, 200-203.

Eriksson, B.O. Karlsson, J. and Saltin, B. (1971) Muscle metabolites during exercise in pubertal boys. **Acta Paed. Scand.**, 217, 154-157.

Krahenbuhl, G.S. Skinner, J.S. and Kohrt, W.M. (1985) Developmental aspects of maximal aerobic power in children. **Exerc. Sports Sci. Rev.**, 13, 503-538.

Kobayashi, K. Kitamura, K., Miura, M., Sodeyama, H., Murase, Y., Miyashita, M. and Matsui, H. (1978) Aerobic power as related to body growth and training in Japanese boys: a longitudinal study. **J. Appl. Physiol.**, 44, 666-672.

Mayers, N. and Gutin, B. (1979) Physiological characteristics of elite prepubertal cross-country runners. **Med. Sci. Sports**, 11, 172-176.

Tanner, J.M. (1980) Some methodological problems in the analysis of human growth, in **"The Biology of Normal Human Growth" (ed. M. Ritzen)**, Raven Press, New York, pp. 309-315.

Vaccaro, P. and Clake, D.H. (1978) Cardiorespiratory alterations in 9 to 11 year old children following a season of competitive swimming. **Med. Sci. Sports**, 10, 204-207.

Van Den Eynde, B. Van Gerven, D., Vienne, D., Vuylsteke-Wauters, M. and Ghesquiere, J. (1989) Endurance fitness and peak height velocity in Belgian boys, in **"Children and exercise XIII",(eds. O. Seid and K.-H. Carlsen)**, Int. Series Sport Sci., 19, 19-28.

THE RELATIONSHIP BETWEEN PHYSIOLOGICAL CHARACTERISTICS OF JUNIOR SOCCER PLAYERS AND PERFORMANCE IN A GAME SIMULATION.

DOUGLAS TUMILTY.
Department of Physiology and Applied Nutrition, Australian
Institute of Sport, Canberra, Australia.

1 Introduction

In assessing the physiological characteristics important for
the soccer player two approaches have frequently been taken.
Physiological tests have been performed to determine those
characteristics which differentiate the good player from the
less able. A second approach has been to film games and by
analysis of them in terms of distances covered at various
speeds, to assess the involvement of the energy systems of
the body.

To relate physiological characteristics more directly to
game performance, the present study utilised a simulation,
based on game analysis, and compared the performance of
players on the simulation with their results in laboratory
and field tests. A simulation was used in order to
standardise the workload for all players, and to regulate,
and increase the range of, the measures taken.

2 Methods

Subjects (n=16) were members of the Australian Institute of
Sport Junior Soccer Squad for 1990. They were well-
conditioned and skilful for their age (16.1 ± S.D.=0.7
years). Their basic characteristics were :- body mass 71.3
(±6.7) kg, and height 177.6 (±7.3) cm.
The following tests were performed:

Anaerobic Power: 1. Maximal sprint over 20 m, time being
recorded electronically. 2. Maximal 10 s effort on an
Exertech air-braked cycle ergometer.
Anaerobic capacity: Whereas anaerobic power is generally
agreed to be dependent principally on the phosphagen energy
system and so to be most appropriately measured by short-
duration maximal tests, anaerobic capacity is more difficult
to define and measure. Operationally it may be assessed by
tests requiring a high intensity effort lasting
approximately 1 minute. Such tests ensure the full
engagement of both the phosphagen and lactic acid energy
pathways, though it is likely that the aerobic system is
increasingly involved as test duration increases. The test
chosen involved a treadmill run to exhaustion at 12.9 km/h
up a 20% incline (Cunningham & Faulkner, 1969).
Repeatability: The ability to repeat brief, high
intensity efforts with minimal deterioration in speed is

crucial in soccer, though there are neither standard tests to assess the ability, nor as yet complete understanding of the physiological basis for the deterioration, or for local muscle fatigue in general. The two repeatability tests performed were: six 35 m maximal effort sprints on the 30 s mark, and, on the air-braked cycle ergometer, 5 repetitions of 6 s maximal efforts on the 30 s mark. Performance decrements were assessed by summing the percentage deterioration of each effort compared to the best effort.

Aerobic power: A maximal oxygen uptake test on the treadmill with gas analysis was performed.

Simulation: This consisted of a sequence of movements which the player executed according to taped instructions. In total, there were four segments of about five minutes each with a rest of one minute between segments. Segments 1 and 4 were identical to each other and of higher intensity than segments 2 and 3, which were also identical to each other; Table 1 contains details. The simulation was intended to realistically represent a vigorous portion of a game and was based on data from several game analysis studies (Van Gool et al., 1988; Mayhew and Wenger, 1985; Reilly and Thomas, 1976; Withers et al., 1982). The speed of all actions was controlled by the tape, except for intermittent 12 or 20 m sprints, in which the subject was encouraged to make a maximum effort. The simulation was run indoors round a 25 m by 35 m rectangle with cones placed at the corners and midway along the sides. As a player approached a cone the tape would inform him of the action to carry out to get to the succeeding cone. No ball work or jumping was included.

Heart rates were monitored throughout. Earlobe blood samples were taken before and after the test and during the three rest breaks. Sprints were timed electronically.

Table 1. Details of simulation test

| | Distance | | Time | | Speeds |
	m	% total	s	% total	m/s
Stationary	-	-	248	17.5	-
Walk	670	17.6	356	25.1	1.88
Jog	1648	43.3	434	30.6	3.80
Stride	808	21.2	186	13.1	4.34
Sprint	352	9.2	56	3.9	6.29
Back	230	6.0	100	7.0	2.30
Side	100	2.6	40	2.8	2.50
	3808		1420 (23 min 40 s)		

(90 minute equivalent distance - 14 481 m)
Ratio of low intensity (stationary, walk, jog, back, side) to high intensity (stride, sprint) distance - 2.28:1; time - 4.87:1

3 Results

Table 2 gives means and standard deviations of results for laboratory and field tests. Table 3 gives the results of the simulation test by segment. A repeated measures ANOVA with a Tukey post-hoc test was applied to the results of each segment, and where applicable to resting values, to determine significance at the 0.05 level.

Table 2. Test results

```
--------------------------------------------------------------
Anaerobic Power
10 s cycle ergo. Work done        9.1(1.1)kJ  126(13)J/kg
                 Peak power    1168(150)W        16.0(1.7)W/kg
Sprints.         Time at 20 m     3.02(0.11)s
Anaerobic capacity
Treadmill run duration            73.5(8.4)s
Repeatability
5x6 s cycle ergo.Total work      24.8(2.3)kJ  345(33)J/kg
                 Decrement        42(15)%
              Mean peak power   1094(118)W        15.2(1.6)W/kg
                 Decrement        32(14)%
6x35 m sprints.  Fastest time     4.77(0.16)s
                 Total time      29.37(0.95)s
                 Speed decrement 16(7)%
Aerobic power
Treadmill V̇O₂ max                 61.4(4.0)ml/kg/min
--------------------------------------------------------------
```

Treadmill $\dot{V}O_2$ max — 61.4(4.0)ml/kg/min

Table 3. Simulation results (with standard deviations)

	pre-test	Segment 1	2	3	4	sign. dif.
Heart rate		170	175	177	181	4 cf. 1,2,3
(beats/min)		(7)	(5)	(4)	(6)	1 cf. 2,3
Lactate		6.7	6.0	4.8	5.9	1 cf. 2,3,4
(mM)		(1.7)	(2.0)	(1.4)	(1.2)	3 cf. 1,2,4
pH	7.47	7.30	7.36	7.39	7.35	pre cf. 1,2,
	(0.08)	(0.11)	(0.09)	(0.06)	(0.08)	3,4. 1 cf. 2,
						3,4. 4 cf. 3.
HCO₃	18.7	12.4	13.1	14.0	11.5	pre cf. 1,2,
(mM)	(4.0)	(2.7)	(3.0)	(2.9)	(3.6)	3,4. 4 cf. 3.
Mean sprint						
time (s) 12 m		2.24	2.19	2.20	2.23	n.s.
		(0.10)	(0.08)	(0.09)	(0.07)	
20 m		3.31	3.17	3.21	3.41	1 cf. 2,3.
		(0.07)	(0.12)	(0.10)	(0.14)	4 cf. 2,3.

Table 4 gives the significant correlations found between performance decrement on 12 m and 20 m sprints during the simulation and results of the laboratory and field tests.

Table 4. Simulation performance decrement v. lab./field
tests - significant correlations
----

	12 m decrement	20 m decrement

Anaerobic power
Cycle - total work-abs.   0.75+
        -rel. to weight   0.57*
      - peak power-abs.   0.73+
        -rel. to weight   0.58*
Sprints - 20 m time   -0.80+   -0.86+
Repeatability
Cycle - total work-abs.   0.56*
      - mean peak power   0.64*
Sprints - total time   -0.71*   -0.74+
Aerobic power
Treadmill $\dot{V}O_2$ max.   -0.59*   -0.74+

* sign. at 0.05 level.   + sign. at 0.01 level.
----

4 Discussion

Because of the fluctuating intensity in the simulation a
gradual increase in sprint times did not occur (see Table
3). Rather the times varied as the players were able to
partially recover. Therefore the performance decrement
measure used was the total fractional increment in time for
the 12 m and 20 m sprints relative to the best times
obtained by a subject during the separate sprint test. These
measures were compared with others found within the
simulation and in other testing to try to isolate the
factors important for performance.

The high level of intensity overall (ie. including the 1
minute breaks between segments) is indicated by a mean heart
rate of 173 beats/min, which was 87% of maximum heart rate.
This is comparable with those found in game measures by
others (Van Gool et al., 1988), and by the author in
monitoring the present group. Lactate levels also are
comparable with those reported elsewhere (Gerisch et al.,
1988), though considerably lower than peak values recorded
in top level overseas games (Ekblom, 1986).

In the first segment, the low heart rates, high lactates
and low blood acidity measures indicate the extra load
placed on the anaerobic system before the aerobic system has
become fully activated.

Segments 2 and 3 were slightly easier than 1 and 4,
resulting in stable heart rates, declining lactates,
increasing pH and bicarbonate levels, and faster 20 m
sprints in the middle two segments.

The final hard segment produced a slower time over 20 m
compared with the middle two, as well as higher heart rates
and lactates and reducing pH and bicarbonate. However,

there was no significant deterioration in any measures (except heart rate) between the two hard and identical segments 1 and 4.

The results indicate that players can maintain reasonable equilibrium over prolonged periods of activity of high though fluctuating intensity with lactate levels above the 4 mM considered as the threshold level in steady- state activities. Muscle fibre changes have been found in soccer players indicating adaptations to both aerobic and anaerobic training (Kuzon jr. et al., 1989), consistent with the performance characteristics found here.

Somewhat contrary to the game situation, the simulation subjects were not able to adopt their own recovery strategy and so the reduction in their sprint speed compared with their best efforts may have been due to genuine physical fatigue and/or a conscious or unconscious attempt to pace themselves to try to keep fatigue to an acceptable level.

Correlations were done between sprint performance decrement and mean heart rate as a percentage of maximum, mean lactate, and mean decline in pH and bicarbonate during the test compared with pre-tests values, but none of significance was found. This may be due to the manipulation of sprint speed suggested in the previous paragraph, or because this was a physiologically homogeneous group.

The direction of the significant correlations between performance decrement and the results of the other tests (Table 4) indicates that the better the anaerobic power and speed in single or repetition efforts, the larger was the simulation performance decrement. An explanation for this may lie in the fibre type profile of subjects, though that could not be determined in this study. Quicker subjects may have a higher proportion of fast twitch fibres and experience greater fatigue in this type of high intensity test. This is supported by the significant negative correlation between maximum oxygen uptake and performance decrement. More aerobic individuals, perhaps with a higher proportion of slow twitch fibres, were better able to maintain their sprint speed, possibly due to greater capillarisation of the muscles and a superior ability to utilise lactate aerobically, both mechanisms allowing swifter clearance of the metabolite from muscle fibres. No significant correlation existed between fastest single sprint times and mean simulation sprint times over 12 m or 20 m, so faster players would seem to have no advantage when required to work continuously at high intensity, unless they also have a good enough aerobic capability to enable them to maintain work rate.

Contrary to other findings (Balsom, 1986), no significant correlation was found between the anaerobic capacity test and simulation performance decrement. This may be due to different simulation protocols, or the differing levels of fitness or degree of homogeneity of the groups. It may be that the Cunningham test requires a high muscle buffering capability, while the current simulation allowed dissipation of lactate by aerobic means (Brooks, 1987).

5 Conclusions

Based on the simulation, soccer players seem able to maintain a high mean level of intensity of work output, provided that recovery periods of lesser, though still high intensity, are allowed.

Good aerobic capability is important for continuous high intensity performance, especially since more powerful and fast players seem more susceptible to fatigue.

6 References

Balsom, P.D. (1986) The relationship between aerobic capacity, anaerobic power, anaerobic capacity, anaerobic threshold, and performance decrementation in male collegiate soccer players. M Sc. thesis, Springfield College, Springfield, Massachusetts.

Brooks, G. A. (1987) Lactate production during exercise: oxidizable substrate versus fatigue agent, in **Exercise: Benefits, Limits & Adaptations** (eds D. McLeod, R. Maughan, M. Nimmo, T. Reilly, and C. Williams), E. & F. N. Spon, London, pp. 144-158.

Cunningham, D.A. and Faulkner, J.A. (1969) The effect of training on aerobic and anaerobic metabolism during a short exhaustive run. **Med. Sci. Sports**, 1, 65-69.

Ekblom, B. (1986) Applied physiology of soccer. **Sports Med.**, 3, 50-60.

Gerisch, G., Rutemoller, E. and Weber, K. (1988) Sportsmedical measurements of performance in soccer, in **Science and Football** (eds T. Reilly, A. Lees, K. Davids, and W. J. Murphy), E. & F. N. Spon, London, pp. 60-67.

Kuzon jr., W.M., Rosenblatt, J.D., Huebel, S.C., Leatt, P., Plyley, M.J., McKee, N.H. and Jacobs, I. (1990) Skeletal muscle fiber type, fiber size, and capillary supply in elite soccer players. **Int. J. Sports Med.**, 11, 99-102.

Mayhew, S.R. and Wenger, H.A. (1985) Time-motion analysis of professional soccer. **J. Hum. Mov. Stud.**, 11, 49-52.

Reilly, T. and Thomas, V. (1976) A motion analysis of work-rate in different positional roles in professional football match-play. **J. Hum. Mov. Stud.**, 2, 87-97.

Van Gool, D., Van Gerven, D. and Boutmans, J. (1988) The physiological load imposed on soccer players during real match-play, in **Science & Football** (eds T. Reilly, A. Lees, K. Davids, and W.J. Murphy,), E. & F. N. Spon, London, pp.51-59.

Withers, R.T., Maricic, Z., Wasilewski, S. and Kelly, L. (1982) Match analyses of Australian professional soccer players. **J. Hum. Mov. Stud.**, 8, 159-176.

THE EVIDENCE OF SPORTANTHROPOLOGY IN TRAINING OF YOUNG SOCCER PLAYER

K.-P. HERM
Institut of Sports Medicine, Leipzig, Germany

1 Introduction

Carter (1985) stated "but what is so empirically obvious has not been so easy to quantify, and little has been done to directly relate characteristics of physique in theoretical and experimental studies with performance".

For young soccer players the research area of sportanthropology postulates that: (1) the components of body composition are fundamental for performance; (2) training influences body development which is affected also by genetic factors; (3) there is a dynamic process of changing development of body composition (Herm, 1986; 1988) and short term and long term rhythms in the development of body structure.

Measurement of morphology of athletes has largely developed during the past century. An essential part of talent promotion is the diagnosis of athletes' development which should include physical development, personality formation and the evaluation of the results in training and competition. Although there is a general maturity factor underlying the tempo of growth and maturation during adolescence in both sexes, there is variation, so that no single system (i.e. somatic growth, skeletal maturation or sexual maturation) provides a complete description of the tempo of growth and maturation of the individual boy or girl during adolescence (Malina, 1988).

For young soccer players there are few experimental models developed for testing the contributions of physique to performance. Timely specialisation requires the attainment of a performance level which allows for optimal development. This level is seldom reached before puberty (Herm, 1988; Kemper, 1985, Malina, 1988).

The aim of this investigation was to examine the relation between short term growth dynamics and the performance of young soccer players.

2 Material and Methods

Altogether 82 soccer players, aged between 11 to 15 years, regularly participating in active and specific soccer training, were investigated in a longitudinal study between 1986 and 1990. Anthropometric measurements, and some performance tests (running about 10 and 30 metres, the agility test, the speed power test and

also a lactate test) were employed.   Three months separated each
series of measurements.
    The interpretation employed the following:

    1. Growth dynamics were calculated according to the velocity of
    growth (cm/year) and the estimation of growth types (Type 1 =
    stable, Type 2 = dynamic).   The formula for the estimation of
    growth type is according to the discrimination function DF 1 and
    DF 2 (Herm, 1988).   For example, at the beginning of training (14
    years old boys):
    DF 1 = 0.0296 body mass (kg) - 0.14 body height (cm)
         - 0.313 muscle mass (kg) - 0.0919 skeletal mass (kg)
         + 0.358 biological age (years)
    and then: growth type 1 = DF 1 < -23.5 and
              growth type 2 = DF 1 > -23.5
    or start of training (15 years old boys):
    DF 2 = - 0.183 body mass (kg) - 0.0922 body height (cm)
         - 0.127 muscle mass (kg) + 0.451 skeletal mass
         + 0.45 biological age (years)
    and then: growth type 1 = DF 2 < -16.9 and
              growth type 2 = DF 2 > -16.9
    2.   The body mass relations according the normal body mass
    estimation with this formula:

    $$\text{normal body mass} = \frac{\text{individual body mass} * 100}{107.68 - 1.6622 * \text{height} + 0.008 * \text{height}^2}$$
    (boys)
    3.   The muscle mass and skeletal mass were estimated according to
    Matiegka (1921).
    4.   The adipose tissue was calculated according to Parizkova
    (1962).
    5.   The biological age was measured according to the body
    development index (Wutscherk, 1981).
    6.   Methodical advice to coaches was given as a result of growth
    and development characteristics.
    7.   Some performance tests were used such as running about 10 and
    30 m, the agility test, the speed power test and also the lactate
    response test.

The means and standard deviations were computed for the growth
velocity and the growth type.   Discrimination analyses were performed
as well as correlation analyses.

3 Results and discussion

3.1 Physique (see table 1)
The biological age of the young soccer player was delayed by one year
in development.   The first pubertal growth spurt started at the age
of 13 years.   The highest growth velocity, 7.4 cm/year, was found at
the age of 13 to 14 years, but it is lower than 9.6 cm/years as an
average of the normal population.   According to the estimation of the
growth types, the young soccer players conform to growth Type 2
(dynamic growth type).
    The muscle mass developed quite poorly (44%) but increased after

14 years. The adipose tissue was relatively high at 14% and
increased at the age of 14 years. We found a late developing,
relatively low growth velocity of body height and body mass, and a
relatively long stagnation of muscle development. The pubertal
growth spurt showed a maximum at the age of 14-15 years.

Table 1   Average of body parameters of young soccer players,
          investigated in a longitudinal study

age (years)		Body mass (kg	Body height (cm)	Growth velo- city (cm/year)	Muscle (kg) (%)		Adipose tissue (kg) (%)	
chrono- logical	biolo- gical							
11	09	32.1	142.2	5.4	14.1	44.0	4.3	13.2
12	11	35.6	148.0	5.3	15.8	44.8	5.1	14.1
13	12	44.1	158.3	7.4	19.5	44.6	5.9	12.6
14	13	47.9	161.2	7.4	21.0	43.6	7.1	14.5
15	15	50.3	164.0	6.3	23.2	46.1	6.6	13.3

3.2 Relation between physique and performance
It has been observed that less speed and power training provides an
intensive growth spurt in body height (Table 2). Development of body
weight was also affected by the highly intensive speed and power
training.
    The young soccer players showed poor performance (running) when
their growth was very fast. Better running velocity was found when
the young players had intensive muscle growth.
    We noted a better performance according to the lactate response,
if the boys had a young biological age, a small body height and a
better muscle mass development. The anaerobic alactacid energy
metabolism develops with increasing biological age.
    Body composition, body size and shape in young athletes are topics
of great interest and controversy. Whether the anthropometry of
growing children is suitable for indicating normal and abnormal
growth is still in question.
    Table 2 summarises the significant correlations between selected
body dimensions and performance tests. The results reflect the
different relations between training and growth dynamics.
Correlation coefficients varied from r = 0.40 to r = 0.92.
    Correlation coefficients between growth velocity of height and
weight illustrated that if we have an intensive growth velocity we
have a lower speed for 30 m running. We have to ask if we did have a
workload that was too high with respect to one of the criteria. The
results of Kemper (1985), Bruggemann and Albrecht (1988), Carter
(1985) and Malina (1988) in different investigations about body
composition and exercise in childhood point in the same direction.
A great emphasis is given to questions arising for young sportsman
regarding the effects of training on growth and maturation. The
dynamics of growth as a new aspect for describing the estimation of
performance of growing children can provide a better basis for
understanding the limits related to biological and physiological
aspects of performance.

Table 2. Significant correlation coefficients between physique and performance of young soccer player (r > 0.44)

height : biological age	r =	0.65
body mass : biological age	r =	0.75
body mass : height	r =	0.82
muscle (kg) : biol. age	r =	0.78
muscle (kg) : height	r =	0.87
muscle (kg) : body mass	r =	0.92
muscle % : calend. age	r =	0.48
adip. tissue (kg) : biol. age	r =	0.51
adip. tissue (kg) : body mass	r =	0.77
adip. tissue (%) : calend. age	r =	-0.69
adip. tissue (%) : biol. age	r =	0.85
speed power : calend. age	r =	0.49
30 m (s) : biol. age	r =	-0.55
30 m (s) : body mass	r =	-0.49
30 m (s) : muscle (%)	r =	0.63
30 m (s) : speed power	r =	0.77
30 m (s) : agility	r =	0.65
growth velocity : body mass	r =	0.40
growth velocity : speed power	r =	-0.67
growth velocity : agility	r =	0.72
growth velocity : 30 m (s)	r =	-0.69
velocity weight : speed power	r =	-0.60
velocity weight : agility	r =	-0.69
velocity muscle : biol. age	r =	0.64
velocity muscle : height	r =	0.47
velocity muscle : muscle (kg)	r =	0.61
velocity muscle : adip. tissue	r =	0.56
velocity muscle : 30 m (s)	r =	-0.55
lactate : biol. age	r =	-0.45
lactate : height	r =	-0.61
lactate : body mass	r =	-0.51
lactate : muscle (kg)	r =	-0.53
lactate : velocity muscle	r =	-0.50

The results show that it is possible to establish different growth types with the help of specific growth velocities over a year (Herm, 1986, 1988). Lenz (1971) demonstrated that the body growth developed allometrically; this means the whole body and body parts develop with different specific growth velocities. It is evident that with sportsmen aged 14 years, a majority of important body composition parameters (54%) change significantly in a one month period. On this ground, anthropometric measurements in longitudinal investigations must be carried out in short intervals.

4 References

Bruggemann, D. and Albrecht, D. (1988) Modernes Fußalltraining. Hoffmann Verlag, Schorndorf, p. 344.

Carter, J.E.L. (1985) Morphological factors limiting human performance, in Limits of Human Performance (eds D.H. Clarke and H.M. Eckert). American Academy of Physical Education Papers, No. 18, Human Kinetics, Champaign, Ill.

Herm, K.-P. (1986) The problem of analysis and interpretation methods in longitudinal research studies, in Growth and Ontogenetic Development in Man, III. Charles University, Prague, p. 265-273.

Herm, K.-P. (1988) Wachstumsdynamik und sportliche Leistung. (Growth Dynamic and Sport Performance.) DHfK Leipzig, Diss.B, p. 154.

Kemper, H.C.G. (ed) (1985) Growth, Health and Fitness of Teenagers. München, p. 263.

Lenz, W. (1971) Physiologie und Pathologie der Entwicklung. (Physiology and pathology of development), in Geschichte der Kinderheilkunde I/1 Springer, Berlin, Heidelberg, New York, p. 903.

Malina, R.M. (1988) Biological maturity status of young athletes, in Young Athletes, (ed R.M. Malina), Human Kinetics Books, Champaign, Illinois, pp. 121-140.

Matiegka, J. (1921) The testing of physical efficiency, in, Amer. J. Phys. Anthropol., Washington 4, 3. pp. 223-230.

Parizkova, J. (1962) Rozvoj Aktivni Hmoty a Tuku u Deti a Mladeje. Praha, p. 132.

Wutscherk, H. (1981) Grundlagen der Sportanthropologie. DHfK Leipzig, p. 163.

SOMATOTYPE, BODY COMPOSITION AND PHYSICAL PERFORMANCE CAPACITIES OF ELITE YOUNG SOCCER PLAYERS

J. GARGANTA, J. MAIA & J. PINTO
Faculty of Sport Sciences and Physical Education. University of Porto, Portugal

1 Introduction

The structure of performance in team sports represents a multifactorial trait. The identification of its components, from a conceptual and operative view, has been a major task in the sport sciences. Several authors have presented the suggestion that somatotype and body composition influence performance (Tanner,1964; Carter & Heath,1989).

Handball, Basketball and Volleyball are examples of team sports where physique and body composition may enhance performance. Soccer playing proficiency seems to present a contradictory position in this regard. Nevertheless, it is our opinion that it is important to draw the attention of coaches and sport scientists to the somatic and motor characteristics of young soccer players for both purposes of profiling and establishing relationships between predictor variables and criteria (specific motor performance, game situations).

The purposes of this study are the following :i) the identification of somatotype and estimation of body composition; ii) the evaluation of flexibility and "general" physical performance capacity; iii) the analysis of relationship between somatotype and body composition with "general" physical performance capacity.

2 Material and Methods

Subjects were young Portuguese soccer players (European champions), age,17.5 ± 0.59 years. height. 174.3 ± 5.9 cm, body mass, 72.1 ± 6.1 Kg.

The somatotype was assessed according to Carter & Heath (1989). The estimation of body composition was done according to the formulae of Siri (1956).

The flexibility was assessed according to Leighton's (1966) procedures for hip flexion with and without a bent knee. abduction and adduction of lower limb. The "general" physical performance capacity was assessed according to:30m dash, shutle run 4 x 5.50 m, medicine ball throw (1 Kg), standing broad jump.

We used parametric descriptive statistics only for illustrative purposes. To test differences between game positions, was used the nonparametric test of Kruskal-Wallis adjusted for small samples (Siegel, 1956).

3 Results

The mean somatotype was 3.0 - 4.0 - 1.76. This characterised players as a whole as endomesomorph.

Table 1. Mean (±SD) of somatotypes according to game position

		Endomorphy	Mesomorphy	Ectomorphy
GoalKeepers	(n = 2)	4.25 ± 0.35	4.05 ± 0.07	2.00 ± 0.71
Half-Backs	(n = 3)	3.00 ± 0.00	4.03 ± 0.06	2.00 ± 0.50
Midfielders	(n = 6)	2.58 ± 0.49	3.97 ± 0.05	1.58 ± 0.58
Forwards	(n = 2)	3.00 ± 0.71	4.05 ± 0.07	1.75 ± 1.06

The somatotypes of the players according to game positions showed some minor differences in the three components. Goalkeepers tend to present greater values in endomorphy.

Table 2. Mean (±SD) of Lean Body Mass (LBM), Percent body fat (% fat) and sum of skinfolds (Σ Skf) according to game position

		LBM	% fat	Σ Skf
GoalKeepers	(n=2)	66.1 ± 2.2	16.1 ± 0.9	91.6
Half-Backs	(n=3)	66.8 ± 8.3	10.9 ± 0.3	64.3
Midfielders	(n=6)	62.5 ± 2.3	9.3 ± 1.6	57.4
Forwards	(n=2)	61.7 ± 7.1	12.6 ± 3.9	78.4

No differences were found, among all game positions, for flexibility and physical performance capacity (Table 3 and 4).

Table 3. Mean values (±SD) of flexibility according to game position

		Hip flexion 1	Hip flexion 2	Abduction	Adduction
GoalKeepers	(n=2)	99.0 ± 1.4	79.0 ± 19.8	18.0 ± 1.4	51.0 ± 2.8
Half-Backs	(n=3)	95.3 ± 15.5	87.3 ± 22.0	23.3 ± 3.1	55.0 ± 3.0
Midfielders	(n=6)	96.6 ± 9.3	74.0 ± 5.6	25.5 ± 10.6	59.0 ± 5.8
Forwards	(n=2)	103.5 ± 6.3	81.6 ± 5.6	21.1 ± 5.1	56.5 ± 19.1

Table 4. Mean values (±SD) of "general" tests according to game position

	30 m dash (")	Shuttle run (")	Throw (m)	SBJ (m)
GoalKeepers (n=2)	4.46±0.30	7.53±0.08	17.6±1.2	2.53±0.04
Half-Backs (n = 3)	4.34±0.01	7.60±0.29	14.8±1.7	2.29±0.08
Midfielders (n = 6)	4.45±0.21	7.36±0.33	13.9±0.9	2.28±0.09
Forwards (n = 2)	4.46±0.01	7.48±0.33	13.5±2.6	2.26±0.15

4 Conclusions

1) At this age group, in this sample, no particular physique was found to be associated with game position.
2) Goalkeepers and forwards evidenced greater values in fat weight as well as in all skinfold sites.No significant difference was found in LBM according to the game position.
3) Further research in developing specific testing is needed. This implies the identification of discriminators between elite and non-elite young soccer players.

5 Ackowledgements

The authors ackowledges the contribuition of the Sub-16 National Team Head Coach Carlos Queiroz and Assistent Coaches, Nelo Vingada e Rui Caçador, for the present study.

6 References

Carter, J.E.L. and Heath, B.H. (1989) Somatotyping - Development and Applications .Cambridge University Press. Cambridge
Leighton, J.R. (1966) The Leighton flexometer and flexibility test. J. Ass. Phys. and Mental Rehabil.. 15, 85 - 89.
Siegel, S. (1956) Nonparametric Statistics for the Behavioral Sciences. McGraw-Hill Book Company. New York.
Siri, W.E. (1956) Growth and composition of the body. In Biological and Medical Physics. Vol. 4. (eds. J.H. Lawrence and C.A. Tobias), New York. Academic Press.
Tanner, J. M. (1964): The Physique of Olimpic Athlete. George Allen and Unwin. London.

PHYSIOLOGICAL PROFILE OF PROSPECTIVE SOCCER PLAYERS

S. JANKOVIC, N. HEIMER AND B.R. MATKOVIC
Faculty of Physical Education, University of Zagreb, Croatia.

1 Introduction

Presence of children in sport today is more obvious than ever. World
and Olympic champions, especially in some sports (gymnastics, tennis,
swimming, ice skating), are younger and younger. This makes the
problem of selection in sport even more important. In soccer, boys
are involved in specific training programmes also very early. For
that reason it is important to establish physiological characteristics of young players and to see whether these characteristics can
help in the process of selection. This study is concerned with this
problem.

2 Methods

The investigation was carried out on a sample of 47 soccer players
within the age span of 15 to 17 years. These were prospective
players according to the opinion of their coaches and the experts in
the Croation Soccer Federation.
    Maximal oxygen intake and other cardiorespiratory variables were
measured directly during a continuous progressive test on a treadmill. Spirometric variables (forced vital capacity, forced expiratory volume in the first second and Tiffeneau's index) were measured
with a Vitalograph Wedge Bellows spirometer. The strength of four
attempts was measured as well as the speed of the dominant hand and
leg. According to the Rohrer and Kahlstorf's method (modified
according to Musshoff and Reindell - see Medved, 1987) heart volume,
absolute and relative, was determined.
    The data obtained were submitted to the standard statistical
methods to determine descriptive parameters. The sample was divided
into two subgroups: one consisted of the players who are currently
members of the first national league teams and the other of those now
in regional leagues. The differences between these two groups were
determined by means of analysis of variance (ANOVA).

3 Results and discussion

Basic descriptive parameters of the observations are presented in
Table 1. Average height of the young players was 175.7 cm and they
were 66.2 kg in weight which are in agreement with the norms for this

age. Spirometric values observed are significantly above the values
predicted from height and age of players using a standard nomogram
(Heimer et al., 1985). Several authors reported previously that
pulmonary function measures are superior in athletes compared with
non-athletes and some of them (Vaccaro et al., 1979) suggested that
sport training provokes hypertrophy of respiratory musculature which
can increase values of forced vital capacity and FEV_1, because both
of these parameters depend a great deal on the strength of the
respiratory muscles. Of course, the real answer to the question
whether this is a result of training or whether these boys enter the
training programme with greater lungs dimensions can be given only
with objective longitudinal investigations.

The average value for heart volume is above the average values of
non-athletes. This is particularly evident in the values of relative
heart volume which is 13.3; this is significantly greater than in untrained subjects. The average value of the heart volume quotient is
very good (42.1) and significantly lower than the norms by Reindell
et al. (1967), which indicates good economy and functional capability
of cardiovascular and cardiopulmonary systems.

Absolute and relative maximal oxygen intakes are significantly
higher than mean values in the normal population of the same age
span. The values are also at the upper limit of those reported by
some other researchers who have investigated young sportsmen in other
sports (Caru et al., 1970). It is interesting to note that young
players have almost the same aerobic power as their older colleagues
in our country in absolute terms, but when expressed relative to body
weight young players are significantly better. This may reflect a
trend towards increased training intensity and conditioning
programmes, of course not at the level of endurance sports but which
is in accordance with the demands of soccer play.

The results for the strength measures show that the arm strength
of young players is very good and is near the upper limits of average
values in young sportsmen and above the average values in the normal
population (Montoye and Lamphiear, 1977). Total anti-gravitational
strength is significantly above the average values both in sportsmen
and the normal population. Concerning the rather inconsistent
measuring criteria and standardisation from laboratory to laboratory,
it is practically impossible to make any appropriate comparison with
the scarce data about the strength of young sportsmen.

In agreement with the strength values are the measures of hand and
leg speed. The speed of the dominant hand is within the normal range
while the leg speed is significantly above the average values of the
normal population and of sportsmen.

The sample was divided into two subgroups: one consisted of the
subjects who are now members of the first national league teams and
the other of those who are in regional leagues. On comparing the
mean values of the measured variables, it is obvious that boys who
are today in the higher level of competition are taller and heavier,
they have a better aerobic power and measures of respiratory
function, their heart volume is greater and they have greater leg
speed. Using analysis of variance, it was shown that only the
differences in height and aerobic power were statistically
significant. It can be concluded that aerobic power may be a useful
tool in the selection of soccer players at the age span of 15 to 17.

Table 4.   Functional characterstics of soccer players

	$\bar{X}$	SD
Age (years)	16.0	0.5
Body mass (kg)	66.2	5.6
Height (cm)	175.7	5.2
Heart volume (ml)	871.6	89.9
Rel. Heart vol. (ml/kg)	13.3	1.6
Heart quotient	42.1	5.8
FVC (1)	5.3	0.6
FEV_1 (1/s)	4.9	0.5
Tiff (%)	92.2	5.0
$\dot{V}O_2$max (1/min)	3.99	0.6
$\dot{V}O_2$max (ml/kg/min)	59.9	6.3
HRmax (beats/min)	197	9
O_2 pulse (ml O_2/beat)	21.0	3.4
Grip strength (N)	1008.2	238.3
Leg extension (N)	2890.0	749.6
Forearm extension (N)	368.9	86.8
Trunk extension (N)	1612.0	410.1
Arm speed (m/s)	5.5	2.0
Leg speed (m/s)	9.2	2.2

4 References

Caru, B. Le Coultre, L. Aghemo, P. and Pinera Limas, F. (1970)
    Maximal aerobic and anaerobic muscular power in football players
    J. Sports Med. Phys. Fit., 10, 100-103.
Heimer, S., Matkovic, B., Medved, R., Medved, V. and Zuskin, E.
    (1985) Praktikum kineziolska fiziologuije, FFK, Zagreb.
Medved, R. (1987) Sportska medicina, JUMENA, Zagreb.
Montoye, H.H. and Lamphiear, D.E. (1977) Grip and arm stsrength in
    males and females, age 10 to 69. Res. Quart., 48, 109-120.
Reindell, H. Konig, K. and Roskamm, H. (1967) Funktionsdiagnostik
    des gesunden und kranken Herzens. Georg Thieme, Stuttgart.
Vaccaro, P. Clarke, D.H. and Wrenn, J.P. (1979) Physiological
    profiles of elite women basketball players. J. Sports Med. Phys
    Fit., 19, 45-54.

CARDIORESPIRATORY FITNESS IN YOUNG BRITISH SOCCER PLAYERS

A.D.G. JONES AND P. HELMS
Training of Young Athletes (T.O.Y.A.) Study, Institute of Child Health, University of London, London, England

1 Introduction

During the last decade there has been a substantial increase in the number of children participating in organised sport in the UK. Concern has been expressed about the effect that intensive training may have on the physical and psychological growth and development of the young athletes. For this reason the Sports Council commissioned the Training of Young Athletes (T.O.Y.A.) Study (Rowley, 1986). This study has used a longitudinal method, measuring the same individual at intervals over a certain period of time, to make it possible to separate the effects of training from those of growth and development. Four sports were selected, a racket sport (tennis), a contact team sport (soccer), a sport which requires local muscular endurance and stamina (swimming) and a sport which requires flexibility and explosive strength (gymnastics). These sports also have the following in common: a large number of young athletes participate, they start training before puberty and have organised systems of intensive training and standardised age-groups for competition.

It has long been recognised that fitness plays an important part in determining performance. Fitness is not a single simple attribute, it contains elements of cardiorespiratory function, local muscle endurance, muscle strength and speed, joint mobility and body composition. Cardiorespiratory fitness is a measure of maximum aerobic performance ($\dot{V}O_2$ max). This is the highest rate of oxygen consumed by the body in a given period of time during exercise involving a significant portion of the muscle mass. It provides a gross measure of the state of the gas transport system and reflects pulmonary, cardiovascular and muscular components. Maximal aerobic power ($\dot{V}O_2$ max) has been extensively studied because it is considered to be the best single index of health related physical finess. It is also a good indicator of fitness in soccer players as it has been shown that soccer is predominantly an aerobic sport.

Numerous studies have shown that maximal aerobic power (l/min) increases with chronological age (Seliger et al., 1971; Rutenfranz et al., 1981; Kemper et al., 1983) showing that VO_2 max is related to the maturity of the child. At any given chronological age, however, there exists a great deal of variation, not only in $\dot{V}O_2$ max, but also in such physical dimensions as height and body mass. Therefore $\dot{V}O_2$ max has been traditionally expressed relative to body mass (ml/kg/min), and in boys it has been shown to be fairly stable from childhood through adolescence (Malina, 1990).

In this paper aerobic power, defined as peak oxygen uptake (peak $\dot{V}O_2$), in intensively trained soccer players is related to their pubertal stage of development and a comparison is made with a reference group of non-intensively trained British children. Conclusions are drawn as to the effects of specific physical training before puberty.

2 Methods

2.1 Subjects
The basic criteria for inclusion in the study was that the boys were affiliated with an English football league club (they had signed schoolboy forms) and that they trained for a specific number of hours per week and/or that they had performed successfully to a specified level in the past or were expected to achieve it in the future. A random sample of 64 soccer players aged between 11 and 17 years old was recruited from clubs within a 250 mile (400 km) radius of London. The reference grups consisted of 75 British school children aged between 11 and 16 years (Armstrong et al., 1991).

2.2 Measurements
Body height, body mass, pubertal rating and maximal aerobic power of the subjects were measured. Puberty was determined by assessment of stages of genitalia and pubic hair development with Tanner's criteria (1962). Tanner's stage ratings of I to V were assigned by a trained rater and a mean value for sexual maturity was recorded.

Maximal aerobic power (maximal oxygen uptake) was measured whilst the subject ran on a motor-driven treadmill (P.K. Morgan Instruments Inc., Rainham, U.K.). The subjects ran at an individually predetermined rate, on a 3.4% grade, for 1 min followed by increments of 0.5 km/h every minute until complete exhaustion was reached (Åstrand and Rodahl, 1970). The initial rate was chosen to produce a testing time of within 5-7 min.

Gas exchange parameters were measured by standard open circuit techniques. Subjects breathed through a Speak-Easy II face mask (Respironics Inc., Monroeville, USA). Ventilation was derived through a turbine volume transducer attached to a control unit with digital display. Analysis of expired oxygen was carried out with a Model QA 500D paramagnetic analyser and expired carbon dioxide by an 801D analyser (P.K. Morgan Instruments Inc., Rainham, U.K.). This equipment was interfaced with a Sperry/Unisys Micro IT (286) computer, and gas concentration data averaged every 10 s, with subsequent calculation of oxygen uptake ($\dot{V}O_2$), carbon dioxide output ($\dot{V}CO_2$), expired ventilation ($\dot{V}E$), and respiratory exchange ratio (RER), using Wyvern software (P.K. Morgan Instruments Inc., Rainham, U.K.). The system was calibrated before each session with standard gases of known oxygen and carbon dioxide concentration. Heart rate was continuously recorded during exercise.

Maximal oxygen uptake was accepted as maximal aerobic power if a plateau occurred in oxygen uptake, i.e. an increase less than 2 ml/kg with an increase in work load. If this was not achieved peak oxygen uptake was accepted if one of two criteria was met: a heart rate of greater than 95% of the predicted maximum corrected for age, or an RER over 1.0 (Bunc et al., 1987).

2.3 Statistical methods
Descriptive statistics of mean and standard deviations were calculated for all variables measured. Statistical significance of the differences were tested using Kruskal-Wallis analysis of variance of ranks (Campbell, 1974). All procedures were performed with the assistance of SAS software on a P.C.. Group differences were considered significant at a level of P<0.05.

3 Results

Physical characteristics and peak oxygen uptake in relation to sexual maturity are presented for soccer players and the reference group in Table 1. Comparison of the two populations showed that they were of similar chronological age, height and body mass. In the more mature boys the soccer population had higher values of absolute peak oxygen uptake than the reference population.

Soccer players peak $\dot{V}O_2$ in relation to body mass was superior to the reference group at all stages of maturity (Fig. 1). In the soccer players body mass related peak $\dot{V}O_2$ was shown to be significantly related to sexual maturity (P<0.01). No significant differences were found between stages 1 and 3 or between stages 4 and 5. There was however a significant difference in peak $\dot{V}O_2$ related to body mass between sexual maturity stages 3 and 4 (P<0.01). The more mature boys (stage 5) demonstrated a significantly higher (P<0.01) peak $\dot{V}O_2$ (ml/kg/min) than the less mature boys (stage 1).

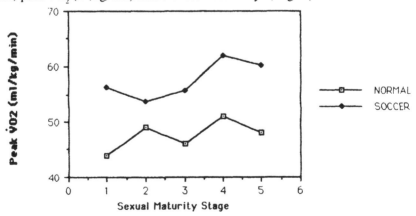

Fig. 1. Peak relative oxygen uptake in relation to sexual maturity.

Table 1. Physical characteristics and peak oxygen uptake with reference to sexual maturity

Sexual Maturity Stage	N	Age (yr)	Height (cm)	Body Mass (kg)	Peak $\dot{V}O_2$ (l/min)	Peak $\dot{V}O_2$ (ml/kg/min)
Soccer						
1	10	12.6	150.2	39.1	2.2	56.2
		0.1	2.9	4.1	0.2	3.7
2	11	12.8	151.0	39.3	2.1	53.7
		0.3	3.8	4.5	0.3	9.8
3	7	13.7	157.1	44.1	2.4	55.6
		1.1	4.4	4.2	0.1	4.7
4	13	14.9	167.9	55.4	3.4	62.0
		1.2	7.7	8.3	0.6	6.2
5	23	15.8	174.9	66.3	4.0	60.2
		1.1	5.5	7.3	0.5	6.0
Normal (Armstrong et al., 1991)						
1	7	11.9	148.0	41.5	1.8	44.0
		0.8	7.0	13.7	0.4	7.0
2	28	12.2	149.0	40.3	2.0	49.0
		0.7	7.0	7.6	0.4	7.0
3	13	12.9	153.0	41.0	1.9	46.0
		1.0	7.0	5.6	0.4	8.0
4	14	14.6	167.0	53.4	2.8	51.0
		1.0	10.0	11.6	0.6	6.0
5	15	14.4	170.0	60.4	2.9	48.0
		1.2	9.0	9.8	0.3	7.0

Values are means and SD

4 Discussion

The problems of studying the effects of training in children are that the simultaneous effects of growth, development and maturation may mask or be greater than those brought about by a particular training programme. It has been found in comparisons between active and inactive untrained subjects that relative $\dot{V}O_2$ max declines with decreasing activity (Mirwald & Bailey, 1986). This would indicate that the reduction in $\dot{V}O_2$ max is an effect of physical inactivity rather than an effect of changes occurring in growth and maturation. In studies of early and late maturing active boys it was found that they both reached similar values of $\dot{V}O_2$ max at maturity (Cunningham and Paterson, 1988).

In the soccer and the reference populations (Armstrong et al., 1991) absolute peak $\dot{V}O_2$ followed a similar pattern and corresponded to previous data which have shown that boys increase their absolute peak $\dot{V}O_2$ with age between 6 and 16 years (Wells, 1986). If data are presented in relative terms, peak $\dot{V}O_2$ in ml of oxygen per kg of body weight, it is immediately clear that there are differences between the two groups. This observed difference, agrees with the majority of investigations which have shown that in children peak VO_2 increases with cardiorespiratory training (Krahenbuhl, Skinner & Kohrt, 1985). Although it is not clear whether training before puberty is as effective as training following puberty, our results indicate that the most pronounced change in relative peak $\dot{V}O_2$ occurred towards the end of puberty. These findings agree with the work done by Mirwald and Bailey (Mirwald et al., 1981). There was also an observed increase in the later stages of puberty in the reference population, although this was not found to be statistically significant.

Aerobic training in pre- and post-pubertal youth footballers appears to have a marked effect on cardiorespiratory fitness levels when compared to untrained children of the same sexual maturity stage. In the more mature boys there is a further significant increase in fitness levels which is probably a result of growth and maturation rather than training. It is important therefore that sports scientists, physical educators and coaches take sexual maturity into account when evaluating physical performance capacity of young soccer players.

Analysis of the longitudinal data will make it possible to take in to account the effects of growth and development so that changes brought about by training alone can be investigated. The initial results from this cross-sectional study suggest that aerobic training before puberty does have a beneficial effect which is further improved as the individual reaches the end of maturity.

5 Acknowledgements

This work was funded by the Sports Council Research Unit.

6 References

Armstrong, N., Williams J., Balding, J., Gentle, P. and Kirby, B. (1991) The peak oxygen uptake of British children with reference to age, sex and sexual maturity. **Europ. J. Appl. Physiol.**, 62, 369-375

Astrand, P., and Rodahl, K. (1970) **Textbook of Work Physiology**. McGraw-Hill Kogakusha Ltd., Tokyo, pp. 1-669.

Bunc, V., Heller, J., Leso, J., Sprynarova, S. and Zdanowicz, R. (1987) Ventilatory threshold in various groups of highly trained athletes. **Int. J. Sports Med.**, 8, 275-280.

Campbell, R.C. (1974) **Statistics for Biologists.** Cambridge University Press., Cambridge, pp 61-63

Cunningham, D. and Paterson, D. (1988) Physiological characteristics of young active boys, in **CompetitiveSports forChildren and Youth: An Overview of Research and Issues.** (eds E.W. Brown and C.F. Branta) Human Kinetics Books, Champaign, Illinois, pp. 159-169.

Kemper, H., Dekker, H., Ootjers, M., Post, B., Snel, J., Splinter, P., Storm-van Essen, L. and Verschuur, R. (1983) Growth and health of teenagers in the Netherlands: survey of multidisciplinary studies and comparison to recent results of a Dutch study. **Int. J. Sports Med.**, 4, 202-214.

Krahenbuhl, G., Skinner, J. and Kohrt, W. (1985) Developmental aspects of maximal aerobic power in children. **Exerc. Sport Sci. Rev.**, 13, 503-538.

Malina, R. (1990) Growth, exercise, fithess, and later outcomes, in **Exercise, Fitness and Health.** (eds C. Bouchard, R.J. Shephard, T. Stephens, J.R. Sutton and B.D. McPherson), Human Kinetics Books, Champaign, Illinois, pp 637-653.

Mirwald, R., Bailey, D., Cameron, N. and Rasmussen, R. (1981) Longitudinal comparison of aerobic power in active and inactive boys aged 7.0 to 17.0 years. **Ann. Hum. Biol,.** 8, 405-414.

Mirwald, R. and Bailey, D. (1986) **Maximal Aerobic Power.** Pear Creative Ltd., London Ontario, pp. 1-80.

Rowley, S. (1986) The effect of intensive training on young athletes: A review. **Sports Council Publication Unit,** London, England.

Rutenfranz, J., Andersen, K., Seliger, V., Klimmer, F., Berndt, I. and Ruppe, M. (1981) Maximum aerobic power and body composition during the puberty growth period: similarities and differences between children of two European countries. **Europ. J. Pediatrics ,** 136, 123-133.

Seliger, V., Cermak, V., Handzo, P., Horak, J., Jirka, Z., Macek, M., Pribil, M., Rous, J., Skranc, O., Ulbrich, J. and Urbanek, J. (1971) Physical fitness of the Czechoslovak 12- and 15-year-old population. **Acta Paed. Scand Suppl.**, 217, 37-41.

Tanner, J. '(1962) **Growth at Adolescence**. Blackwell Scientific Publications Inc., Boston. ed 2.

Wells, C. (1986) The effects of physical activity on cardiorespiratory fitness in children. in **Effects of Physical Activity on Children.** (eds H.A. Stull and H.M. Eckert) Human Kinetics Publishers, Champaign, Illinois, pp114-124.

A COMPARATIVE STUDY OF EXPLOSIVE LEG STRENGTH IN ELITE AND NON-ELITE YOUNG SOCCER PLAYERS

J. GARGANTA ; J. MAIA ; R. SILVA & A. NATAL
Faculty of Sport Sciences and Physical Education. University of Porto, Portugal

1 Introduction

Motor and mental performance, in soccer , are affected by a variety of factors. During play, a single action is affected by the presence of opposing and supporting players, in such a way that it is difficult to recognize and rank a single task in the whole. Nevertheless, it seems that there are important characteristics that contribute to the competitive success in a soccer match , such as neuromuscular performance, especially during the various sprints and jumping activities taking place repeatedly during competitive soccer games (Bosco, 1980).

Little regard has been devoted to the fitness status of young soccer players. Therefore, the purpose of the present study was to evaluate and compare neuromuscular performance characteristics of explosive leg strength in young soccer players of different competitive levels.

2 Material and Methods

The sample comprised 40 athletes divided in two groups: 23 national team soccer players (Elite) and 17 regional soccer players (Non-Elite). Table 1 shows the characteristics of the sample.

Table 1. Physical characteristics of the young soccer players according to competitive level: Elite and Non-Elite

Variables	Elite (n = 23)	Non-Elite (n = 17)
Age (yrs)	16.1 ± 0.4	15.6 ± 0.6
Height (cm)	171.1 ± 4.5	166.7 ± 5.4 *
Body mass (kg)	65.8 ± 5.1	60.1 ± 8.7 *
Endomorphy	2.3 ± 0.5	2.2 ± 0.8
Mesomorphy	4.9 ± 0.7	5.1 ± 0.8
Ectomorphy	2.5 ± 0.5	2.7 ± 0.9

* $P < 0.05$

Testing procedures consisted of:

i) Shuttle run
In the shuttle run the subjects run a 4 x 5.50 m distance at maximal speed from a standing position.
ii). Jumping performance
The jumping test consisted of a maximal vertical squat jump from a static semi-squat position (SJ) and a maximal counter-movement jump (CMJ) on a force platform. This was performed according to Bosco (1980).

3 Results

Results are shown in Table 2.

Table 2. Mean (±SD) values for Shuttle run, SJ and CMJ

Variables	Elite (n = 23)	Non-Elite (n = 17)
Shuttle run (s)	7.2 ± 0.2	7.6 ± 0.3 **
SJ (cm)	33.3 ± 3.5	30.3 ± 3.4 ‡
CMJ (cm)	34.7 ± 3.4	31.6 ± 3.5 ‡

** $P < 0.0001$; ‡ $P < 0.01$

All the results demonstrating significant differences in the three tests, favoured elite players.

4 Discussion

Raven et al. (1976) and Thomas & Reilly (1979) found no differences in explosive leg strength between professional soccer players of different levels. The same trend occurred in the study of Luhtanen (1984) when he compared elite and non-elite young soccer players. The present findings demonstrated the opposite: elite young soccer players evidenced more significant results in sprinting time, squat jump and counter-movement jump than the non-elite ones.
Although soccer presents a complex performance model, this study shows that at this age and competition level, it seems possible to differenciate two kinds of players according to their explosive leg strength level. This implies that greater demands on explosive strength are probably placed upon elite players according to the structure of modern soccer.

5 Ackowledgements

The authors ackowledges the contribuition of the Sub-16 National Team Head Coach, Carlos Queiroz and Assistent Coaches, Nelo Vingada e Rui Caçador, for the present study.

6 References

Bosco, C. (1980) Elasticity and Football, in First Int. Congress on Sports Medicine Applied to Football . Proceedings. vol. II. ed. Vechiet L. Roma, pp 629 - 637.

Luhtanen, P. (1984) Evaluación fisica de los jugadores de futbol. Apunts . XXI, 99-102.

Raven, P.B. Gettman, L.R. Pollock, M.L. and Cooper, K.H. (1976) A physiological evaluation of professional soccer players. Brit. J. Sports Med., 10, 209-216.

Thomas, V. and Reilly, T. (1979) Fitness assessment of english league soccer players through the competitive season. Brit. J. Sports Med., 13, 103-109.

THE APPLICATION OF THREE MODES OF GOAL SETTING TO GOAL SHOOTING WITH SCHOOLBOY SOCCER PLAYERS

S. FISHER[1], R.D. THORPE[2], and A. CALE[3]

[1]   West London Institute of Higher Education, London, England
[2]   Loughborough University, Loughborough, England
[3]   Staffordshire Polytechnic, Stoke-on-Trent, England

1   Introduction

Recent theoretical and empirical studies into goal setting have questioned the transferability and applicability of research findings obtained in organisational and industrial settings to the sporting environment (Hall and Byrne, 1988). It has been suggested that teachers and coaches may have prematurely, albeit intuitively, accepted such findings and this may account for the lack of literature concerning the effect of goa setting in the realm of sport, and specifically soccer. The purpose of this study was to evaluate whether theory taken from organisational and industrial settings would be applicable in a soccer situation.

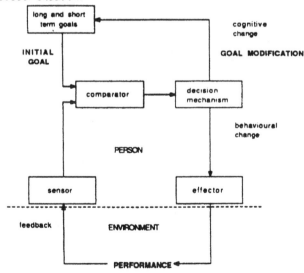

Fig.1. <u>An adapted control systems model of motivation:
modelled after Powers (1973).</u>

The theory under investigation was based around a control systems model of motivation first outlined by Powers (1973). The model begins with a goal that is set, for example, by the coach or teacher. This may be a long or a short term goal. This information is fed into what is termed a "comparator". This is essentially the "thinking part" of the individual or player, where a perception is formulated as to how easy or difficult the goal that has been assigned will be. At this point s/he will either "accept" or "reject" this goal. If s/he rejects it, there may be some form of cognitive change and the goal may be modified to something more suitable. If s/he accepts the goal, signals will be sent to the effector system where muscle actions are determined and executed to allow performance to take place. Once the performance is over, feedback from the environment will be used to assess whether s/he has achieved the particular goal. This process can obviously be repeated as long as some form of original goal is present. The purpose of this particular study is to establish whether such a model can be applied to a soccer situation under three different modes of initial goal setting.

2   Method

The present study used 30 schoolboy association footballers aged between 11 and 13. All 30 subjects were allowed 6 warm up attempts followed by 20 practice trials on a soccer shooting task with their preferred foot. The task was constructed and validated by the English Football Association in 1987 and was subsequently used in its Coca Cola Award schemes.

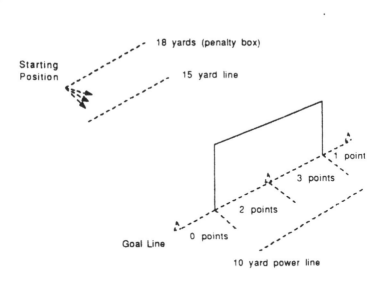

Fig.2. The goal shooting task.

The task required subjects to begin from a starting position to the left hand side of the penalty area. The ball was played in front of the player and they were required to shoot for goal before they got to a line 15 yards (13.72m) away from goal. They received points for each shot, provided it ended up beyond the "10 yard power line" behind the goal. This was to ensure that the players did not simply roll the ball into the goal. If the shot missed at the near post 0 points were scored. If the shot went into the goal in the near-post half of the goal 2 points were scored. If the shot went into the goal at the far-post half of the goal a maximum 3 points were awarded. If they just missed at the far post 1 point was scored but a shot anywhere else received 0 points.

After an initial warm-up, each player had 20 shots in a practice condition with no particular goal assigned to them. The sum points for the 20 shots were calculated for each individual and the players ranked on the basis of this ability score. The players were then assigned into one of three goal setting groups in an attempt to equate the three groups in terms of original ability on the shooting task.

All the subjects returned the day after their practice condition and were assigned to their experimental groups. All subjects in the first group were assigned individual goals. A specific, difficult goal was assigned that was set at 30%* above each individual's practice score. The second group was also assigned a specific goal, but this time the goal was based on the group mean score, rather than the individual score. The mean score of the 10 subjects was calculated and then a goal 30%* above this mean was assigned to all the subjects in that group. The third and final group were simply set a vague, "do your best" goal. (*A goal 30% above the criterion score was selected because this had been reported as being perceived as "very difficult" and therefore challenging.)

All subjects were informed of their goal immediately prior to performing 6 warm-up trials and then proceeded to perform their 20 shots in their experimental condition. Immediately after performance the subjects were required to respond to a question relating to goal modification.

Did you stick to the goal given to you?   Yes or No.

If the answer was no, there were further questions which identified whether the new goal was higher or lower than that which was originally assigned.

3   Results

The most obvious question the soccer coach will ask is - "Does it work, do certain procedures produce higher scores?"

Because of the way subjects were assigned to groups, "practice scores" were similar between conditions. However, differences did emerge when the groups performed under the experimental conditions.

The setting of "do your best goals" appears to have caused a slight reduction in performance when compared with the practice trials, but this difference was not statistically significant (p>0.05). Similarly, although there was a slight increase in performance when a "group goal" is set, this was again not statistically significant

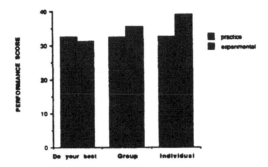

Fig.3. Performance scores on the soccer shooting task.

(p>0.05). However, in the third group in which specific goals were "individually assigned", performance was greater when compared to the practice condition (p<0.05). When comparisons were made between group scores obtained on the experimental conditions, there appeared to be a trend for the scores to increase as the more specific goals were assigned. The performance scores rose from the rather vague "do your best" to the more focussed "group goal" and then again to the specific "individually assigned goal". Whilst this trend is in keeping with the findings in the literature it is important to note that only the difference between "do your best" and "individually assigned" goals reached statistical significance (p<0.05).

Having assessed the effects of different goal setting procedures on his/her players the coach may ask the question "Are my players accepting the goals I set?"

Turning to the results relating to goal modification, all of the subjects in the "do your best" group reported that they did not stick to the goal that had been set for them. Eight out of ten subjects assigned the group goal also reported modifying their goal. In contrast, only one subject in the individually assigned goal condition modified his goal. It would appear, on the basis of these results, that individuals did modify their goals to varying extents depending on the nature of the initial goal that was assigned to them. Interestingly, all the subjects who modified their goals in both the "group" and "do your best" groups reported that their modified goal was higher than that originally assigned.

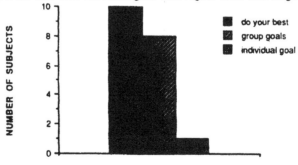

THREE GOAL SETTING GROUPS
Fig.4. Extent of goal modification across three goal setting groups.

310

4   Discussion

It would appear that different modes of goal setting have differing effects in terms of both goal modification and eventual performance outcome, at least on a soccer shooting task in schoolboy soccer players. The individualised, specific and difficult goals do seem to facilitate performance better than vague, "do your best" instructions. Perhaps more importantly, these results provide some evidence that goal setting should be viewed as a dynamic process, with the individual being seen as an active processor of information, who monitors the environment, assesses the situation and has the capability to assign modified self-set goals. It is important that teachers and coaches understand such processes since the issue of introducing specific and difficult goals on an individual basis, in order to maximise performance, is based upon them. To emphasize this importance, let us relate these results back to the theoretical model outlined earlier. What implications do they have for the practitioner?
Firstly, if at all possible, the teacher or coach should aim to set specific, difficult goals based around the ability of each individual in the group. Having assigned such goals, the teacher or coach should expect each individual to assess whether this goal is suitable to his/her level of ability and should not be surprised if the individual decides to modify the goal which has been set. If the performer modifies the goal, but sees this as contrary to the aims of the teacher or coach, then a potential source of conflict may result. It would seem wise for the coach to consider involving the performer in the goal setting process so that modifications, if necessary, occur in a supportive environment.
It should be noted that it is the perceived ability of the individual that is important and not necessarily the actual ability level. It may well be that the goal is an appropriate one for the individual but that the individual perceives it as too difficult. In these circumstances, the coach may have to "persuade" the individual that he/she do possess the necessary ability or reduce the goal to something that is perceived to be within reach. The interaction of goal setting and self-confidence is central to effective teaching and coaching but outside the remit of this paper.
Finally, the effectiveness of both short and long term goal setting is dependent upon the appropriate feedback being available to the individual. If particular goals have been assigned, the coach should ensure that feedback that is directly relevant to these goals is extracted from the environment for immediate use by the individual.
The original purpose of this study was to evaluate whether theory taken from organisational and industrial settings would be applicable in a soccer situation. Hopefully, the reader can now see how such a theoretical model may have some relevance to the real world and how it may be used by the coach or teacher in applied settings.

5.   References

Hall, H. K. and Byrne, A. T. J. (1988) Goal setting in sport: Clarifying recent anomalies. J. Sport and Exerc. Psychol. 10, 184-198.

Locke, E. A., Saari, L. M., Shaw, K. N. and Latham, G. P. (1981) Goal setting and task performance. Psychol. Bull., 90, 125-152.

Powers, W. T. (1973) Feedback: Beyond Behaviourism. Science, 179, 351-356.

Russell, R. (1988) Coca-Cola Football Association Soccer Star. English Football Association, London.

SOCCER SKILLS TECHNIQUE TESTS FOR YOUTH PLAYERS: CONSTRUCTION AND IMPLICATIONS

J.H.A. VAN ROSSUM & D. WIJBENGA
Department of Psychology, Faculty of Human Movement Sciences,
Free University, Amsterdam, the Netherlands

1 Introduction

Junior soccer players are being educated into real soccer players. They have to learn the ingredients of the game during their junior years. According to 56 Dutch soccer trainers of junior youth teams a series of characteristics is important to achieve success as a soccer player (the trainers were asked to do so in a questionnaire which purported to describe various aspects of their training during the soccer season, cf. Van Rossum & Kunst, this Volume). On a scale of 0 to 10 they rated the importance of each of the following characteristics (mean rating between brackets): physical fitness (7.96), social guidance (7.23), mental fitness (8.14), natural endowment (7.48), technique (8.30), tactical ability (8.30), intensity of practice (7.96), social interaction with trainer, coach etc. (8.14), social interaction with team mates (8.66). If the trainer should try to incorporate each of these characteristics in his training according to their rated importance, the number and length of training sessions would drastically increase!

In the questionnaire study, one of the findings with respect to technique was that about half of the trainers would want to measure it; those trainers who did measure technique all used a self-devised task/test (Van Rossum & Kunst, this Volume). In the present study the scientific literature has been surveyed for soccer skills technique tests; some empirical work has subsequently been carried out in order to adapt/change an existing test for usage with junior soccer players.

2 Existing soccer skills technique tests

An examination of the scientific literature on sport skills tests yielded 21 soccer tests measuring technique. Of these, 11 tests are unacceptable from a scientific point of view, as no information is available about their objectivity, reliability and validity. In the remaining 10 tests, only one matches each of these scientific standards well: a German test designed for sport-students (Kuhn, 1978).

Kuhn's (1978) test comprises the five following tasks: (a) goal-kicking for accuracy (distance to goal: 16.5 m); (b) passing for accuracy (distances: 30 and 40 m); (c) slalom dribble (9 flag staffs); (d) juggling ('keep the ball in the air'; 2 versions); (e) a circuit task, combining dribble and goal-kick (timed). Task (a) and (b) are carried out with the preferred as well as non-preferred foot; the score is the summed total across both feet.

In order to ascertain the ease of administration of Kuhn's (1978) test, the test was administered to the junior A-1 selections of two professional soccer clubs (Ajax, Amsterdam and PSV, Eindhoven). It was concluded that some tasks needed revision ('goal-kicking for accuracy' - adaptation of scoring procedure; 'passing for accuracy' - too easy; 'slalom dribble' - too easy) and that the dribble-goal-kick task should be abandoned (apparently measuring technique as well as aspects of physical fitness).

3 Method

On the basis of pilot-work with several versions of particular tasks (amateur soccer club, Amsterdam) six tasks were chosen for the final version of the soccer test. The tasks included in the final version of the soccer test are:
a. goal-kicking for accuracy (distance to goal: 16.5m)
            5 times preferred foot (max: 15 points)
            5 times non-preferred foot (max.: 15 points)
b. (ground) passing for accuracy
            (A or B juniors 30m; C juniors 20m)
            5 times preferred foot (max: 15 points)
            5 times non-preferred foot (max.: 15 points)
c. (air) passing for accuracy
            (A or B juniors 30m; C juniors 20m)
            5 times preferred foot (max: 5 points)
            5 times non-preferred foot (max.: 5 points)
d. dribbling (slalom; 9 staff flags)
            (distance between flags 1.5m)
            2 trials
e. juggling-1 (all parts of body permitted, except hands/arms)
            (each ball-contact 1 point, max.: 100 points)
            2 trials
f. juggling-2 (identical to task e. except that the
            ball may not hit the same part of the
            body twice in succession)
            (each ball-contact 1 point, max.: 100 points)
            2 trials

The test was evaluated in three stages. The first stage was the administration of each of the tasks to junior soccer players of three amateur clubs in the vicinity of Amsterdam, each of which was known for their well-organized youth training and each had teams at the highest competition level at each age-level (A, B and C juniors; age 17-18, 15-16 and 13-14, respectively). In total 116 players were tested (A-1: n=36; B-1: n=35; C-1: n=45). The data of this first stage were analysed in order to determine the distribution of individual scores (discriminability of test scores), the scoring procedure (summation of scores for tasks using preferred and non-preferred leg; summation of scores for tasks with two trials), and the differences of mean scores between players at A, B and C-level (validity of test scores).

The second stage consisted of a repeated administration of the tasks after 4 weeks (1 amateur club: A, B and C juniors: n=24) in order to determine the reliability (stability) of the scores.

For the <u>third</u> stage in the evaluation of the test data, each of the trainers was asked to indicate which three of his players would obtain the best and worst scores at each of the tasks. Differences of mean scores between the best and worst players, who had been pointed out by their trainers, would yield indications on the content-validity of test scores.

4 Results

4.1 Administration of tasks

Each of the tasks was administered to junior players (n=116), of three different age-levels (A, B, and C juniors). The distribution of individual scores proved to be satisfactory for each of the tasks with the exception of 'passing for accuracy through the air' (most players obtain very low scores).

The scoring procedure is evaluated on the basis of the product-moment correlation coefficient. For the tasks using both preferred and non-preferred leg, values ranging from 0.007 (p>0.05) to 0.17 (p>0.05) were obtained, suggesting that scores of both versions should better be analysed separately instead of being summed. For tasks with two trials, values between 0.33 (p<0.005) and 0.63 (p<0.005) were found, suggesting scores of both trials should be summed and divided by two to obtain final score.

The differences of mean scores between A, B and C-level players were analysed for each of the tasks. For tasks with identical versions for A, B, and C-level players significant statistical differences between levels (3 groups) were found, using ANOVA ('goal-kicking for accuracy': F (2, 113) = 3.21; p=0.04; 'dribbling': F (2, 113) = 5.59; p=0.005; 'juggling-1': F (2, 113) = 20.43; p=0.0001; 'juggling-2': F (2, 113) = 7.28; p=0.001) (see Figure 1).

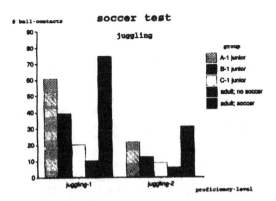

Figure 1.
Mean score at tasks "juggling-1" and "juggling-2" for A, B and C juniors (present study) and adults (Kuhn, 1978; in this study one group of adults did not have any regular soccer experience, the other group practised soccer in regular clubs. (Cf. section 3 for description of both tasks.)

For tasks with identical versions for A and B-level players significant statistical differences between levels (2 groups) were obtained, using ANOVA ('passing for accuracy on the ground': $F (1, 69) = 4.13$; $p=0.046$; 'passing for accuracy through the air': $F (1, 69) = 4.52$; $p=0.037$ (see Figure 2), except for (ground) passing with preferred leg ($F (1, 69) = 1.82$; $p=0.18$).

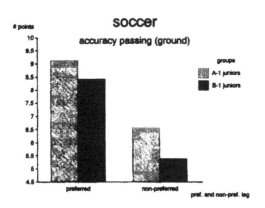

Figure 2.
Mean score at task "passing for accuracy on the ground" for A and B juniors, separately for the preferred and non-preferred leg. Distance is 30m.

4.2 Repeated administration of tasks
A second administration of the tasks was carried out four weeks after the first one. Pearson product-moment correlation coefficients between scores obtained at the first and the second administration were calculated for each of the tasks. Values vary between 0.63 ($p<0.005$) and 0.88 ($p<0.005$), indicating reasonably reliable scores.

4.3 Content-validity of tasks
The scores of the best and worst players according to the trainer were compared at each of the tasks.
At A-level, 5 of 6 mean scores were significantly lower for the worst players compared to the best players, using ANOVA (goal-kick, passing for accuracy ('ground' as well as 'air'), juggling (both 1 and 2); F-values $(1, 14)$ ranging from 5.61 ($p=0.03$) to 28.50 ($p=0.0001$). No significant difference was found at 'slalom dribble' task ($F (1, 14) = 1.58$; $p=0.23$).
At B-level, 3 of 6 mean scores proved significantly different. Differences were obtained for goal-kick, juggling-1 and juggling-2 (F-values $(1, 14)$ ranging from 12,87 ($p=0.003$) to 19.46 ($p=0.001$)). No difference were found for passing for accuracy (both 'ground' and 'air') and slalom dribble (F-values $(1, 14)$ ranging from 0.88 ($p=0.36$) to 2.68 ($p=0.12$)).

At C-level, all 6 mean scores were significantly different between worst and best players in the expected direction (F-values (1, 14) ranging from 4.75 (p=0.045) to 18.28 (p=0.001).

5 Discussion and conclusions

For the measurement of soccer technique, various instruments are available. Although many tests should be avoided from a scientific point of view (lacking information on the reliability and validity of the test) several tests do match scientific standards. It is relevant, however, to evaluate tests also on their usefulness (ease of administration by trainers, cf. Bös, 1984). An adaptation of Kuhn's (1978) soccer test was suggested in pilot-work.

The six tasks of the final version of the soccer test were administered to 116 junior players. While it appeared that the tasks yielded reliable and valid scores, the necessity to separate scores for preferred and non-preferred leg was also apparent. The tasks appear to indicate proficiency of fundamental soccer techniques (tasks discriminate between players within a team and between teams at different age-levels), except for the task 'air passing for accuracy'. For this latter skill very low scores were obtained by the Dutch players (see Figure 3), compared to the East-German norms (Rogalski & Degel, 1990) for the same age-levels. This task obviously needs further empirical work and/or practice by players of the investigated teams.

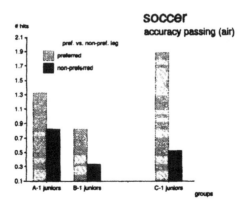

Figure 3.
Mean number of hits at task "passing for accuracy through the air" for A, B and C juniors, separately for the preferred and the non-preferred leg. Distance is 30m for A and B juniors, 20m for C juniors.

A test measuring aspects of soccer technique might be used for several reasons. From the perspective of the trainer the scores might inform him about the present performance level of players, and/or, with repeated administration, about the performance changes within players. Test scores might also indicate to the trainer which player(s) might need specific (extra) practice. Further, scores (at the team-level) might be used as a measurement of a set goal for practice, and/or an refinement of a practice goal.

From the perspective of the player, test scores might stimulate or motivate players (to increase individual practice; increase of inter-individual competitiveness). The scores obtained with a test provide objective feedback to players about their present status and/or effect of (extra) practice.

It is claimed that the test is a valuable tool in the context of the motor learning process since it conveys direct and comparable feedback information to the players, while it also hands objective information to the trainer, enabling him to measure and chart the technical improvement of individual players and improving, eventually, the process of selection as a whole over a period of years.

6 References

Bös, K. (1984) Testanwendung in der Trainingspraxis. Lehrwesen, 37 (17 Oktober), 23-27.

Kuhn, W. (1978) Leistungsverfassung im Sportspiel: Entwicklung einer Fussball-Spezifischen Testbatterie. Verlag Karl Hofmann, Schorndorf.

Rogalski, N. & Degel, E. (1990). Soccer for youth: Fundamental techniques and training routines. Sport Books Publisher, Toronto.

Van Rossum, J.H.A. & Kunst, R. (1991) The usage of skills tests by trainers of youth teams: tests of physical fitness and technique. Paper presented at the Second World Congress on Science and Football (Veldhoven, The Netherlands: May, 1991).

THE USAGE OF SKILLS TESTS BY TRAINERS OF YOUTH TEAMS: TESTS OF PHYSICAL FITNESS AND TECHNIQUE

J.H.A. VAN ROSSUM & R. KUNST
Department of Psychology, Faculty of Human Movement Sciences,
Free University, Amsterdam, the Netherlands

1 Introduction

In empirical studies on the usage of skills in the context of sport (Bös, 1984; 1987), it was found that if trainers obtain information on the level of physical fitness and technique (motor skills), they do so mostly by way of self-constructed tests; of course, this results in problems when comparing data collected earlier and later, for example. Another finding in these studies is that if trainers do not employ scientific tests, this is mainly because of practical reasons (test takes too long to administer, and so on).

In this paper some results are reported of a replication of these studies with soccer trainers of youth teams. Against the background of the basic assumption that junior soccer players are being educated into real soccer players and that they, therefore, have to learn the ingredients of the game, several questions have been put to soccer trainers about the importance of measuring relevant skills. The present paper adresses some of these questions regarding physical fitness and technical ability.

2 Method

Questionnaires to obtain information about the structure and content of the training during the soccer season 1989-1990 were sent to eighty-seven trainers of first teams at A-level (17-18 years), B-level (15-16 years) and C-level (13-14 years) of 29 amateur clubs in the soccer districts of Amsterdam and Haarlem. The questionnaires were sent by mail. Response was obtained from 56 trainers (64%); from pilot-work it was estimated that completing the questionnaire takes about one hour.

Each of the responding trainers was male; each trainer turned out to have been active as a soccer player; 39 trainers (70%) were officially qualified (KNVB-certificate). In Table 1 some background information on the trainers is presented (age of the trainers, number of years active as soccer player and number of years active as soccer trainer).

Nearly every team at each age-level has two practice sessions per week; the length of the session increases with age (total mean practice time per week in hours for A-, B- and C-teams turned out to add to about 3.5 hours, 3.0 hours and 2.5 hours, respectively).

Table 1. Age, number of years active as soccer player and active as soccer trainer of the responding trainers (n=56).

	age (yrs)	years soccer-player	years soccer-trainer
A-1 level: 20 trainers	36.4	21.8	10.8
B-1 level: 17 trainers	32.9	20.7	8.5
C-1 level: 19 trainers	36.6	23.7	9.9

3 Results

3.1 Importance of physical fitness and technique
In order to get an indication of the importance of several characteristics, the trainers were asked to rate each of nine characteristics on a 0-10 scale for their importance for success in soccer. Each characteristic proved to be important: no characteristic obtained a mean rating less than 7. Physical fitness received a mean rating of 7.96, technique of 8.30 (for a complete overview of the rated characteristics, see Van Rossum & Wijbenga, this Volume). It can be concluded, therefore, that the trainers regarded physical fitness and technique as important characteristics for success in soccer.

3.2 Measurement of physical fitness and technique
Several questions were asked about the measurement of both characteristics. Is it important to measure physical fitness and technique, has each characteristic been measured during the recent soccer season and if so, what has been measured and which instrument has been used? In Table 2 the number is presented of those trainers who positively answered the questions, firstly, about the importance of measuring and, secondly, about their use of measurements during the season.

Table 2. Number of yes-answers on the questions 'Is it important to measure physical fitness and technique?' and 'Did you measure physical fitness and technique?' (n=56).

	physical fitness		technique	
'important...'	26	(46%)	31	(55%)
'did measure...'	26	(46%)	23	(41%)

From the figures in Table 2 it can be concluded that those who viewed it as important to measure did indeed measure the characteristic. With respect to technique, eight trainers (all but one at C-level) reported not to have measured, mainly because 'there was no assistance with measurements', 'there was not enough time in practice sessions' and 'it does not match my way of operating'.

3.2.1 Measurement of physical fitness

Physical fitness is commonly distinguished into four components: stamina, strength, flexibility and speed. The trainers who said they measured physical fitness (n=26) were asked if they measured aspects of each of these components. The results showed that not each component was measured to the same extent: while all trainers claimed to have measured stamina (26, 100%) and a large majority claimed to have measured speed (22, 85%), both strength and flexibility turned out to have been measured by 12 trainers (46%).

The next question addressed the manner (instrument) that was employed. To measure stamina, the Cooper-test was mentioned by most trainers (n=11), while some stated they employed an endurance run (n=7; no standardized distance or time). Measurement of speed was in most cases done by a sprint (n=17), with varying distances (ranging from 20 to 300 metres).

3.2.2 Measurement of technique

To measure technique several motor skills should be considered. A list of 13 fundamental soccer skills was included in the questionnaire. The trainers indicated which of these were measured (cf. Table 3).

Table 3. Number of trainers who indicated having measured the motor skill during the soccer-season (n=23).

motor skill	#	%
passing	19	(83%)
dribbling	16	(70%)
circuit (various skills)	16	(70%)
heading	15	(65%)
goal-shot	14	(61%)
deception	9	(39%)
kicking (non-preferred leg)	9	(39%)
long pass	8	(35%)

Further, skills such as accuracy-kick, corner-kick, ball juggling, throw-in and tackling were ticked by less than 20% of the trainers.

With respect to the way in which the characteristic had been measured, the trainers were unanimous: each of the various skills was measured by a task devised by the trainer himself; none of the trainers employed a scientifically constructed test as a measuring device.

3.3 Why measuring physical fitness and technique?

If the trainer answered that he regarded it as important to take measurements of physical fitness or technique, he was asked to indicate the reasons for measuring. Whereas two different questions were asked (one for physical fitness measurements and one for measuring technique), the reasons given by the trainers were essentially the same for both characteristics. The following list succinctly reproduces the

reasons mentioned by the trainers (n=43):
- it stimulates or motivates players;
- it informs the trainer about performance level of players;
- it informs the trainer about performance changes within each player (increase or drop);
- it indicates which player might profit from specific and/or extra practice;
- it can be used as a measurement of targets for purposes of training and practices (at the team level);
- it can be used to attune practice activities.

Those trainers who answered that taking measurements of physical fitness or technique was not considered important, were also asked to indicate their reasons for abstaining from measuring. Again, both the reasons for not measuring were largely identical for physical fitness and technique. This group of trainers (n=42) stated the following reasons:
- the trainer is able to evaluate such things without help;
- differences in performance levels are easily detected;
- measurements stress differences between players too much;
- it is a waste of time;
- there are not enough people to help administer the test;
- the characteristic is not or is difficult to measure;
- measurement does not inform about match-performance.

In sum, while those in favour of measuring emphasized both the relevance for the teacher, the curriculum and the pupil, the group of trainers who did not take measurements appear to base it partly on practical arguments and mainly on an attitude opposing measuring.

4 Discussion and conclusions

From the data presented it can be concluded that nearly 50% of the trainers of junior soccer teams think that it is important to measure physical fitness; a similar figure was found with respect to the importance of measuring technical aspects. The majority of those who regard it important to measure, also does measure these characteristics.

With respect to measurement, trainers employ in most cases a self-devised task and not a scientifically constructed test. Regarding the measurement of physical fitness, most trainers limit themselves to measuring stamina and speed. Those trainers who think that it is important to use measuring instruments claim that it helps the trainer as well as the players by providing feedback. Those trainers who think it is not important to take measurements claim to do so partly because of a negative attitude towards measuring and partly because of practical problems with taking the measurements.

In general, therefore, the investigation supports and extends the findings of earlier German studies on the usage of measuring instruments in the context of sport. The present results indicate that the measurement of central aspects of youth training (physical fitness and technique) does hardly profit from scientifically constructed instruments. Of the group of 56 trainers, only 14 regarded it important to measure both physical fitness and technique!

The findings have been presented for the group of 56 trainers, although 3 sub-groups of trainers were involved, engaged in teams at A, B and C level. Occasionally, the results should have been distinguished for each of these sub-groups. For example, in response to the question about the importance of measuring physical fitness, only 37% of the C level trainers answered 'yes', while 74% did so in response to the same question regarding technique (at A and B level about 50% of the trainers answered positively on each of the questions).

The importance of physical fitness and technique is rated relatively high by the trainers (cf. Introduction). This finding is supported by answers to other questions of the questionnaire. In response to the question 'do you pay explicit attention to physical fitness in practice sessions?' a large majority of the A and B level trainers confirmed this, whereas less than 50% of the C level trainers stated they had done so. The overwhelming majority of the trainers at each level claimed to have paid explicit attention to technique. The answers to yet another question corroborates this. Indicating how much of the training sessions is spent on physical fitness/technique, only 10 trainers responded they spent more than 50% of practice time at physical fitness aspects, whereas 25 trainers claimed to do so for technique. From the answers to various questions, then, the inevitable conclusion is that control over the fundamental motor skills is the central theme during the formative years of soccer players. Nevertheless, the trainers hardly use scientifically constructed tests in order to determine improvement in a more objective way. This study, then, suggests that the training process of Dutch youth soccer players is generally not approached by the trainers from a strict learning point of view, but appears to be based on a rather global and superficial view, possibly best expressed in the phrase "practice makes perfect".

5 References

Bös, K. (1984) Testanwendung in der Trainingspraxis. **Lehrwesen**, 37 (17 Oktober), 23-27.

Bös, K. (1987) **Handbuch Sportmotorischer Tests**. Verlag für Psychologie-Dr. C.J. Hogrefe, Göttingen.

Van Rossum, J.H.A. & Wijbenga, D. (1991) Soccer skills technique tests for youth players: Construction and implications. Paper presented at the Second World Congress on Science and Football (Veldhoven, The Netherlands: May, 1991).

PHILIPS, UW PROFESSIONELE PARTNER IN DE GEZONDHEIDSZORG

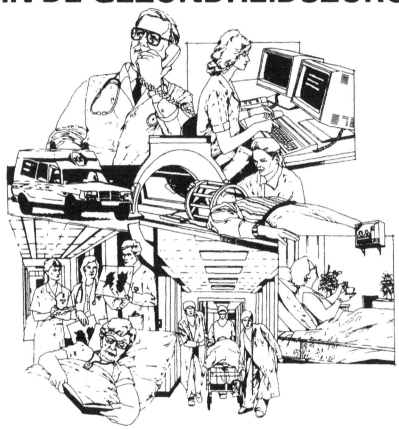

Philips weet de weg in het ziekenhuis. Kent de specifieke eisen op het gebied van medische apparatuur, automatisering, verlichting, telecommunicatie, oproepsystemen, beveiligings- en bewakingssystemen, gebouwenbeheer en distributie van radio- en TV-signalen. Heeft daar ook een antwoord op. Voor elk type ziekenhuis kan Philips een breed pakket voorzieningen aanbieden dat perfect aansluit op uw werkwijze. Compleet met de benodigde infrastructuur.

Philips brengt er lijn in. Want met apparatuur die dezelfde taal spreekt is het immers goed werken!

Uw partner voor advies, levering, begeleiding, ondersteuning en service.

Philips Nederland B.V.,
Medical Systems, Postbus 90050, 5600 PB Eindhoven,
Telefoon 040- 782715.

Philips Medical Systems

PHILIPS

PHILIPS

PART NINE

Biomechanics

THE BIOMECHANICS OF FOOTBALL

A. Lees

Sports Biomechanics Laboratory, School of Health
Sciences,Liverpool Polytechnic, Liverpool, U.K.L3 3AF.

1 Introduction

Biomechanics can be defined in general terms as a study of
the mechanical functioning of the biological system. This
definition encompasses a wide range of applications
including sports and exercise. Biomechanics applied within a
sports context is termed sports biomechanics and is
concerned exclusively with the human body as the biological
system. Further, sports biomechanics is often concerned
with the mechanical factors affecting sports and exercise
participation. These mechanical factors often relate to the
design of equipment or other apparatus used in the
performance of a sport, or the effect of environmental fluid
forces, and may encompass such activities as modelling and
computer simulation of motion. Sports biomechanics
therefore has a focus wider than the biological system as
implied by the definition at the start of this paragraph.
     When sports biomechanics is applied to football there
are a number of major areas which are of interest. Firstly
there is the equipment used in the game which covers
functional and protective clothing, including boots,
equipment such as the ball, and playing surfaces. A major
factor in the development of these products comes from
economic considerations. Parallel with this is a
concern over their functional characteristics. Therefore
biomechanics looks at these products from their ability to
provide both performance and protection. The cost may
determine the selection of a product, but does not affect an
assessment of its biomechanical effectiveness. Secondly,
biomechanics is concerned with the performance of skills and
techniques. Biomechanics offers methods by which the very
fast actions which occur in football can be recorded and
analysed in detail. There are various considerations here.
One is the general mechanical effectiveness of the movement,
another is the detailed description of the execution of the
skill, yet another is an analysis of the factors underlying
successful performance. A third major area of concern in
the biomechanics of football is with an understanding of the
causative mechanisms of injury so as to better understand

the principles of injury prevention and rehabilitation. This interest links very closely with that of medical practitioners, but while their role is in the provision of effective treatment for problems which players sustain, biomechanics attempts to form the basis of sound knowledge and understanding which can support successful medical practices. In this context medical scientists also use and apply biomechanics.

This paper attempts to look at these three major areas in turn, with illustrations from the literature.

2 Equipment

There has been much controversy in Britain concerning the use of artificial turf for playing soccer. It has been more readily accepted in North America, Scandinavia and the Middle East where there has not been the same longstanding traditions associated with the game, or where environmental considerations are important. In other parts of Europe particularly, there is little contemplation of anything other than a natural turf surface. The use of artificial turf is an issue in soccer not least because of the economic benefits that may accrue from its use, but also the impending World Cup in the USA in 1994.

There is much conjecture and opinion concerning the merits of artificial surfaces, but only a little scientific evidence. Much of this was collected in England by a commission headed by Winterbottom (1985) and supported by the English Football Association and the Sports Council. The first artificial pitch was installed in the UK in 1971, and the first Football League artificial pitch was installed at Queens Park Rangers (then in the second division) in 1980. The opinions of players, managers and club chairmen were that soccer to a high standard could be played on artificial pitches but necessitated a modification to the playing of the game which often did not suit the 'British' game. Therefore a three year moratorium was placed on the installation of artificial pitches for League football until Winterbottom's report had been considered fully. The report attempted to obtain scientific data on the comparative performance of both natural and artificial pitches. The author took several examples of each class of pitch from various levels of play and conducted a series of tests of performance characteristics. The tests were concerned with aspects of ball-surface interaction, player movement, and player-surface interaction.

The general conclusions of Winterbottom's Committee were that in some respects there were little differences between the two types of surface, but in other important respects there were. In these respects artificial surfaces could be designed to make their performance within that acceptable for natural surfaces, and the performance

of pitches already laid could be controlled by the use of
water to deaden a lively pitch and to provide a better
energy absorbing surface. Although artificial surfaces
could be tailored to suit playing requirements, one feature
of their performance does not readily match that of real
turf, and that is its variability. Generally a natural
surface is more varied both between surfaces and within an
area of a pitch, and this is thought to be a crucial element
in the game of soccer. The Football League in 1989 published
its final report after the period of moratorium and
concluded that artificial surfaces were not suitable for the
playing of the game at high level in the English League.
This unsuitability was as much to do with the subjective
judgements of how the game should be played as to the
performance, economic or injury characteristics of
artificial surfaces. In this case biomechanics furnished the
methods and techniques for evaluating the surfaces but could
not influence the final decision.

Another important aspect of equipment is that of the
soccer ball. Levendusky et al.(1988) investigated the impact
characteristics of a stitched and moulded soccer ball and
measured the force of impact using a force platform. They
found that for velocities of impact of about 18 m/s the
force of impact was about 6% higher in the stitched rather
than the moulded ball. This finding has implications for the
injury of players when heading a ball. Armstrong et al.
(1988) continued this investigation by considering the
effect of ball pressure and wetness on the impact force.
They found that if a ball was wet it could increase the
impact force by about 5% due to the extra weight as a result
of water retention, and if a ball had a pressure increase
from 6 to 12 psi (1 psi=6.975 kPa) there would be an
increase in impact force of about 8%. These results clearly
show the effect that poor combinations of conditions could
have for the impact load sustained by the head during
heading.

Biomechanics then has provided the techniques and
methods for evaluating equipment not only in terms of its
immediate physical characteristics but also in terms of its
effect on playing performance and its implication for
injury.

3 Technique analysis

Biomechanics provides methods for investigating the
performance of a skill. The skill itself can be considered
from the point of view of correct mechanical performance,
and many of the common skills in football are judged
subjectively in this way. Biomechanics also provides the
means for detailed analysis, and the detailed aspects of
performance can be related to other characteristics (such as
strength) in order to infer causation.

Kollath and Schwirtz (1988) investigated the long throw-in action of skilled players with and without a run up. They used high speed video analysis to record the action. The resultant image was digitised in order to record the position of each joint and the ball. This is a typical approach to a detailed biomechanical analysis of a skill. From the resultant data many kinematic and kinetic parameters were obtained. They found that angles at the joints did not correlate well with performance, indicating that the ranges of motion moved through were not important performance parameters. However, they did find significant correlations between time taken to cover a distance (i.e. speed of movement) and distance of the throw. These correlations had higher significances the closer the distance to the release point, indicating that the build up of speed or acceleration in the final phase of the movement is important. Although they did not measure muscular strength characteristics for their throwers, one might expect that this would relate to the increase in speed over the latter part of the movement. This relationship with muscle characteristics is something that has been found in studies relating to kicking.

Another example of a biomechanical analysis of skilled activity is that of the diving motions of a goal-keeper investigated by Suzuki et al. (1988). They analysed two skilled and two less skilled goalkeepers in terms of their ability to dive and save. They found that the more skilled keepers dived faster (4 m/s as opposed to 3 m/s) and more directly at the ball. They also presented a pictorial display of the body positions for each keeper. It was possible to detect other differences between the keepers not evident from the quantitative data. In this case the skilled keeper was able to perform a counter-movement jump and launch himself into the air and then turn to meet the ball. The less skilled keeper failed to perform a counter-movement, thereby restricting his take-off velocity and failed to turn his body effectively to meet the ball. Such qualitative analyses of technique are possible from the single picture representation of a complete action and form a valuable tool in biomechanics.

There are many skills in football, and none has been the subject of analysis more than the kicking action. This, like many of the skills in football, is developmental in nature and develops from an early age. Biomechanical techniques have been used by Elliot et al. (1980) to analyse the punt kicking action of young boys from the age of 2 to 12 years. They looked at various indicators of performance and were able to characterise six levels of development. These ranged from level 1 (average age 3.1 years) where the children often hit the ball with their knee or leg, to level 6 (average age 9.9 years) where the mature kicking pattern had been achieved by 80% of the children. The intermediate ages for levels 2 to 5 were 4.6, 4.7, 4.8, and 5.2 years.

Although chronological age was not found to be a good predictor of level of skill development, the age ranges suggest that the skill develops rapidly between the age of 4 and 6 years. This has implications for skill development and illustrated the role biomechanics can have in this area.

The relation between muscle strength and performance has been referred to above for throwing. This relation has been investigated for kicking by several researchers. Cabri et al. (1988) found that there was a high correlation between knee flexor and extensor strength as measured by an isokinetic muscle function dynamometer and kick distance. There was also a significant relationship between hip flexor and extensor strength but this was lower than that for the knee. Similar results were found by others. If muscle strength is correlated with performance then it would be expected that training should show positive effects, and this has been shown by De Proft et al. (1988).

This evidence suggests that there is a good relationship between muscle strength and performance. However, there are other factors which affect successful kick performance. These factors can be appreciated from a consideration of the relationship between foot and ball velocity. Following the treatment of Plagenhoef (1977), this can be stated as :-

$$V(ball) = V(foot).\frac{[M + m].[1 + e]}{M}$$

where V = velocity of ball and foot respectively, M = effective striking mass of the leg; m = mass of the ball; and e = coefficient of restitution. The effective striking mass is the mass equivalent of the striking object (in this case the leg) and relates to the rigidity of the limb.

The term [M + m] / M gives an indication of the rigidity of impact and relates to the muscles involved in the kick and their strength at impact. Therefore one would expect that the best correlations with performance would be with eccentric muscle strength, and the data from Cabri et al.(1988) suggest that this is the case.

The term [1 + e] relates to the firmness of the foot at impact. Because the ball is on the ground, the foot contacts the ball on the dorsal aspect of the phalanges and lower metatarsals. The large force of impact serves to forcefully plantar flex the foot and it will do so until the bones at the ankle joint reach their extreme range of motion. At this stage the foot will deform at the metatarsal-phalangeal joint. There is little to prevent considerable deformation here and this will affect the firmness of impact and the value of 'e'. Asami and Nolte (1983) measured the amount of deformation at both the ankle and the metatarsal-phalangeal joint and found that while the change in ankle joint angle did not correlate at all with ball velocity, the change in angle at the metatarsal-phalangeal joint correlated highly significantly with ball velocity. The conclusion from this is that the deformability of the foot should be reduced for powerful ball kicking and that this deformability is related to the deformation at the front of the foot.

4 Sports injury

Injury generally originates from physical causes and arises due to excess force or stress in the musculo-skeletal system over and above that which can be tolerated by the biological structures. The stress on the musculo-skeletal system can be described by forces, load rate, and frequency of application. A level of stress is necessary in order to develop structural strength, and should be a part of a training or injury rehabilitation programmes.

A question which is often asked concerning possible injuries in soccer is about the danger of heading the ball. Is the severity of impact such that it may cause short or long term injury? Levendusky et al. (1988) gave examples from the literature of where heading the ball can cause damage due to (i) surface deformation leading to broken nose, eye damage, and lacerations (ii) damage due to direct impact causing compression waves travelling through the brain creating high internal pressures, and (iii) rotational accelerations causing shearing between the brain and the skull. The levels of impact which are likely to cause injury are about 80 g for loss of consciousness and 200 g for fatalities. For rotational accelerations values greater than 5500 rad/s/s are likely to lead to a loss of consciousness.

Burslem and Lees (1988) investigated the acceleration on the head during a modest speed header (ball velocity about 7 m/s) and found that accelerations were about 60 g, and rotational accelerations about 200 rad/s/s. Clearly there is more danger from the direct impact. In a mathematical simulation of impact Townend (1988) estimated that the average acceleration of impact was about 25 g, but increased with the reduction of mass of the player and the increase in mass of the ball, supporting the results of Armstrong et al. (1988). The conclusion which can be drawn here is that although heading is below the injury threshold, it is sufficiently close to it for care to be needed, particularly in dealing with young children in the development of the skill. The skill of heading can lead to greater head and neck rigidity thereby reducing the effect of the impact. This skill must be taught properly and carefully, and a reduced ball mass should be used for younger players.

The ankle joint is one of the most vulnerable joints for a soccer player, and the boot is often relied upon to protect this joint from an inversion/eversion sprain or more serious damage. The role of the boot in protecting the ankle joint was investigated by Johnson et al. (1976). They investigated the torsional stiffness of different design boot uppers. They modelled the lower leg by a mass-spring-dashpot system which gave the joint its characteristic features with response to load. The boot added another resistive layer to the outside of the ankle allowing the natural stiffness of the joint to be supplemented by the properties of the boot. The low cut boot protected the subtalar joint, while the higher cut boot protected both this and the ankle joint. In a simulation of the effect of using materials of different stiffness, they found that if a low cut boot was used it should be made of low-stiffness material. This was because the subtalar joint had a certain amount of mobility, and if the ankle was turned a low cut boot would allow the subtalar joint to accommodate most of the movement. If the low cut boot was of stiff construction, then the boot would transfer some of the load away from the subtalar joint to the ankle joint. As this does not have any degree of flexibility in the inversion/eversion direction the additional load would be taken up by the collateral ligaments, leading to a greater likelihood of ligament damage. On the other hand the high cut boot should be made with stiff material because it already has a protective function with regard to the ankle joint and collateral ligaments. The stiffer the material, the more the load is taken by the boot material rather than the ligaments themselves. It should be noted that the high cut boot with stiff material has only about twice the stiffness of the low-cut, low-stiffness material boot, and that for a severe inversion movement even the high cut boot would be insufficient to prevent damage occurring.

5 Conclusions

This overview has shown different ways in which biomechanics can be applied to football. Many features of the games of football are amenable to mechanical treatment, and this applies not only to the body but also to equipment and the environment. There are still many opportunities for biomechanists to have a role in football science, and it is hoped that this overview will help to direct future investigations.

6 References

Asami, T. and Nolte, V. (1983) Analysis of powerful
    ball kicking, in Biomechanics VIII-B (eds H. Matsui and
    K. Kobayashi), Human Kinetics, Champaign, Illinois, pp.
    695-700.
Armstrong, C. W., Levendusky, T. A., Spryropoulous, P.

and Kugler, L. (1988) Influence of inflation pressure and ball wetness on the impact characteristics of two types of soccer balls, in Science and Football (eds T Reilly, A.Lees, K.Davids and W.J.Murphy), E. & F. N. Spon, London, pp.394-398.

Burslem, I. and Lees, A. (1988) Quantification of impact accelerations of the head during the heading of a football, in Science and Football (eds T. Reilly, A. Lees, K. Davids and W.J. Murphy), E. & F. N Spon, London, pp.243-248.

Cabri, J. De Proft, E. Dufour, W. and Clarys, J. P. (1988) The relation between muscular strength and kick performance, in Science and Football (eds T. Reilly, A. Lees, K. Davids and W.J. Murphy), E. & F. N Spon, London, pp.186-193.

De Proft, E. Cabri, J. Dufour, W. and Clarys, J. P. (1988) Strength training and kick performance in soccer, in Science and Football (eds T. Reilly, A. Lees, K. Davids and W.J. Murphy), E. & F. N. Spon, London, pp.108-113.

Elliott, B. C. Bloomfield, J. and Davies, C.M. (1980) Developmentof the punt kick: a cinematographical analysis. J. Human Movement Stud., 6, 142-150.

Football League (1989) Commission of enquiry into playing surfaces - Final Report. The Football League, Lytham St. Annes.

Johnson, G., Dowson, D. and Wright, V. (1976) A biomechanical approach to the design of football boots. J. Biomech., 9, 581-585.

Kollath, E. and Schwirtz A. (1988) Biomechanical of the soccer throw-in , in Science and Football (eds T. Reilly, A. Lees, K. Davids and W.J. Murphy), E. & F. N Spon, London, pp.460-467.

Levendusky, T.A. Armstrong, C.W. Eck, J.S. Spryropoulous, P.Jeziorowski, J. and Kugler, L. (1988) Impact characteristics of two types of soccer balls, in Science and Football (eds T. Reilly, A. Lees, K. Davids and W.J. Murphy), E. & F. N. Spon, London, pp.385-393.

Plagenhoef, S. (1971) The Patterns of Human Motion. Prentice-Hall,New Jersey.

Suzuki, S. Togari, H. Isokawa, M. Ohashi, J. and Ohgushi T.(1988) Analysis of the goalkeeper's diving motion, in Science and Football (eds T. Reilly, A. Lees, K. Davids and W.J. Murphy) E. & F. N. Spon, London, pp.468-475.

Townend, M. S. (1988) Is heading the ball a dangerous activity?, in Science and Football (eds T. Reilly, A. Lees, K. Davids and W.J. Murphy), E. & F. N. Spon, London, pp.237-242.

Winterbottom, Sir W. (1985) Artificial ,grass surfaces for Association Football - Report and Recomendations. The Sports Council,London.

THE DEMANDS ON THE SOCCER BOOT

A. Lees and P. Kewley
Sports Biomechanics Laboratory, School of Health
Sciences,Liverpool Polytechnic, Liverpool, U.K. L3 3AF.

1 Introduction

The soccer boot has evolved along traditional lines with
features being added gradually to take account of the
requirements of players and the trends within the game.
Although manufacturers take a systematic approach to boot
design, there have been few reported scientific
investigations of boot performance which have then been fed
back into design. Notable exceptions are the work reported
by Valiant et al. (1988) and Rodano et al. (1988).
    Both of these studies have presented data on the
vertical and horizontal forces. Essentially the vertical
force serves to compress the boot whereas the horizontal
forces serve to deform the boot by the action of the foot
on the boot. This could lead to deformation of the heel
cup, stretching of the boot material or even splitting of
the boot. The presentation of force data in these two
studies does not indicate how the forces will lead to boot
deterioration and have not been related to the many
different actions performed with the boot during the game.
    The actions made by a player in soccer are many and
varied and each is likely to put a unique demand on the
strength of the boot. In order to obtain an indication of
the role the boot has in the game it is necessary to
investigate the types and numbers of actions which are made
during the game. In an early study Reilly and Thomas (1976)
performed a motion analysis of the different positional
roles in professional soccer. Although differences were
found between positions of play the authors averaged the
distances covered among the different positions to give the
data shown in Table 1. Also in this table are further
comparative data from Withers et al. (1982). Both sets of
data show differences, but the general trends in distances
covered, and their respective percentages, for each
activity can be clearly seen. In addition to this
perspective both studies reported on the frequency of
occurrence of some other more specific movements. Reilly
and Thomas reported that the average number of jumps per
individual per game was 15.5 and shots was 1.4. Withers et

al. reported that the average number of tackles per individual per game was 13.1, jumps 9.4, turns 49.9 and contacts with the foot 26.1. Despite the differences between the two studies, the general trends are evident.

Table 1. Distances(m) of major movement categories
----

activity	Reilly & Thomas		Withers et al.	
	m	%	m	%
walking	2150	24.7	3026	27.0
jogging	3187	36.8	5139	45.8
cruising	1810	20.8	1506	13.4
sprinting	974	11.2	666	5.9
backing	559	6.5	874	7.9
total distance	8680		11211	

It might be expected that the more forceful actions (i.e. jumping, turning, sprinting) would be the actions putting the greater strain on the boot. Although small in number the intensity of the actions could well be a critical factor which determines the life of the boot. However, no study has been reported which attempts to combine the requirements placed on the boot in terms of playing action with the stress imposed upon it by that action. This present study attempts to investigate the physical demand which is placed on the boot during soccer playing and training. It does this by identifying the major categories of movements made during a game of soccer, and recording their frequency of occurrence. An estimate of the demand put on the boot can be obtained by measuring the physical stress (or horizontal force) on the boot during each of the categories of movements.

2 Methods

Three major procedures were used. Information on the problems associated with soccer boots was sought from both professional and amateur players using a questionnaire; data on the occurrence of key actions were collected by using a notational analysis technique; the data on the frictional force values produced during each of these key actions were obtained from the use of a Kistler force platform. The data from the latter two approaches were then combined to give an overall estimate of the demand on the boot, and related to the problems experienced by the players. The questionnaire requested players to indicate any problems they had had with their boots. In all 37 professional players (all second or third division English League) and 40 skilled amateurs were used as subjects.

From inspection of video recordings of soccer matches, ten playing actions were identified which were thought to put a high level of stress on the boot. These were turning, jumping, trapping the ball, dribbling, tackling, being tackled, hard pass, medium pass, soft pass, and shooting. The frequency of these ten playing actions was recorded over a series of games for both professional and amateur players. Professional match-play was recorded from televised broadcasts of six different English League first and second division teams. In all 12 hours of play were analysed, and the number of each playing action was recorded by reviewing the video from each game. The amateurs consisted of the Liverpool Polytechnic first team. Altogether a total of 4.5 hours of play were analysed. Twelve hours of professional training were analysed. The professionals used were from the first team members of English League second and third division teams.

Force data were collected from the supporting foot during each playing action using a Kistler force platform which was sited indoors. Some of the playing actions could not be reasonably duplicated in this manner and so were not included in the remainder of the analysis. One subject was asked to perform each of the playing actions several times on the force platform. The horizontal data were presented as a vector plot together with a 'stress-clock' (Fig. 1). The stress clock was produced by adding up the magnitudes of the force during foot contact which appeared in each of twelve 30 degree or 'hourly' segments. The 'hour', total stress and number of counts were given on the graphical output, together with their total and the sample rate.

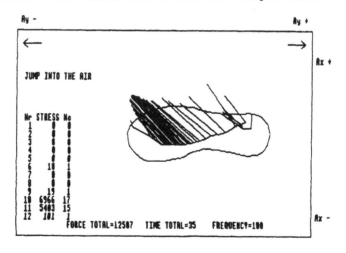

Figure 1. A stress clock for the horizontal friction force vectors acting on the shoe.

3 Results

The responses to the questionnaire are given in Table 2. All video data recorded (Table 3) were converted to an equivalent number of actions per individual per game.

Table 2   The results from the questionnaire analysis
----

	professionals	amateurs
N	37	40
age (yrs)	26.2 +/- 4.4	20.3 +/- 1.7
% sample with problems	65%	65%
splitting	27% (10)	15% (6)
soles leaving uppers	-	18%
stretching	16%	-
location of split-front	4	4
-outside	3	2
-rear	1	0
-inside	2	0

The accumulated force can be easily converted to impulse by multiplying by the sample rate (0.01 s used in this study). The accumulated impulse gives a measure of the stress applied to the boot for a given playing action. The average impulse acting on the boot can be calculated by dividing the total impulse by the duration of the action. This gives an average force acting on the boot, and is used as a 'severity index' for each of the playing actions. The mean of three trials of force data is presented in Table 4, together with the 'severity index'. The direction of force was not quantified specifically in this experiment, but a subjective impression of its direction was obtained from an inspection of the shoe stress plots similar to Figure 1. It was observed that in all cases except starting, the stress was directed primarily to the front and lateral side of the shoe. In starting it was directed to the rear and marginally to the lateral side.

4 Discussion

Although the directions of stress were not quantified in this study, a subjective evaluation has provided a useful insight into the nature of the directions of stress on the shoe.
    The occurrence of splits in the forefront and outside regions correspond very well with the main directions of the stress on the boot. Some of the playing actions identified were not amenable to the measurement of force

(eg. dribble, trap and tackles) and so these were omitted
from the analysis. Others were more relevant and were
included (e.g. locomotor actions). The average stress level
on the boot which serves as a severity index can be
integrated with the number of actions of each type
occurring during both playing and training. If this is done
the accumulated severity for 90 minutes of activity is :-

professional training	161 kN
professional match-play	58 kN
amateur match-play	50 kN

Table 3. The number of occurrences of each action per
individual per game

		full back	centre back	mid field	forward	mean
turn	prof.train	37.3	34.8	41.4	24.7	34.6
	prof.play	5.1	2.8	6.6	5.8	5.1
	amat.play	2.7	1.2	4.9	6.5	3.8
jump	prof.train	46.1	36.4	39.9	36.8	39.8
	prof.play	6.2	14.7	6.2	13.9	10.3
	amat.play	7.4	8.5	8.6	15.8	10.1
trap	prof.train	16.8	20.7	15.8	16.0	17.3
	prof.play	9.0	5.3	8.0	7.1	7.4
	amat.play	5.9	3.9	7.4	6.4	5.9
dribble	prof.train	7.9	15.4	17.0	8.5	12.4
	prof.play	11.6	6.3	12.4	8.7	9.8
	amat.play	5.8	3.3	7.6	8.6	6.4
tackle	prof.train	3.8	5.4	2.6	3.9	3.9
	prof.play	4.3	5.9	5.7	2.9	4.7
	amat.play	4.6	5.4	6.4	4.4	5.2
tackled	prof.train	1.3	0.3	2.7	1.3	1.4
	prof.play	1.3	0.4	3.5	3.8	2.6
	amat.play	1.9	1.4	2.8	4.2	3.3
hard pass	prof.train	4.3	3.6	3.6	1.5	3.3
	prof.play	6.9	6.7	3.7	0.6	4.8
	amat.play	7.3	4.1	4.0	0.8	4.1
mod. pass	prof.train	18.0	17.7	16.1	9.9	15.4
	prof.play	14.0	8.4	10.7	3.4	9.1
	amat.play	14.3	11.4	11.4	6.0	10.8
soft pass	prof.train	28.6	53.2	29.1	32.2	35.8
	prof.play	18.1	14.0	18.8	16.4	16.8
	amat.play	9.8	9.5	12.3	12.8	11.1
shot	prof.train	4.7	1.1	4.5	7.3	4.4
	prof.play	0.6	0.1	1.6	1.6	1.0
	amat.play	0.8	0.2	1.6	2.4	1.3

While these data must be interpreted with care as they
cover only a selection and not all of the actions occurring
in the game, results illustrate that the demand put on the

boot is likely to be considerably (i.e. 3 times) more severe in training than in match-play.

It may be concluded that this approach to the assessment of the demand on the boot is useful, and one which has not previously been described in the literature. From the results obtained here this would seem to correspond well with the general expectations of the locations of boot problems. A full picture of the demand on the boot during a game has not been produced here because the actions used were only those which were thought to present the more demanding stresses on the boot. Some of the more general locomotor actions and those involving sharp turning were not integrated into the final approach. Further, the stress on the boot was obtained from just one player and a greater selection of individual actions should be used.

Table 4. The mean (n=3) of boot parameters

playing action	total force (N)	duration (ms)	severity index (N)
turn	15640	37	423
run & jump	9646	29	333
hard pass	13950	108	129
mod. pass	16041	115	139
soft pass	15552	109	143
shot	10624	91	117
start	9963	23	433
walking	2629	76	35
jog	3975	22	181
backwards walk	4649	80	58

5 References

Reilly, T. and Thomas, V. (1976) A motion analysis of work rate in differential roles in professional football match play. J. Human Movement Stud., 2, 87-97.

Rodano, R., Cova, P. and Vigano, R. (1988) Design of a football boot: a theoretical and experimental approach, in Science and Football (eds T. Reilly, A. Lees, K. Davids, and W.J. Murphy), E & F. N. Spon, London, pp. 416-425.

Valiant, G.A. Ground reaction forces developed on artificial turf, in Science and Football (eds T. Reilly, A. Lees, K. Davids, and W.J. Murphy), E & F. N. Spon, London, pp.406-415.

Withers, R.T.,Maricic, Z.,Wasilewski,S. and Kelly, L.(1982) Match analyses of Australian professional soccer players. J. Human Movement Stud., 8, 159-176.

THE FOOT-GROUND REACTION IN THE SOCCER PLAYER

R. SAGGINI, A. CALLIGARIS, G. MONTANARI, N. TJOUROUDIS, and L. VECCHIET
Postgraduate School of Sports Medicine, University of Chieti, Medical Section of F.I.G.C., Coverciano (FI), Italy

1 Introduction

Soccer is a sport of movement and contact where the basic aim is to gain possession of the ball, with which the principal act of the game must to be accomplished. This refers to the scoring of a goal. Soccer play entails periods of running with the ball, but for much of the time there is no contact with it.

During the game, the player performs different technical actions such as running, jumping, gaining possession of the ball, receiving, 'conducting', passing and shooting. All of this is carried out with or without the ball in a continual series of accelerations and decelerations of pace, of vigorous and rapid sprints, and continual changes in direction. Very rare, however, are the moments when the run is completely free, that is an expression of the simple action of transferring the body from one point of the field to another. When this happens, it is at most a rapid reverse or advance and can no longer be compared to the run of the track athlete. It is a technical device to position the player in the best possible way to receive a pass, to prepare him for a tackle, for dribbling the ball, or for a shot at goal.

The composition of the actions is therefore very complex, both so far as the neuromotor content is concerned, and relative to the metabolic-energetic involvement. The complexity of the actions places the sport amongst those which require a prevalently technical qualification (Saggini and Calligaris, 1989).

The body's motion is a succession of elementary movements that are possible to study like synthesis of translation and rotation movements. The development possibility of a motor action at any frequency is strictly correlated to the balance between internal and external forces. The internal forces are the muscular forces, the bone-articular forces, the intersegmental forces; the external forces are the force of gravity, the inertial force and ground: the first impose on the ground the body's weight while the second responds with an equal and opposite force during the stance phase. This phenomenon is the foot-ground reaction. The vector and numerical characteristics of the reaction are correlated to the physical and mechanical characteristics of the bodies which are in relationship.

This reaction has been analysed and studied with the use of force platforms. Those are constituted by sluggish material with transducers which function to translate the stress into an electrical impulse.

341

The ground reaction is characterised by an R vector applied to the ground at the point P; this vector is broken down into the three spatial components Rx, Ry, Rz. On the transverse plane it is possible to recognize also the Cz moment.

In the present work the characteristic ground reaction force of the soccer player was studied.

2 Methods and Materials

The analysis was performed during the normal 'foot strike' and running of the soccer player. A dynamometric platform and another plate composed of 1024 piezoelectric pressure sensors were used. Usually, from 3 to 5 recordings were used for each trial condition, so as to pinpoint the most recurrent and representative characteristics of the dynamics of the lower limb and the relative foot-ground reaction.

The podobarographic plate is provided by 1024 piezoelectric sensors and it is able to describe the assessment of the foot in the stance phase during locomotion. The system defines the vertical force that is applied per unit of time on each contact point of the foot's surface during locomotion. The Kistler dynamometric plate provides the complete progression of the foot-ground reaction which develops during the stage of placing the foot on the ground (Kistler Instruments, 1975).

During the placement stage of each step cycle mechanical actions are developed by the foot on the placement surface, which vary rapidly in time. These may be analysed in terms of the different components of force and moment which result. There are three components in particular for the resulting force (vertical, horizontal on the progression plane, and horizontal on the frontal plane, respectively), and three components for the resulting moment.

As far as the elaboration and presentation of the data are concerned, apart from the simple analysis of the components of the placement reaction and the application point in operation of time, the vector diagram represents the placement reaction by dynamic characteristics.

Twenty four soccer players of the Italian national team and forty soccer players with high ability and performance were examined. The tests were correlated with a control reference group of normal subjects.

3 Results

The analysis of the foot-ground reaction on the sagittal plane revealed that during the normal strike an impact phase was characterised by high force both maximum (148 ± 3% of the body weight) and medium (126 ± 4% of the body weight) and high velocity of progression of the point of application. During the support phase the progression of the application point demonstrated a lower velocity compared to the velocity during the impact. In the same phase the vectors showed a completely backward inclination. A guidance phase had a peak of force lower than the first one in the contact phase and with rotational moment significantly increased compared to the normal

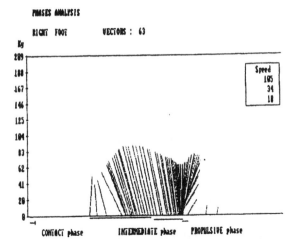

Fig. 1. Foot-ground reaction on the sagittal plane.

(Fig. 1). The medium centres of the application point of the forces
showed a wider extension of internal rotation during the contact
phase and movement with a predominance of external rotation during
the support phase (Fig. 2).

The morphology of the ground reaction of the soccer player was
different only for the goalkeeper. The specific action of the goalkeeper differed both for the spatial conditioning to which he is
subject and also for the better degrees of articular mobility
compared to other soccer players (Oberg et al., 1984).

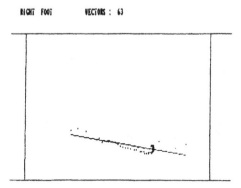

Fig. 2. Foot-ground reaction: trace diagram on the
        transverse plane.

4 Conclusions

The body's structure is solicited during locomotion in soccer by
force phenomena during the impact phase and during the propulsive
phase. In particular during the stance phase the body produces a

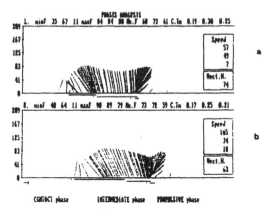

Fig. 3. Foot-ground reaction on the normal group (a)
compared to the soccer group (b).

ground reaction force composed of vertical and horizontal forces.

The instrumentation useful and necessary to represent this reaction is formed by dynamometric or strain-gauged platforms and by a platform of piezoelectric sensors. Our approach foresees the simultaneous use of these two types of platforms. We have defined the standard parameters for the single analysis and for the comparison of intraindividual and interindividual data.

The ground reaction pattern of the professional soccer player is repetitive, typical and different from that of the control group (Fig. 3).

5 References

Kistler Instruments A.G. (1975) Multicomponent measuring platform for biomechanics and industry. Type 9261A, Amherst, New York.
Oberg, B., Ekstrand, J., Moller, M. and Gillquist, J. (1984) Muscle strtength and flexibility in different positions of soccer players. Int. J. Sports Med., 5, 213-216.
Saggini, R. and Calligaris, A. (1989) Analysis of running in soccer players, Symposium of Biolocomotion, Formia.

THE EFFECT OF THE REPLACEMENT OF THE ANTERIOR CRUCIATE LIGAMENT (ACL) ON TRANSLATION AND KINEMATICS OF THE KNEE JOINT.

R.J. van HEERWAARDEN, T.N.M. LEK, J.J. de BRUIJNE, A.H.M. LOHMAN and
L. POLIACU PROSÉ
Dept. of Anatomy and Embryology, Free University, Amsterdam, Netherlands.

1 Introduction

Seventy percent of knee instabilities (grade II and III) caused by sport activities are the result of injuries to the anterior cruciate ligament (ACL); football and soccer account for 25 % of the pathologic anterior tibial translation due to acute rupture of the ACL (Hirshman et al., 1990). This is in accordance with the notion that the ACL functions as the primary mechanical restraint of anterior tibial displacements (Hsieh and Walker, 1976; Markolf et al., 1976; Piziali et al., 1980) and that in almost all cases of ACL-insufficiency an instability of the knee joint develops (Müller, 1983). The anterior displacement of the tibia is best measured by means of the Lachman test with the knee positioned at $20°-30°$ of flexion (Donaldson et al., 1985; Askew et al., 1990; Daniel, 1990).

According to Biden et al. (1990), the significant role played by the knee ligaments in gait justifies the development of surgical procedures to repair or replace injured ligaments in order to restore the normal muscle-ligament interactions that guide knee motion.

The aim of this study is to evaluate the effect of replacement of the ACL with an artificial ligament (placed between the centres of the attachment sites of the ACL, according to the findings of Odensten and Gillquist, (1985) on the anterior translation of the tibia and the kinematics of the knee joint. It is assumed that the length-pattern of the artificial ligament should reproduce that of the central bundle of the initial ligament during knee joint movement (Poliacu Prosé et al., 1992). The attachment sites and the distances between the centres of attachment of the ACL (ACL-length) were three-dimensionally (3-D) recorded at knee joint angles ranging from $0°-140°$ similar to the studies of Poliacu Prosé et al. (1987, 1989).

2 Material and Methods

Ten embalmed human cadaver knees were used. The knees were excised approximately 15 cm above and below the joint line and were then dissected, leaving intact the menisci and the collateral and cruciate ligaments. In each femur and tibia, two steel pins of 100 mm length were drilled into the shafts of the bones. The pins represent the local orthogonal axis systems of the bones.

At 10 knee joint angles, ranging from $0°$ to $140°$ of flexion, the positions of the femur against the fastened tibia (given by the local orthogonal axis system) were recorded three-dimensionally (3-D) by means of a measuring frame consisting of a Sony LM12S-31T Magnescale Computer Digital System with three perpendicular oriented axes, each formed by a SR-1711 scale of 450 mm effective length (accuracy ± 0.01 mm). By measuring the positions of the pins, 3-D data were collected, offering the possibility to reconstruct three-dimensionally the positions of the femur relative to the fastened tibia.

In addition, the magnitude of the anterior displacement of the tibia against a fastened femur was measured. An apparatus was constructed to simulate the clinical Lachman test. The femur was fixed at 30° of flexion and the tibia was clamped to a sliding frame which enabled antero-posterior displacement in the sagittal plane only. Two forces, 8 lbs (3.6 kg) and 16 lbs (7.2 kg), were applied to the tibia by means of a Tension Isometer (MEDmetric). This isometer was also used for measuring the anterior displacement with an accuracy of 0.25 mm. After cutting the ACL, the anterior translation of the tibia relative to the femur was again measured.

After the measurements, the ACL was removed and replaced by an artificial ligament whereby the femoral and tibial bone tunnels were positioned at the geometrical centres of the attachment sites of the ACL. A "Dyneema" artificial ligament with a cross-section area of 40 mm^2 and approximately twice the stiffness of the ACL was inserted with a preload of 4 lbs (1.8 kg) at 0° of flexion. The knees were first placed in the Lachman test simulation apparatus and the anterior translation was measured with the same procedure as described above. The positions of the femur against the fastened tibia were then recorded with the "Sony" measurement frame, again at 10 knee angles ranging from 0° to 140° of flexion.

Finally, the attachment sites, the geometry of the articular surfaces defined by the coordinates of arbitrarily chosen points at the femur and tibia contours, and the location of the drill holes were recorded relative to the coordinate systems of the femur and tibia with the "Sony" measurement frame. From the 3-D coordinates, the positions of the bones were reconstructed and the magnitudes of the attachment sites and the geometric midpoints of the attachments together with the distances between the drill-holes were calculated for each position of the knee joint. In addition, the cross-section area of the ACL was measured (IBAS system).

3 Results

The mean value of the anterior displacement of the tibia in the 10 knees with intact ligaments is 1.4 mm (SD 0.3) at 8 lbs and 3.0 mm (SD 0.6) at 16 lbs (Fig. 1-A). In correspondence to the observation of Donaldson et al. (1985), all knees were considered to be stable. Cutting the ACL results in an increase of the anterior displacement of the tibia of 3.5 mm (SD 2.3) at 8 lbs and of 9.2 mm (SD 3.8) at 16 lbs (Fig. 1-B). The replacement of the ACL with the artificial ligament placed between the geometric midpoints of the attachment sites with a preload of 4 lbs results in an anterior displacement of the tibia which is comparable to the anterior displacement measured in the knees with intact ligaments: 1.7 mm (SD 0.8) at 8 lbs and 3.9 (SD 1.2) at 16 lbs (Fig. 1-C).

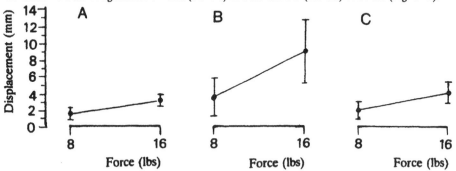

Fig.1. The mean anterior displacement of the tibia measured at 8 lbs and 16 lbs in 10 knees.
A. knees with intact ligaments; B. knees with cut ACL; C. knees in which the ACL is replaced by an artificial ligament.

In all knees with intact ligaments, the distance (Lo) between the drill holes is maximal (29.5 mm;

SD 3.6) at 0° of flexion. As shown in Fig. 2-A, the distance decreases during flexion, being minimal (about 90% of Lo) between 105° and 140° of flexion. In knees in which the ACL is replaced by an artificial ligament, the distance (Lo) between the drill holes is also maximal (27.9 mm; SD 3.2) at 0° of flexion. This distance behaves isometrically between 0° and 90° and decreases to a small extent (maximal 5% of Lo) between 105° and 140° of flexion (Fig. 2-B).

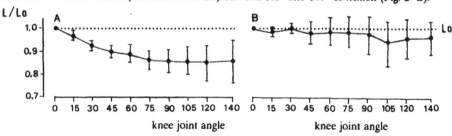

Fig.2. Graph representing the relative distances (L/Lo) between the drill holes at different knee joint angles in 10 knees with intact ligaments (A) and in the same 10 knees in which the ACL is replaced by an artificial ligament (B).

The positions of the femoral and tibial condyles at different knee joint angles was studied by recording the coordinates of the arbitrarily chosen points on the contours of the femur and the tibia and by projecting these values in the sagittal, transversal, and frontal planes. As shown in Fig. 3-B and D (0° flexion), the intra-articular placement of the artificial ligament through the bone tunnels drilled approximately at the geometric midpoints of the attachment sites with a preload of 4 lbs results in an compression of the articular surfaces and an anterior displacement of the femur relative to the fastened tibia. Not shown in figure 3 is that the femur displaces medially and endorotates.

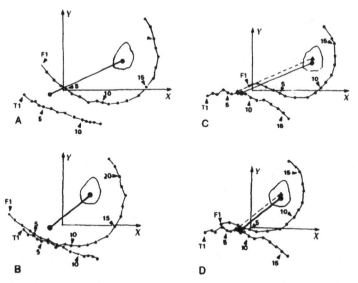

Fig.3. Plot-drawing illustrating the effect of the replacement of the ACL by an artificial ligament on the position of the femur against the fastened tibia projected in the sagittal plane at 0° of

flexion.

A. the position of the drill holes (●) and the reference points on the medial femoral (F) and tibial (T) condyles in knees with intact ligaments;

B. the position of the drill holes (●) and the reference points on the medial femoral (F) and tibial (T) condyles in knees in which the ACL is replaced by an artificial ligament;

C. the position of the drill holes (●), the geometric midpoints (▲) and the reference points on the lateral femoral (F) and tibial (T) condyles in knees with intact ligaments;

D. the position of the drill holes (●), the geometric midpoints (▲) and the reference points on the lateral femoral (F) and tibial (T) condyles in knees in which the ACL is replaced by an artificial ligament.

The cross-section area of the ACL (measured in the midpart) was 38.0 mm^2 (SD 0.16).

4 Discussion

In this study we have made two simplifications. Firstly, the ACL was represented by one line element connecting the centres of the attachment sites of the ligament. This representation of the ACL is often used because of the inaccessibility of the ACL for direct measurements in intact knees. Secondly, for defining the positions of the bones we measured the coordinates of the contours of the bones in the middle of the femoral and tibial condyles. Because we only measured the position of the femur relative to the tibia this simplification of the geometry of the bones was considered by us to be permitted.

When the ACL is replaced by an artificial ligament, the graft should preferably have approximately the same cross-sectional area as the ACL because of bending of the ACL over bone structures during flexion of the knee (Poliacu Prosé et al., 1989, 1992). The cross-sectional area of the graft we used was 40 mm^2. We measured a cross-sectional area of 38 mm^2 of the ACL in the 10 knees used in this study.

Detenbeck (1974) found in his study on the function of the cruciate ligaments in knee stability that the anterior cruciate ligament remains taut during flexion of the knee. The lower limit of tension was 4 pounds. We applied 4 lbs preload on the artificial ligament before fixation which resembles this lower limit of tension of the ACL as found by Detenbeck (1974). It should be noted that in ACL reconstructions artificial ligaments with comparable stiffness characteristics are sometimes preloaded with twice the preload used by us.

Markolf et al. (1978) reported that the forces manually applied by the clinical examiner during a Lachman test vary from 45 to 90 N. Therefore, we have chosen to put an anterior load of 8 and 16 lbs to cause anterior displacement of the tibia relative to the fastened femur in the simulation of the clinical Lachman test.

According to Donaldson et al. (1985) and Daniel (1990), the anterior displacement of the tibia in the sagittal plane, measured with the instrumentalised Lachman test at 30° of flexion, shows that all knees with intact ligaments are stable. Cutting of the ACL resulted in all knees studied by us in an increased anterior displacement of the tibia (Grade II and III instability). The artificial ligament that was inserted with 4 lbs preload completely prevents anterior translation of the tibia in all knees and thus restores the stability of the knees.

The length-pattern of the central bundle of the ACL, represented in this study by means of the distance between the holes drilled approximately in the geometric midpoints of the attachment sites of the ACL, is not isometric in knees with intact ligaments. This is similar to the results reported recently by Sapega et al. (1990) and Poliacu Prosé et al. (1992). By contrast, the length of the artificial ligament placed between the same points with a preload of 4 lbs shows an isometric pattern.

In this study, an important observation was made as regards the effect of replacement of the ACL on the positions of the bones. It appears that the kinematics of the "stabilised knees" changes to a great extent after ligament replacement. We found not only a compression of the articular surfaces at all knee joint angles but, in addition, the femur endorotates and translates medially and anteriorly. Lewis et al. (1989) reported similar findings in their reconstructions of the ACL with two autologous grafts. After loading, the tibia of some of the reconstructed knees was positioned posterior and was rotated externally relative to the normal knee (= knee with intact ACL). They introduced the term "over-corrected knees" for this group of reconstructed knees. We found the same changes when describing the position changes of the femur (antero-medial translation and endorotation of the femur). Lewis et al. (1989) stated that the over-correction of the knees was probably due to variations in the relative position of the tibia and femur at the moment of graft fixation, which in turn changes the initial graft length. We used an artificial ligament and propose that the following factors influence the over-correction: the stiffness characteristics of the artificial ligament compared to the stiffness of the intact ACL, and the preload applied to the ligament.

We conclude that a reconstructed knee may exhibit normal anterior displacements (as we found in the Lachman-test that we applied; the anterior translation of the tibia was completely prevented) but that the kinematics of the knee has changed considerably. This implies that the status of a replaced ACL, tested with the usual clinical laxity examinations, is an insensitive measure for assessing the status of an ACL reconstruction.

5 References

Askew, M.J. Melby, A. and Brower, R.S. (1990) Knee mechanics – a review of in vitro simulations of clinical laxity tests, in Articular Cartilage and Knee Joint Function (ed J.W. Ewing), Raven Press, New York, pp. 249–266.

Biden, E. O'Connor, J. and Collins, J.J. (1990) Gait analysis, in Knee Ligaments (ed D. Daniel), Raven Press, New York, pp. 291–314.

Daniel, D.M. (1990): Diagnosis of a ligament injury, in Knee Ligaments (ed D. Daniel), Raven Press, New York, pp. 3–10.

Detenbeck, L.C. (1974) Function of the cruciate ligaments in knee stability. Am. J. Sports Med., 2, 217–221.

Donaldson, W.F. Warren, R.F and Wickiewicz, T. (1985) A comparison of acute ACL examinations. Am. J. Sports Med., 13, 5–9.

Hirshman, H.P. Daniel, D.M. and Miyasaka, K. (1990) The fate of unoperated knee ligament injuries, in Knee Ligaments (ed D. Daniel), Raven Press, New York, pp. 481–504

Hsieh, H.H. and Walker, P.S. (1976) Stabilizing mechanisms of the loaded and unloaded knee joint. J. Bone Jt. Surg., 58–A, 87–93.

Lewis, J.L. Lew, W.D. Hill, J.A. Hanley, P. Ohland, K. Kirstukas, S. and Hunter, R.E. (1989) Knee joint motion and ligament forces before and after ACL reconstruction. J. Biomech. Eng., 111, 97–106.

Markolf, K.L. Mensch, J.S. and Amstutz, H.C. (1976) Stiffness and laxity of the knee. J. Bone Jt. Surg., 58–A, 583–594.

Markolf, K.L. Graff-Radford, A. and Amstutz, H.C. (1978) In vivo knee stability. J. Bone. Jt. Surg., 60–A, 664–674.

Müller, W. (1983) The Knee – Form, Function and Ligament Reconstruction, Springer, Berlin.

Odensten, M. and Gillquist, J. (1985) Functional Anatomy of the Anterior Cruciate Ligament and a Rationale for Reconstruction. J. Bone Jt Surg., 67–A, 257–262.

Piziali, R.L. Seering, W.P. Nagel, D.A. and Schurman, D.J. (1980) The function of the primary ligaments of the knee in anterior-posterior and medial-lateral motions. J. Biomech., 13, 777–784.

Poliacu Prosé, L. Lohman, A.H.M. Luth, W.J. and Krick, H.R. (1987) The attachments of the anterior (ACL) and posterior (PCL) cruciate ligaments in man – an anatomical and radiological study. Acta Morph Neerl-Scan., 25, 303–304.

Poliacu Prosé, L. Krick, H.R. Schurink, C.A.M. and Lohman, A.H.M. (1989) The attachments and length patterns of the anterior (ACL) and posterior (PCL) cruciate ligaments in man. Anat Anz., 168, 82.

Poliacu Prosé, L. Krick, H.R. Schurink, C.A.M. and Lohman, A.H.M. (1992) The attachments and length patterns of the anterior (ACL) cruciate ligament in man – an anatomical basis for ligament replacement (in this book).

Sapega, A.A. Moyer, R.A. Schneck, C. and Komalahiranya, N. (1990) Testing for Isometry during reconstruction of the anterior cruciate ligament. J. Bone Jt. Surg., 72–A, 259–267.

ISOKINETIC ASSESSMENT OF UNINJURED SOCCER PLAYERS

E.C. BRADY, M. O'REGAN, B.McCORMACK(*)
Trinity College Dublin, *University College Dublin, Eire

1 Introduction

The hip adductor, quadriceps and hamstring muscle groups are the most commonly injured muscles in soccer often causing chronic prolonged absence from soccer (Smodlaka, 1979; Muckle, 1981). There are several intrinsic and extrinsic factors which contribute to injury. Although several authors have named likely factors predisposing to injuries, few have actually investigated the relative contribution of various factors towards injuries (Burkett, 1970; Berger-Vachon et al., 1986). Some causative factors are training related, e.g. muscle strength imbalances: (a) over-emphasis on one-sided activities such as kicking may lead to asymmetry or dominance of one leg, i.e. greater than normal differences in strength between contralateral muscle groups; (b) an unfavourable difference between agonist and antagonist muscle groups is considered to leave the weaker muscle group at a disadvantage, e.g. hypertrophy of the quadriceps perhaps at the expense of the hamstrings may be a factor in hamstring injuries. If these factors are identified as responsible for injury, then injuries may be effectively reduced or prevented by appropriate modifications to training regimens.

Isokinetic dynamometry offers an accurate method of measuring the strength of large muscle groups. However, research to date is characterised by differences in protocols. For example, in many studies the subject groups are different or their characteristics are not fully stated, i.e. the mean, standard deviation and range of values for age, height and body mass of subjects, the level of soccer playing and hours of activity per week of soccer players or control subjects. Since muscle strength is a product of the cross-sectional muscle area and body leverage, omission of details of height and mass may lead to inappropriate conclusions and difficulty in comparing results of different studies. Some investigators have compared the strength of left and right legs without stating whether the subjects were predominantly left or right footed (Ekstrand, 1982). Other studies tested the dominant side only, failing to clarify the question of muscle imbalance (Poulmedis, 1988). Most studies only note the peak torque or moment of the range tested. It may be equally important to look at the shape of the strength curve when comparing groups or individuals, e.g. to note where the peak moment occurs, and the presence of any unusual peaks or dips in the curve.

1.1 Hamstring/Quadriceps Ratios

Burkett (1970) described a Hamstring/Quadriceps (H/Q) ratio of less than 60% as predisposing to injury. This work has not been adequately substantiated by later writers. Poulmedis (1988) reported a correlation between low H/Q ratio and hamstring muscle strains, but did not state what the low H/Q ratio was. At slow speeds of isokinetic testing (0.52 or 1.04 rad/s), the H/Q ratios of soccer players are around 60% (Agre and Baxter, 1987; Poulmedis, 1988). These studies compared peak moment of concentric hamstrings strength to peak moment of concentric quadriceps strength. In the final part of the swing phase of gait, the hamstrings extend the hip and decelerate knee extension (acting eccentrically), while the quadriceps are about to act concentrically to extend the knee. Therefore, it would be more appropriate, when discussing H/Q ratios, to compare the eccentric hamstrings strength to the concentric quadriceps strength (and vice versa), and since the hamstrings are working in outer range and the quadriceps in inner range at the end of swing phase/heel strike, it is also proposed that the strength at these parts of range should be compared and not just peak moment, which occurs in middle range.

The aim of the current study was to investigate muscle strength differences/leg dominance and H/Q ratios in soccer players and non-soccer players and thereby attempt to describe the normal strength curves for these groups.

2 Materials and Methods

Sixty one adult males underwent isokinetic testing of the quadriceps, hamstrings and hip adductor muscle groups of both lower limbs, concentrically and eccentrically at slow speeds (1.04 rad/s for the quadriceps and hamstrings; 0.52 rad/s for the hip adductors). The group was divided into experimental (38) and control subjects (23). The control group were (1) not actively involved in sport and (2) had no injuries to the lower limbs. The mean, standard deviation (SD) and range of values for age, height and body mass of the control subjects were:- age 22±3 (18-29), height 177±6 (166-190)cm, mass 83±7 (60-87)kg. The experimental subjects were non-professional soccer players, members of 4 Dublin clubs. Their age, height and mass values were:- age 22±4 (18-31), height 176±6 (165-190)cm, mass 72±7 (58-95) kg. All the soccer players trained at least two nights per week and played a match at weekends. The Kin Com II isokinetic dynamomenter (Chattecx Corp 1986) was used. All subjects were questioned on their soccer and injury history and where indicated, underwent examination to assess any injuries present. Only the results of uninjured subjects were statistically analysed. The protocol for isokinetic testing is described elsewhere (Brady, 1991). The results were corrected for gravity and normalised by dividing an individual's moment score by his weight (Nm/kg). For the soccer players, the dominant leg was compared to the non-dominant leg. The control subject's left and right legs were compared. Strength curves rather than peak moments were analysed. Using ANOVA the following comparisons were made for and between the experimental and control groups:- (1) concentric and eccentric strength curves, (2) dominant and non-dominant muscle groups (left and right for the control subjects), (3) hamstrings and quadriceps of the same leg (eccentric hamstrings effort compared to concentric quadriceps effort). None of those tested became injured in the 18 month follow-up period. The mean strength curves were analysed. The relative differences (as a percentage) between dominant and non-dominant and between concentric and eccentric were also calculated.

3 Results

There was no statistically significant difference (P>0.05) in strength between the soccer players and the control group for any of the muscle groups tested, but in every case the soccer players were between 5% and 10% stronger than the control subjects.

There was no significant difference in contralateral thigh muscle strength among either group. A further ANOVA, carried out on the results for the experimental group only, supported this finding (see Figure 1).

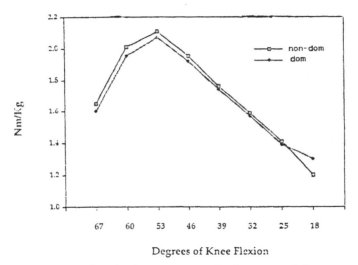

Fig. 1. Means for dominant vs non-dominant quadriceps strength curves (concentric)

The concentric-eccentric ratio was slightly lower for the soccer players than for the controls; average 74% (experimental) compared to 86% (controls), (N.S.; P>0.05). There was no difference in the concentric-eccentric ratios for dominant and non-dominant sides.

The HQ ratio was higher throughout range for the soccer players (average 84%) in comparison to the control (average 77%) (not significant). There was no difference between the H/Q ratios of dominant and non-dominant legs.

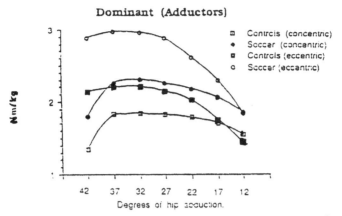

Fig. 2. Hip adductor concentric and eccentric strength curves.

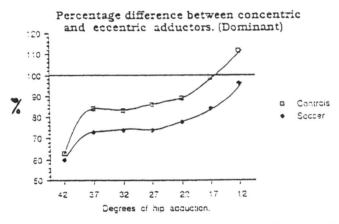

Fig. 3. Concentric strength as a percentage of eccentric strength
through range, (dominant adductors).

4 Discussion

The shape of strength curves was the same for both the experimental
and control groups but varied according to the muscle group tested.
Strength curves for the quadriceps and hip adductor muscles were very
similar in shape, with a steep build up to a peak at mid-range and a
less rapid fall off towards inner range. The hamstrings strength
curve was much flatter with a less dramatic peak moment. The
differences in shape may reflect the endurance and anti-gravity
function of the hamstrings or perhaps the position and/or the

velocity of testing. Further study is required to investigate the effect of these factors on the shape of strength curves.

The present study showed no significant difference between the thigh muscle strength of soccer players and control subjects. This may be due to close similarity in age, height and mass of each group, since muscle strength is a product of muscle bulk and leverage as mentioned above. Since there was quite a large range or variation of values for these parameters, the results of isokinetic testing also show a large range of values within each group. Therefore statistical analysis could not claim significant differences between either group. Closer matching of groups and sub-groups according to height and mass and testing of power or endurance or use of a higher velocity may have shown greater differences in musculoskeletal profiles of the two groups.

There was no significant evidence of leg dominance among either group, indicating that, for these soccer players, training and matches include sufficient bilateral exercises to prevent the development of muscle imbalances. This agrees with findings of Agre and Baxter (1987).

The slightly greater eccentric strength of soccer players compared to non-soccer players is probably due to the effects of training and the requirements of the game. These include rapid accelerations, decelerations and so on.

Unlike previous studies the current study also compared eccentric hamstrings as well as concentric quadriceps strength curves. The resulting H/Q ratio was slightly higher throughout range for the soccer players than for the control subjects. Thus, among the soccer players, there was no evidence of over-emphasis on quadriceps strengthening at the expense of the hamstring muscles. The H/Q ratio is lowest at mid-range and approaches unity at inner and outer ranges, where equal strength may be more functionally relevant since it is in outer/inner range that these two muscle groups may be acting in opposition/co-contraction as described above.

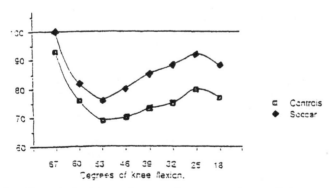

Fig. 4.   Eccentric hamstrings and concentric quadriceps strength; soccer players' dominant leg.

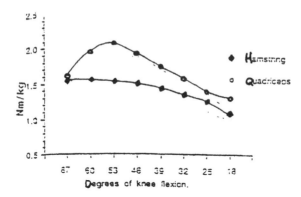

Fig. 5. Hamstrings-Quadriceps ratio (%) through range.

5 Conclusion

Amateur soccer players are not significantly stronger than an age
matched group of sedentary subjects. There was no evidence of muscle
imbalances in the current study. Since the soccer players did not
become injured in the follow up period, it is possible that their
moment values and strength ratios are "normal" or not predisposing to
injury. Further study is required to analyse trends for injured
subjects and to assess whether these findings for amateur soccer
players also apply to professional players.

6 References

Agre, J.C. and Baxter, T.L. (1987) Musculoskeletal profile of male
    collegiate soccer players. Arch. Phys. Med. Rehabil. 68, (March)
    147-150.
Berger-Vachon, C., Gabard, G. and Moyen, B. (1986) Soccer accidents
    in the French Rhone-Alps soccer association. Sports Medi., 3,
    67-77.
Brady, E.C. (1991) The incidence, and factors involved in soft tissue
    injuries in 82 Dublin soccer players. Doctoral thesis, Trinity
    College, Dublin, Ireland.
Burkett, L.S. (1970) Causative factors in hamstring strains. Med.
    Sci. Sports, 2, 39-42.
Ekstrand, J. (1982) Prevention of injuries in soccer. Linkoping
    University Medical Dissertation No. 130, Linkoping, Sweden.
Muckle, D.S. (1981) Injuries in professional footballers. Brit. J.
    Sports Med., 16, 37-39.
Poulmedis, P. (1988) Muscular imbalance and strains in soccer.
    Proceedings, Council of Europe Meeting: "Sports injuries and their
    prevention", Papendal, The Netherlands, 53-57.
Smodlaka, V.N. (1979) Rehabilitation of injured soccer players.
    Phys. Sports Med., 7, (8) 59-67.

THREE-DIMENSIONAL ANALYSIS OF INSTEP KICK IN PROFESSIONAL SOCCER PLAYERS

R. RODANO * and R. TAVANA **
* Politecnico di Milano, Dept. of Bioengineering, Milano, Italy
** Milan A.C., Milano, Italy

1 Introduction

When examining the complex system of motor actions used in a game of football, kicking obviously occupies a place of fundamental importance where, by definition, the player tries to impress different levels of speed and trajectories on the ball, all with a high level of precision. The chosen objective is reached by controlling the kinematic variables, the dynamic and motor coordination of joints and body segments, especially the lower limbs.

Many researchers have dedicated their time to studying the art of kicking with all its complexities, including Roberts and Metcalfe (1968), Macmillan (1975), Stoner and Ben Sira (1981) and Asami and Nolte (1983) who examined the kinematics as applied to kicking, Luhtanen (1988), who measured ground reaction. Other dynamic readings (inertial force, reactions and use of the limbs) were calculated by Putnam (1983), Luhtanen, (1989), Narici et al. (1988).

The purpose of this study is to provide a three-dimensional description of the kinematic variables that come into play in the art of kicking, and the ground reaction force on the supporting limb seen in relation to ball speed during instep kicking carried out by a group of professional footballers.

2 Method

2.1 Subjects

The experiment was carried out using 10 professional football players (Body mass = 72.4, S.D. = 7.7 [kg], age = 17.6, S.D. = 0.5 [years], height = 1.79, S.D. = 0.07 [m]) belonging to AC Milan football club.

2.2 Equipment

For collecting data on five points of anatomical reference on the kicking limb (iliac crest, greater trochanter, knee, external malleolus, 5th metatarsal head) the optoelectronic ELITE system was used (Ferrigno and Pedotti, 1985). The above points were marked by applying passive markers, half spheres of a diameter of 10 mm covered by reflecting material. Three markers were fixed on the ball to establish the coordinates of the centre by way of a computer program especially developed for the purpose.

The ELITE system was made up of the following: two TV cameras, 100 Hz sample frequency, 1.66 mm of accuracy on movements in three-dimensional displacements. A force platform (Kistler 9281B) was used for measuring the ground reaction force. The platform data were sampled at the same frequency and at the same instance as the kinematic data.

2.3 Protocol

The footballers, after a warming up phase, carried out a series of five instep kicks with a two pace run-up, wearing standard professional soccer footwear. The experiment was carried out in an area covered by artificial grass, the platform being covered with the same material. The data were registered once the trainer confirmed that the kick had been carried out correctly.

3 Results

3.1 Three-dimensional versus bi-dimensional analysis

Generally speaking, instep kicks are studied on the flat, at least concerning the phase where the foot hits the ball. In order to check this approach the modulus of the linear speed of the five markers was calculated considering both the coordinates X,Y,Z and the coordinates X,Y corresponding to the plane XY of the reference system lined up with the trajectory of the ball. Similarly the modulus of the joint speeds defined by the segments that join the markers on the joints was compared.

As far as the linear speed was concerned, the error margin varied from 0.12 m/s, (ankle) to 0.28 m/s (hip) with a standard deviation of the same proportion. The degree in percentage of error, referring to the absolute speed value, was over 10% as regards the marker on the iliac crest, hip and knee, while as regards the foot it was negligible (0.9-1.1 %). The errors carried out on the angular speed varied from 2.25 rad/s (knee) to 0.92 rad/s (ankle). The highest average error (expressed in percent) was registered in the ankle (83.9%). Readings for the hip (43.8%) and the knee (12.8%) should not be underestimated in particular when reading the data on the flat to calculate variables like kinetic energy of the different segments.

3.2 Kinematics

The ball speed data, ranging between 22.3 and 30 m/s, reflect the ability of the players. The difference between the average value and the best performance for each the players is under 6-7%, once again confirming the participants' kicking skills. The two best results (30 and 28.8 m/s) were obtained by the two forwards identified by the trainer as the most powerful players in the group.

Fig.1 shows figures for the speed modulus of each marker at the moment of impact. The speed increases in the more distal anatomical point. There aren't any significant differences between the average values taken from the entire test and those calculated considering only the best performance.

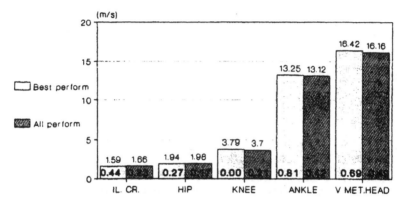

Fig.1. Speed modulus of the markers and r coefficients with the speed of the ball.

Few of the variables considered showed a good correlation and it is surprising to note that the linear speed of the malleolus and of the fifth metatarsal head, even though being the most highly correlated variables, generally were at r=0.42 and 0.49. These values were relatively low for an impact between rigid bodies, thus supporting the idea that other factors like the state of rigidity of the limb to the impact and the relative position between the foot and the ball, greatly influence the speed of the ball.

This idea was also confirmed by the fact that on considering the data relative to the best performance, when it is possible to hypothesize the most favourable mechanical condition of impact between foot and ball, the correlation coefficient of the speeds of the ball and the malleolus increased (r=0.81) as well as the correlation coefficient of the speeds of the ball and the 5th metatarsal head (r=0.69).

The angular settings of the lower limb at the moment of impact, seen as a deviation from the standing position, were as follows: hip flexed at 8.6 [°] (S.D.=7.1), knee flexed at 41.1 [°] (S.D.=8.6) and ankle plantar flexed at 27.1 [°] (S.D.=10.3). On average the best performance presents values that are slightly higher, (the limb is flexed even further), but these differences do not have any real statistical significance.

The average values of angular speed taken throughout the test are as follows: hip 146 (S.D.=89) [rad/s], knee 1169 (S.D.=211) [rad/s], ankle = -65 (S.D.=74) [rad/s]. The average value relative to the best performance did not show particular variations in the angular speed. There appears to be a weak or indeed non-significant positive correlation between the speed of the ball and the angular speed of the joints in the two given situations.

3.3 Ground reaction force

The test average for the maximum value of the ground reaction force, was 3.20 (±S.D.=0.29) [BW]. The vertical component was 2.69 BW while the horizontal reading was 1.24 BW. The direction of the horizontal reaction was medial and worked against the forward movement. The maximum was reached nearly 130 ms after impact. The average value of the reaction, at the moment the foot hit the ball, was 2.04 (± S.D.=0.33) [BW].

Reaction to impact and maximum of reaction did not change to any great degree during the best performances. The reaction modulus and the components were not correlated with ball speed.

3.4 The analysis of the single player

The kinematic and dynamic data were used to evaluate the existence of a correlation between ball speed, considering each player separately. The results indicate that each athlete's performance is to a greater or lesser degree correlated to one or more readings. However, the number and relative figure for each readings and degree are strictly dependent on the subject considered, and do not lead to the elaboration of general criteria.

This leads one to believe that the method applied enables the establishment of monitoring procedures to be adopted for the individual player, due also to the low interference level and to the immediate availability of the results.

4   Conclusions

The study of instep kicking movements in professional footballers has underlined the fundamental importance of the three-dimensional kinematic analysis with the bi-dimensional, relative to the movement. The secondary result of the study has helped in the identification of the average kinematic state of the lower limb at the moment of impact with the ball.

The increased correlation between ball and foot speed when the footballers kick at their best leads one to believe that performance is highly influenced by minimum variations in motor coordination. This consideration, associated with the general absence of statistical correlation between kinematic and dynamic variables, leads to the conclusion that the act of kicking is governed by the motor characteristics of each player, despite the high technical level of the group studied.

The fact that each individual showed typical correlations, and these between the variables considered and ball speed, means that this study might be useful in establishing a monitoring programme for soccer players' motor skills. This would also seem realistic in view of the low interference level of the equipment used and the possibility of obtaining results in a short space of time.

Acknowledgement

This study was sponsored by the Italian Research Council (CNR). CN 88.01815.04.

5 References

Asami, T. and Nolte, V. (1983) Analysis of powerful ball kicking, in **Biomechanics VIII-B**, (eds H. Matsui & K. Kobayashi), Human Kinetics Publishers, Champaign, Illinois, pp. 695-700.

Ferrigno, G. and Pedotti, A. (1985) ELITE: A digital dedicated hardware system for movement analysis via real time TV-signal processing, in **IEEE Trans. on Biomed. Eng.**, Vol. BME 32, No. 11, pp. 943-950.

Luhtanen, P. (1988) Kinematics and kinetics of maximal instep kicking in junior soccer players, in **Science and Football**, (eds T. Reilly, A. Lees, K. Davids and W.J. Murphy), E. & F.N. Spon Ltd., London, pp. 441-448.

Luhtanen, P. (1989) Biomeccanica del calcio. in **SdS**, No. 15, pp. 61-70.

Macmillan, M.B. (1975) Determinants of the flight of the kicked football. **Res. Quart. Am. Ass. Health Phys. Educ. Recreat.**, 46, 48-57.

Narici, M.V., Sirtori, M.D. and Mognoni, P. (1988) Maximal ball velocity and peak torques of hip flexor and knee extensor muscles, in **Science and Football**, (eds T. Reilly, A. Lees, K. Davids and W.J. Murphy), E. & F.N. Spon Ltd., London, pp. 429-433.

Putnam, C.A. (1983) Interaction between segments during a kicking motion, in **Biomechanics VIII-B** (eds H. Matsui & K. Kobayashi), Human Kinetics Publishers, Champaign, Illinois, pp. 688-694.

Roberts, E.M. and Metcalfe, A. (1968) Mechanical analysis of kicking, in **Biomechanics I**, (eds J. Wartenweiler, E. Jokl and M. Hebbelinck), Basel, Switzerland: S. Karger, pp. 315-319.

Stoner, L.J. and Ben-Sira, D. (1981) Variation in movement patterns of professional soccer players when executing a long range and a medium range in-step soccer kick, in **Biomechanics VII-B** (eds A. Morecki, K. Fidelus, K. Kedzior and A. Wit), PWN Polish Scientific Publishers, University Park Press, Baltimore, pp. 337-342.

A COMPARISON OF THE PUNT AND THE DROP-KICK

M. McCRUDDEN and T. REILLY
Centre for Sport and Exercise Sciences, The Liverpool Polytechnic,
Liverpool, England.

1 Introduction

Kicking actions are common to all the football codes. These include
free-kicks, drop-kicks and punts. In many contexts of open play
there is a choice between drop-kicking and punt-kicking. In games
with the round ball this choice applies to all Gaelic football
players and to the soccer goalkeeper. These skills also apply to the
games with the oval ball.
   Studies of the kicking action have tended to concentrate on limb
torques and angular velocities and to a lesser extent on muscle
activity. De Proft et al. (1988) reported the extent of agonist and
antagonist activity during the soccer kick. They found that extensor
muscles were likely to be active during the flexion movement and that
antagonistic muscle activity was greater in skilled compared to
non-skilled players whereas agonistic activity was dominant in the
non-skilled individuals. These authors referred to the requirement
to train agonist muscles concentrically and antagonist muscles
eccentrically to improve performance. In a separate study they
demonstrated that training muscle strength in fast isokinetic
movements was effective in improving kick performance, using the
maximum distance the ball was kicked as a criterion (Cabri et al.,
1988).
   In this study the punt and drop kick were selected for comparison.
As kicking is a major factor in the football codes, it was thought
that combining a descriptive electromyographic analysis with the
distance of the kick and kinanthropometric factors (isometric leg
strength, anaerobic power, leg volume) would provide basic
information of practical relevance.
   The aims of the study were to:-
   i) compare the performances of drop-kicking and punt-kicking with
      a soccer ball in laboratory and field conditions.
  ii) examine the extent to which kick performance is influenced by
      lean leg volume, muscle strength and anaerobic power.

2 Methods

Twenty undergraduate males, aged 20-29 (mean 22.6 ± 2.4) years,
participated in the study. All had experience of both soccer and
rugby and were familair with both kicking styles. Seven of the
twenty took part in the EMG study : all twenty participated in the
remaining investigations.

A soccer ball (weight 4.5 N) was used in all kicking tests. In the EMG study 9 muscles of the kicking leg were investigated. These were:- M. tibialis anterior, M. gastrocnemius, M. vastus lateralis, M. vastus medialis, M. rectus femoris, M. biceps femoris, M. semimembranosus, M. semitendinosus and M. gluteus maximus. Silver - silver chloride surface electrodes were connected by cable to a multi-channel polygraph (NFC San-ei Instruments, Tokyo) for recording of the raw EMG. The polygraph had bioelectric amplifiers with filters set to record a bandwidth of 10 to 1000 Hz. The electrode arrangement provided a balanced input for the amplifier, minimising 50 Hz artefacts and maximising the signal's common mode rejection ratio.

A series of 12 kicks, alternating every 3 kicks between punt and drop-kick, was performed. Subjects were instructed to take one step from a standing start before producing the striking motion and to kick maximally for distance as they would do outdoors. The cables were held by an attendant while the kick was being performed and the ball was kicked into a golf net.

Film analysis (100 Hz) was used to synchronise EMG recordings and the path of the leg in the kicking action. A switch mechanism was used to mark the recording paper at the time of ball contact and activate a flash unit that was picked up on the film.

The kicks for distance were performed on a hard court outdoors, subjects being instructed as in the laboratory test. Practice kicks were allowed prior to 10 experimental kicks using each of the two styles and kicking into a 45° sector. The maximum distances achieved for both kicking styles were recorded. Wind speed was found to be negligible whilst the kicks were performed.

Anthropometric measures included lean leg volume determined according to the method of Jones and Pearson (1969). Knee extension strength was measured at an angle of 135° using cable tensiometry. Anaerobic power was measured using a modification of the stair-run test of Margaria et al. (1966). The best of 3 trials following warm -up practices was used in each of the muscle performance tests.

3 Results

Muscle activation differed little in duration for the 9 muscles during both kicking styles, with some exceptions. The mean time of activity of M. vastus medialis was longer in the drop than in the punt kick. The timing of the activity on the other muscles was gauged by using this muscle as a reference, as its activity started at the same phase of the kicking action for both styles (Figure 1).

The M.rectus femoris, M.vastus lateralis and M.vastus medialis showed little activity until the drive phase towards the strike. Rectus femoris activity started 50 ms before vastus medialis was activated and stopped (60 ms for the punt, 80 ms for the drop) before M.vastus medialis did. Vastus lateralis started 10 ms (both kicks) into the activity period of M.vastus medialis and finished 40 ms before M.vastus medialis activity stopped. The hamstring group showed opposite tendencies, most activity being noted before M.vastus medialis was activated. Semitendinosus and M. semimembranosus showed the greater activation durations in the punt kick whereas the opposite applied to M.biceps femoris. Activity was first observed in

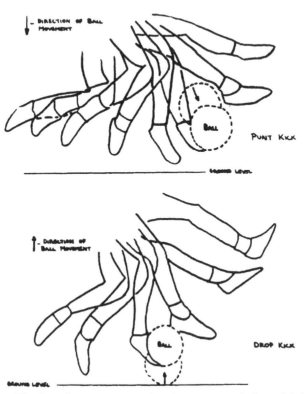

Fig.1. Leg movement in the punt and drop kick

Table 1. Anthropometric and performance data (n=20)

	Mean	S.D.
Height (cm)	177	6.2
Body mass (kg)	75.6	7.2
Leg length (cm	91.3	4.0
Leg volume (1)	9.42	1.17
Volume : muscle + bone (1)	9.05	1.09
Volume : thigh muscle + bone (1)	5.64	0.75
Volume : calf muscle + bone (1)	3.41	0.47
Volume : leg fat (1)	0.37	0.12
Volume : thigh fat (1)	0.22	0.08
Volume : calf fat (1)	0.14	0.05
Stair run (W)	1229.4	137.3
Knee extension (N)	788	130

M.biceps femoris, then in M.semimembranosus (punt) or M.semitendi-
nosus (drop). Biceps femoris ceased activity before activitation of
M.vastus medialis (134 ms for the punt and 76 ms for the drop kick).
The biceps femoris, unlike the other two hamstrings, seemed to be
active through the drive and strike phase of both kicks.

Mean activity patterns of M.tibialis anterior and M.gastrocnemius
indicated activity in a complementary fashion through the whole of
the movements. As the leg was loaded forward the greater activity
(as denoted by % MVC) in M.tibialis anterior was observed in the drop
kick. Activity in the M.gastrocnemius was greater in the drop kick
but was similar in duration during the drive and strike phases of the
kicking motion. Both muscles, along with M.rectus femoris showed
activity after M.vastus medialis stopped, which took place as the leg
moved through the vertical to the top of the swinging action. At
this time the leg was decelerating and the ankle was plantar-flexed.

Gluteus maximus activation preceded M.vastus medialis activity by
120 ms in the drop kick and 30 ms in the punt. The time span of the
movement was similar for the two kicks. Activity was seen as the hip
extended and rotated, and when the ball was struck and the leg
followed through.

Observations corroborate the muscle recruitment patterns and the
'soccer paradox' noted by De Proft et al. (1988) in that muscle
activity, albeit slight, was noted in quadriceps muscles at the
backward loading stage when they are antagonistic to the movement.
During the forward loading drive phase, activity (albeit reduced) was
noted in the antagonist - the hamstrings and M.gluteus maximus. The
main overall difference between the two kicking styles was that in 8
out of the 9 muscles examined, activity in the punt started before it
did at a comparative phase of the drop kick and also ceased before it
did in the drop kick. The exception was M.gluteus maximus. The
distinguishing feature was the exertion of knee extension force later
into the kicking action in the drop kick.

The punt-kick was found to be the most effective technique in
kicking for distance. This result was significant for both the best
kick (mean 40.1 ± S.D. = 4.3 m vs 36.1 ± 3.6 m) and the mean distance
(mean 34.8 vs 30.7 m) for the ten trials (P < 0.01). The
recommendation to use the punt-kick must be tempered by considerations of accuracy (and desired angles of projection) which mostly
prevail in competitive contexts.

None of the anthropometric variables was significantly correlated
with kick performance. Anaerobic power was significantly correlated
with the mean punt distance (r = 0.56; P < 0.05) but the correlation
coefficient for mean drop-kick distance (r = 0.39) was non-
significant. This implies that skill factors were more important in
executing the drop-kick. Although leg muscle volume was
significantly related to time for the stair run (r = 0.60; P < 0.01),
the muscle volume was not significantly correlated with performance
in either kicking style (P > 0.05). These results suggest that
static measures have poor predictive value for kicking actions which
may be determined more by specific technical and kinematic
considerations than kinanthropometric measures. Current observations
suggest that among the array of factors affecting kicking for
distance, muscle force plays a greater part in the punt kick than in
the drop kick.

4 References

Cabri, J. De Proft, E. Dufour, W. and Clarys, J.P. (1981) The
    relation between muscular strength and kick performance. In
    Science and Football (eds T. Reilly, A. Lees, K. Davids and
    W.J. Murphy) pp. 186-193, E. and F.N. Spon, London.
De Proft, E. Clarys, J.P. Bollens, E. Cabri, J. and Dufour, W.
    (1988). Muscle activity in the soccer kick. In Science and
    Football (eds T. Reilly, A. Lees, K. Davids and W. J. Murphy) pp.
    434-440, E. and F.N.Spon, London.
Jones, P.R.M. and Pearson, J. (1969) Anthropometric determination of
    leg fat and muscle plus bone volume in young male and female
    adults. J. Physiol. 204, 63-66 P.
Margaria, R. Aghemo, P. and Rovelli, E. (1966), Measurement of
    muscular power (aerobic) in man. J. Appl. Physiol., 21,
    1662-1664.

PART TEN

Medical Aspects of Football

THE ETIOLOGY AND EPIDEMIOLOGY OF INJURIES IN AMERICAN
FOOTBALL

W.B. SMITH
Blount Orthopaedic Clinic, Milwaukee, Wisconsin, U.S.A.

1 Introduction

The aim of this paper is to give some insight into the
etiology and epidemiology of injuries in American
Football.
    Adequate epidemiological studies are very difficult to
do. These have rarely been accomplished in the past
because of the volume of data required, the previous
necessity to handle the data manually, and the fact that
while colleges usually have trainers, only one of six
high schools in the U.S.A. have trainers. Also, there
are the problems of defining an injury and measuring the
severity of the injury, identifying the total population
at risk, measuring the exposure of the various positions
within that population, and having an available
comparison group. Having accomplished that, you still
need a control group for each compounding factor, and the
players have to be randomized from a large pool.
    Though not based on true epidemiological studies, we
have several large data bases from which we can derive
useful information. The data are not from a random
series and there aren't control groups and comparison
groups, but the large numbers lend some credibility to
our annual surveillance data. There are various surveys,
including the Annual Survey of Football Injury Research,
the Annual Survey of Catastrophic Football Injuries, the
National Athletic Trainers Association's, the National
Collegiate Athletic Association's, and the National High
School Coaches Association annual injury surveillance.

2 Injury Surveys

The National Athletic Trainers Association defines time
loss injury as an injury that required a player to
suspend practice that day or miss the day after. Using
this criterion, over 32,000 players were examined from
1986-1989. In all sports there were 1.3 million injuries
per year. Football had 36 injuries per school per year;
therefore, about 1/3 of players have an injury, and 75%
are "minor", which means they miss less than a week. Hip
and thigh injuries are the most common at 17%, the foot
and ankle 16%, the forearm, hand and wrist 15%, the knee
14.5%, and the shoulder and torso plus the head, neck,
and spine 10% each. The data show that the overall
percentage of surgical cases has remained very close to
4% of all injuries per year and that over these years
about 3% of injuries necessitated surgery on the knee.

369

The defense is hurt more often than the offense.
Linebackers, defensive linemen, and defensive backs make
up approximately 58% of the injuries, while offensive
linemen, running backs, and receivers make up about 42%.
The backfield is the most dangerous place to play--one is
three times as likely to get hurt as the 4 linemen
(centre, down lineman, tight end, wide receiver).

More injuries (about 60%) occur in the second half of
games and practices. This suggests that fatigue is a
factor. More surgical injuries occur in games, with the
knee making up two-thirds; 60% of injuries are in
practice, 40% in games. Therefore, practice scheduling,
techniques, and drills can be altered to decrease the
overall injury rate!

3 Cervical Injuries

From 1960 to 1975 there was an average of 16 serious
cervical spine injuries with paralysis per year. In
1973, Schneider published his monograph "Head and Neck
Injuries in Football". Prior to this time, contact with
the head was common and it was taught by coaches. There
was some awareness that tackling with the neck in flexion
would lead to cervical spine injuries, so athletes were
coached to tackle with the head up. However, there was
little knowledge of axial loading, with the neck straight
or extended, as a cause of major cervical spine fracture
or fracture-dislocation. For the 1976 season, rule
changes in both high school and college had outlawed
"spearing". This referred to use of the top of the
helmet as the initial point of contact for blocking and
tackling.

Torg et. al. (1979) reported 99 permanent cervical
spine injuries from 1971 to 1975. He has maintained the
"National Head and Neck Injury Registry" since then.
Figure 1 shows what has happened to the injury rate to
the cervical spine since that rule change in 1976.

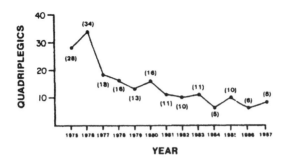

Figure 1. Cervical spine injuries since 1976.

370

Currently cervical spine paralysis occurs in 0.62
players per hundred thousand high school football players
and in 1.85 players per hundred thousand in college.
This is based on roughly a million and a half high school
players and about 75,000 college players in the U.S.A.
There is estimated to be another 225,000 sand-lot and
professional ballplayers. The overall rate for all
players is 0.78 per 100,000. Of the cervical spine
paralysis that occurs, about 80% are to a defensive
player, and in the vast majority of those instances the
player is tackling. About 80% of the injuries have been
in games. Coaches must stress "heads up!" tackling (no
initial contact with the head), and referees should throw
more penalty flags to further discourage the use of the
head (helmet) as the initial point of contact between
players.

4 Fatalities

The following information comes from Mueller in the
annual "Survey of Football Injury Research". There have
been an average of 36 total fatalities in all sports per
year; about 24 are in football. In 1990 that figure
dropped to 9: 6 indirect in high school and 3 in
college. An indirect death is one caused by a physical
defect—aortic stenosis or cardiomyopathy—or one caused
by exertion. This has been a particularly exciting year:
1990 is the first year that there has been no direct
fatality from a football injury.

5 Protection

A "burner or stinger" is a traction injury to the
brachial plexus associated with forced compression of the
shoulder while the head and neck are forced in the
opposite direction. We have had success with decreasing
the incidence of "burners and stingers" by making a
continuum of the helmet, horseshoe collar, and shoulder
pads. Sometimes a posterior strap is added to prevent
excess lateral traction on the neck. We routinely use
elevated shoulder pads and a horseshoe collar in patients
that have had any cervical problem, and they appear to
decrease the recurrence of injury.
The helmet has not been shown to be the cause of
cervical spine injuries. It is a comment on American
society that 50% of the helmet's cost is liability
insurance for the manufacturer. Helmet fit is critical.
Any person with a particularly narrow, thin head needs
special fitting rather than the standard helmet off the
shelf. Deaths from craniocerebral trauma have been
decreasing as a result of improvement in helmet design
and the rule changes implemented in 1976.
Prophylactic knee braces have received a fair amount

of attention in the last 10 years. There are several
studies which suggest that they may be helpful, whereas
others suggest that they may be harmful. The only valid
epidemiological study comes from 8-man intramural
football at West Point, where the Academy has absolute
control over the cadets and the game (Sitler et. al.,
1989). The study shows that there is some protective
benefit from the brace for defensive players. In this
study of about 700 athletes in the braced group and the
control group with approximately 11,000 exposures for
each group, the braced group had 16 injuries and the
control group 37 injuries. The braced group had 12
medial collateral and 4 anterior cruciate injuries, and
the control group had 25 medial collateral and 12
anterior cruciate injuries. The defense was the major
beneficiary. At all positions the defensive players with
braces had fewer injuries than those without braces: 7
defensive backs without braces were injured, and only 2
with braces were injured. Similarly, 7 defensive ends, 8
linebackers, and 3 defensive linemen without braces were
injured, compared to 1 player with the brace in each of
these 3 groups. Also, there was no increase in the
incidence of ankle injuries in the braced group.
Previous studies have also shown no increase in knee
injuries associated with ankle taping.

6 Heat Illness

Heat illness has been fairly well understood in the
United States. This is a result of the military recruit
injuries in the 1940's and 1950's. However, players in
the northern states are more likely to get in trouble
because of less tolerance to heat and less experience on
the part of coaches, trainers, and physicians. A good
example of proper medical supervision was the USA Cup
Youth Soccer Tournament which was held in Minnesota in
July of 1988. The temperature was about 38 degrees
celsius (100 degrees fahrenheit), humidity was 85-90%,
and the wet-bulb globe temperature was 29 degrees celsius
(84 degrees fahrenheit) by noon on all 4 days.
Altogether, 18 of 4,000 soccer players collapsed with
heat exhaustion by noon of the second day. Medical
personnel were worried about heat stroke and they, the
coaches, and the referees shortened the playing time per
half by 3 to 5 minutes, lengthened the half-time, added 2
minute "quarter" breaks and permitted unlimited
substitutions. For the next 4 days, only 14 heat
exhaustions occurred. However, the rate per 1,000
actually increased in the 13 and 14 year old boys--
confirming what we already know, that you can't tell an
early teenager anything!
    An adult takes 10 days to acclimatize to the heat and
a child somewhat longer.
    We recommend practice modification whenever the

humidity is above 95%, regardless of the temperature. If the wet-bulb temperature is greater than 70 degrees fahrenheit or 25-26 degrees celsius, practice should be appreciably modified. With this awareness and using these guidelines, the frequency of heat stroke fatalities has decreased in every decade since 1960. There was one fatality in 1990.

Water is the replacement fluid of choice. Cold water leaves the stomach faster than warm, and large volumes faster than small. It's better to pre-hydrate than to rehydrate. Sugar solutions that are pleasant to taste are acceptable only if very dilute. Soda or other concentrated solutions don't empty from the stomach quickly and are not recommended (Elias et. al., 1991).

7   Recommendations

Firm conclusions may not be drawn from these survey data; however, the amount of data and the year to year similarity of injury patterns in practices, by positions, and in games allow us to make some recommendations:

(1)   Practice schedules should include planned breaks.   Non-contact drills should be scheduled before these breaks and intense contact drills immediately after.
          Since 96% of practice injuries occur on full-pad work-out days, many schools have begun very limited contact practices once games begin.   Some have virtually none, except on game days!   Practices should be less than 2 hours and probably only once a day.   Less contact allows more time to work on conditioning, technique, and mental preparation.
(2)   The head should be kept out of direct involvement in the game of football so that the number of catastrophic injuries can be decreased to 0, just as the number of deaths in 1990.
(3)   Pre-participation physical examinations, off-season weight training programmes, mandatory mouth guards, and certification of coaches have all been stressed as ways to decrease the number of injuries.
(4)   Flexibility is of utmost importance.   A student athlete should be able to sit on the ground and reach his palms past his toes.   Stretching of the calf muscles is strongly recommended.   An additional arc of dorsiflexion allows time to unload the ankle before the inversion torque, which develops at the end of passive extension, tears the lateral ligaments.

This paper has considered football injuries, and these can be put in perspective.   Statistics from the National Data Bank allow us to compare football injuries to other daily activities.   In the United States, about 1000 people are killed per year in bicycle accidents, and

about 50,000 people per year are killed in automobile
accidents. The figures show that not only are you safer
on the football field than you are in your automobile or
in an airplane, but you are also safer on the football
field than you are in the hospital.

8 References

Elias, S.R., Roberts, W.O., and Thorson, D.C., (1991),
   Team sports in hot weather. **Phys. Sportsmed.**, 19,
   67-78.
Schneider, R.C. (1979) **Head and Neck Injuries in
   Football.** The Williams & Wilkins Company, Baltimore,
   MD.
Sitler, M., Ryan, J., Hopkinson, W., Wheeler, J.,
   Santomier, J., Kolb, R., and Polley, D., (1989)
   The efficacy of a prophylactic knee brace to reduce
   knee injuries in football. **Am. J. Sports Med.**, 18,
   310-315.
Torg, J.S., Quedenfeld, T.C., Burstein, A., Spealman,
   A., and Nichols III, C., (1979) National football
   head and neck injury registry: report on cervical
   quadriplegia 1971 to 1975. **Am. J. Sports Med.**, 7,
   127-132.

INJURY PREVENTION IN SOCCER: AN EXPERIMENTAL STUDY.

H. INKLAAR[*], E. BOL[**], S.L. SCHMIKLI[**], H.J.M. BEYER[**] and
W.B.M. ERICH[**].
* KNVB, Zeist; ** University of Utrecht, Holland.

1 Introduction

Prevention of soccer injuries is a major aim in the Dutch
governmental policy directed to the reduction of incidence of
injuries by 25% by the year 2000. Only three controlled
studies on the efficacy of prevention procedures were found
in the literature. Ekstrand (1982) studied the efficacy of a
prophylactic programme consisting of 7 items in a randomized
trial in a male senior soccer division in Sweden. A 75%
reduction in injuries was found.
Tropp et al. (1985) studied the efficacy of an ankle brace and
of ankle disk training on the incidence of sprains to ankles
in a randomized trial amongst 450 soccer players in Sweden.
A significant reduction in sprains to the ankle was found in
comparison with a control group.
Jörgensen (1988) studied the efficacy of free substitution on
the incidence and duration of soccer injuries in a randomized
trial in Danmark. Although no reduction in the incidence of
injuries was found, a significant reduction in the absence
from games was noted.
The results of these intervention studies seem very
promising. Nevertheless, there are questions with respect to
the efficacy of the separate items of the prophylactic
programme and the transfer to the Dutch soccer scene.
The purpose of this study is to investigate the efficacy of
selected preventive measures on incidence, nature,
localization and consequences of soccer injuries.

2 Material and methods

Two Dutch amateur soccer clubs were followed during the
second half of the 1986-1987 competition and the first half
of the 1987-1988 competition.
At the start of the study the population consisted of 475
players, mean age 21.6 ± 8.4 (range 12-60) years. According
to age the population was divided in 243 senior players, 78
boys (aged 17-18 years), 79 boys (aged 15-16 years) and 75
boys (aged 12-13-14 years).

The senior players represented the first nine teams, which were divided into two levels of soccer competition. The junior players in each age group represented the first three teams, which were also divided into two levels of competition. Injuries sustained during official practice and in official soccer competition games causing the end of participating in that practice or soccer game and/or subsequent absence from practice, games and/or work and study as well as a need for medical treatment were registered. By weekly visits to both clubs all of the injured players were examined and questioned with respect to the injury pattern, the injury mechanism, possible risk factors and the consequences of the injury.

In the course of weekly contact, a follow-up of consequences of injuries was administered. Reports of injuries were made by the coach of each team, by the central contact person in each club and/or through a monthly questionnaire filled in by the players.

Practice attendance records kept by the coach of each team and copies of the official game registration forms allowed calculation of the exposure time. Injuries were not treated by the authors and we had no influence on the time of return.

Prior to the start of the study assessment took place of participation in soccer and other sports, previous sports injuries, status of health, sports motivation, and sociographic status. This was done by means of questionnaires.

Also the players were subjected to biometry and medical examination. Finally the behaviour of players and spectators and the number of fouls during games were monitored.

Due to significant differences between both clubs on some variables the comparability of the clubs was not optimal.

During the first half of the 1987-1988 competition one club was subjected to preventive measures. The preventive measures that were selected were easy to implement and consisted of introduction of a standard warm-up modified from the warm-up suggested by Ekstrand (1982), a cool-down programme according to Ekstrand (1982) and exhaustive education and information about various aspects of injury prevention through different channels of communication.

Group differences were tested by the chi-square tests or student's t-tests. Effects of the intervention programme were tested by MANOVA repeated measures (SPSS).

3 Results

The prevalence and incidence of injuries both for the second half of the 1986-1987 competition and the first half of the 1987-1988 competition are shown in Table 1. Although time effects can be detected, there are no significant condition effects.

Table 1. Incidence of injury

	CLUB A. (control club)		CLUB B. (test club)	
	*	**	*	**
PREVALENCE	19	9	28	16
INCIDENCE	33	33	49	55
INCIDENCE/1000 GAME HOURS	14.3 (13.7)	7.8 (6.5)	23.5 (15.8)	16.4 (15.1)
INCIDENCE/1000 PRACTICE HOURS	0.7	0.5	0.8	1.0

* second half 1986-1987 competition.
** first half 1987-1988 competition.
( ) incidence/1000 game hours for 281 players participating in both competitions.

The localization of the injuries are shown in Table 2. During both periods of time most injuries are sustained from the knee down to the foot. Again there are no significant condition effects.

Table 2. Localization of injury

	CLUB A. (control club)		CLUB B. (test club)	
	*	**	*	**
GROIN/THIGH	5	6	15	5
KNEE	4	4	14	13
LOWER LEG	3	7	7	13
ANKLE	11	7	7	14
FOOT	3	4	2	2
OTHERS	7	5	4	7
TOTAL	33	33	49	55

* second half 1986-1987 competition.
** first half 1987-1988 competition.

The nature of injuries is shown in Table 3. More than 80% of the injuries are diagnosed as sprains, strains, and contusions. The condition effects do not reach the level of significance.

Table 3. Nature of injury

	CLUB A. (control club)		CLUB B. (test club)	
	*	**	*	**
SPRAIN	13	8	12	20
STRAIN	5	3	10	5
CONTUSION	8	16	14	20
DISLOCATION	1	1	1	0
FRACTURE	3	1	1	3
BURSITIS/TENDINITIS	1	1	4	4
OTHERS	2	3	7	3
TOTAL	33	33	49	55

* second half 1986-1987 competition.
** first half 1987-1988 competition.

The absence of play in relation to injuries is shown in Table 4. There are no significant condition effects.

Table 4. Absence of play

		CLUB A. (control club)		CLUB B. (test club)	
		*	**	*	**
MINOR	(< 7 DAYS)	20	22	24	38
MODERATE	(7-30 DAYS)	10	7	17	13
MAJOR	(> 30 DAYS)	3	4	8	4
TOTAL		33	33	49	55

* second half 1986-1987 competition.
** first half 1987-1988 competition.

4 Discussion

It turns out that the results of the prophylactic programme are very poor indeed. The following explanations might be considered:
i)   The comparability of both clubs is questionable due to significant differences on some important variables. However, corrections on the basis of analysis of co-variance did not considerably effect the results reported above.
ii)   It is possible that there are major differences between the second half of the 1986-1987 competition and the first half of the 1987-1988 competition of teams regarding type of play, motivation and interests of players, and composition of teams due to factors like illness, injuries, and study.

378

The comparability of both parts of the competition therefore is questionable.
iii)   There might be an information bias due to increasing
        under-reporting of injuries in the course of the study.
        This phenomenon is well known from other studies. In
        the light of this phenomenon the good results from
        other intervention studies can be questioned.
iv)   Selection bias may have influenced the effectiveness of
        preventive measures in this study. We will look into
        this problem more closely. The diagram shows injury
        chances based on the percentages of players injured
        during the 1986-1987 competition within subdivisions of
        groups according to age and level of competition.

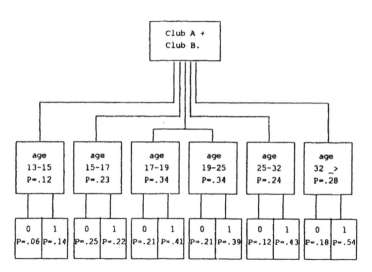

P = percentage score
0 = low level of activity
1 = high level of activity

Fig.1. Percentage of injured players in each subgroup of the
       study population according to age and level of
       activity.

On the level of individual players these two factors are
significantly related to the dependant variable "injury",
explaining 6.6% of the variance. The point is, however, that
the factors age and level are related to selective
characteristics of teams, that is players match certain teams
on the basis of their personal features like age, skill,
speed, strength, motivation, etc., and are selected by
coaches accordingly in a non-random manner.

Teams differ with respect to sports practice like training (content, duration, frequency), preparation (warm-up, stretching), and type of play during games (speed, force, techniques, tactics, actions). We therefore assume that the factors level and age are related to personal features on the one hand, and to team characteristics on the other. Indeed we find that level and age significantly correspond with the personal factors height, weight, ligamentous laxity, health status, and motivation, and with the team characteristics training (duration and frequency), warm-up, and stretching. If each player is described on the basis of these factors, in our study three clearly distinct groups (class 0, 1, and 2) of players can be detected. The factor "**class**" explains 16% of the variance of the dependant variable "**injury**".

So a combination of personal and team factors results into a stronger predictor of injuries than the factors age and level.

If the combination of personal and team factors is relevant with respect to the matching of players and teams we should expect a much higher correlation between the average class score of teams and injuries. By combining teams playing on the same level of competition, 18 groups were formed. During the second half of the 1986-1987 competition the correlation between the groups of teams and the percentage of injured players turned out to be 0.69 (explained variance = 45%). At the beginning of the new 1987-1988 competition many players were selected for other teams. Nevertheless, the new average class scores of the groups of teams correlated even more highly with the percentages of injured players during the first half of that competition: $r = 0.84$ (explained variance = 68%). It seems that injury risk is closely related to personal and team factors.

In order to control for type of play during games agressive behaviour of spectators, agressive behaviour of players with respect to each other and with respect to the referee, the number of fouls, and the number of game hours were calculated during the second half of the 1986-1987 competition. The averages of these game scores of each group of teams were used as co-variates in an analysis of variance with "**class**" as independant and average injury chance (percentage of injured players) as dependant variables.

It turns out that the co-variates explain 65.2% of the variance of "**injury**", and that the independant variable is non-significant. This demonstrates that the features of players and the components "**training and preparation**" of sports practice are closely related to types of play and only indirectly to injuries, while types of play during games correspond with risk factors.

The latter analysis explains why the prophylactic programme did not work. The programme was not aimed at the changing of play during games.

In fact the programme was aimed at activities before and after matches and practices (warm-up, cool-down) and at informing players about various aspects of injury prevention (e.g. taping, sports wear). As a rule the high risk players and teams (high level of competition) applied most of such prophylactic measures already, and these measures seem not very fruitful for low risk players and teams.

Accordingly, the relatively low incidence of muscle tendon injuries in this study population, in comparison with studies of about ten years ago, might reflect the fact that nowadays prophylactic procedures like warm-up and cool-down are well known and generally applied by soccer players as suggested by Ekstrand (personal communication).

This study did show the complexity of the injury problem in soccer. Therefore differentiation is needed in dealing with the prevention of soccer injuries.

Our experimental study has resulted in the following recommendations for programming future research on soccer injuries (Bol et al., 1991):

i)   Prospective studies with respect to mechanisms and risk factors related to incidence, nature, localization and seriousness of soccer injuries have a high priority.

ii) The study of the aetiology of soccer injuries should focus on the selection of homogenous subgroups with respect to the aetiology. As to the aetiology of soccer injuries there should be a clear distinction between these subgroups. Selection of homogenous subgroups at least should be based on age, level of competition and gender.

iii) The study of internal risk factors should be performed within homogenous subgroups.

iv) Future research on the aetiology of soccer injuries should include observation during games and practice and careful registration of the behaviour of players and the circumstances in cases of injury as well as registration of medical care during and immediately after games or practices.

v)   More attention should be paid to the study of diagnosis and treatment of soccer injuries and rehabilitation of soccer players and to the study of the reduction of the social consequences of soccer injuries through improvement of secondary and tertiary prevention.

5 References

Bol E., Schmikli S.L., Backx F.J.G. and van Mechelen W. (1991) Sportblessures onder de knie. National Institute for Sports Health Care, Oosterbeek, Holland.

Ekstrand J. (1982) Soccer injuries and their prevention . Linköping University, Medical dissertations nº 130 Linköping, Sweden.

Jörgensen U. and Sörensen J. (1988) Free substitution in soccer: A prospective intervention study. Proceedings Council of Europe 3rd meeting ed. van der Togt, National Institute for Sports Health Care, Oosterbeek, Holland.

Tropp H., Askling C. and Gillquist J. (1985) Prevention of ankle sprains. Am. J. Sports Med., 4, 259-262.

EPIDEMIOLOGICAL CHARACTERISTICS OF SOCCER INJURIES AND PROPOSED
PROGRAMMES FOR THEIR PREVENTION IN SCHLESWIG-HOLSTEIN 1988

C.RASCHKA and H.deMARÉES
Professorial Chair of Sports Medicine, Ruhr-University, Bochum
Germany

1 Introduction

The study is offered as a perspective into the epidemiological aspects of both indoor and outdoor soccer. This is done in order to
detect a substantial typology of sports accidents and offer special
programmes for their prevention.

2 Methods

The accident-report-sheets of Schleswig-Holstein for the year 1988
were examined. As all soccer club-players have sports-insurance coverage by collective agreements between the regional sports association and the ARAG-sports-insurance company, the sportsmen were
given a second sheet for the present study. This was based on 1664
players (outdoor soccer: goalies n=84, others n=1333; indoor soccer: goalkeepers n=29, others n=218).

3 Results

The following accident-types were discovered. For indoor soccer
the injury rate was: goalies: parrying and blocking 55.2 %, contu-
sion-accidents 24.1 %, falls 10.3 %, ankle sprains 6.9 %, knee-
joint-distorsions 3.4 %. For the others the figures were: contu-
sion-accidents 39.4 %, ankle sprains 28.9 %, knee-joint-distorsions 10.1 %, spontaneous damage of muscles or tendons 9.2 %,
being hit by the ball 5 %, getting hurt because of the inventory
4.6 %, heading-accidents 2.8 %. For outdoor soccer the results
were: goalkeepers: parrying and blocking 39.3 %, contusions 38.1
%, falls 10.7 %, ankle sprains 8.3 %, knee-joint-distorsions 3.6
%; others: contusion accidents 50.1 %, ankle sprains 21.8 %,
knee-joint-distorsions 13.4 %, heading accidents 7.4 %, spontaneous damage of muscles or tendons 3.9 %, being hit by the ball
2.2 %, getting hurt because of the inventory 1.3 %.
When subdividing the most frequent type of accident, the contusion,
we find the following types: indoor soccer: simultaneous kick 36.0
%, collisions 18.6 %, falls, when being pushed by an opponent 14.0
%, blows and kicks 10.5 %, falls without any extraneous influence
9.3 %, collisions with following falls 5.8 %, sliding tackling 3.5
%, foul kick 1.2 %, falling overhead kick 1.2 %. The figures for
outdoor soccer were: blows and kicks 25 %, collisions 20.1 %,
simultaneous kick 13.5 %, falls, when being pushed by an opponent

12.7 %, slide tackling 9.7 %, falls without any extraneous influence 9.6 %, collisions with following falls 3.7 %, outstretched leg 2.8 %, foul kick 1.9 %, falling overhead kick 0.9 %.

4 Proposed programmes for the prevention of soccer accidents

4.1 Physiological taping
This absolutely necessary prophylactic precaution can be defined as invigorating important muscles and stretching their antagonists. The concern should be primarily with the ankle joints, knee joints, finger and wrist joints, where the peroneal muscles, extensor muscles of the hand, M. interossei dorsales, the quadriceps and the internal rotators of the knee joint should be strengthened and their antagonists should be extended.

4.2 Proprioceptor training
Proprioceptive modalities of sensation include the sense of position of the limbs, degree of tension in the muscle-tendons, degree of stretch of the muscle fibres and deep pressure in different parts of the body. This proprioceptive system should be trained by means of ankle disks or wobble-boards for the ankle joints, standardized rotational knee-joint motions on a wave-shaped surface for the knee-joints and exercises of catching a ball, being attached with an elastic rope to the hand of the goalies, for the fingers and wrist joints.

4.3. Suitable equipment
The aim of prophylactic taping is to support externally certain ligamentous structures without limiting the physiological range of function or motion. A common technique for the ankle joint is the 'stirrup and horseshoe'-tape, followed by a figure-of-8-lock round the heel. The frequency of ankle sprains in indoor soccer should be further reduced by wearing high-top shoes. As the tapes provide only significant support for 10 min, but not after 1 h of exercise, different types of semi-rigid ankle guards as reusable lace-on-braces or the pneumatic aircast brace should provide a similar or better and cheaper support. As a desirable, but unrealistic proposal the conventional soccer-type shoe should be improved by minimizing the cleat length and maximizing the number of cleats and their tip diameters. Ideally the cleats should be stabilized only against vertical forces and leap out of the shoe on the impact of strong rotational forces. In general soccer shoes should have low rotational frictional forces. Goalkeepers ought to use protective soft headgear and mouthguards. The shinguards should consist of an inflexible, hard shelf with installed air cushions and be equipped with a cover of the calf, also being provided with protecting caps for the ankles. Catch-gloves might prevent hyperextensions and intense lateral movements of the fingers. Goalies might wear protective armguards.

4.3 Methodology of training

When performing jump training the players should try to land on both feet after jumping. They should also be taught to attract their attention not only to the fly of the ball, but also to the motions of their own and their opponents' feet. An extensive stretching and warming-up programme should be exercised prior to participation in ball games and also before any substitution in indoor soccer. Goalies should hold their arms in a flexed position and the players ought to kick the ball by using the little toe-side of their feet and practise standard evading manoeuvres and falling exercises like judokas.

4.4. The sports medical check-up

An important desirable realizable prophylactic programme might be a comprehensive preventive sports medical check-up concerning the detection and treatment of isokinetic muscle imbalances, increase in relative lean body mass, diagnosis, treatment and training of defects of vision, especially dynamic visual acuity. Players with grave knee instability should be excluded. The medical examination could also include a conscientious sonography of the Achilles tendons.

4.5 Rule changes as desirable, but unrealistic proposals

Slide tackling should be prohibited. Head work should only be allowed, if the player is out of reach of his opponent's legs. In indoor soccer the side-boards should be abolished.

5 Conclusion

Upon using the prophylactic proposals described, the number and the grade of sports injuries could be minimized, if slide tackle was prohibited and if the side-boards in indoor soccer were abolished.

6 References

Raschka, C. (1992) Sportartspezifische Präventivmaßnahmen zur Minimierung der Zahl der Sportunfälle in den großen Ballspielsportarten Fußball, Handball, Volleyball und Basketball, aufgeführt am Beispiel der Sportunfälle im Landessportverband Schleswig-Holstein e.V. des Jahres 1988. Sportwissenschaftliche Dissertation, Ruhr-Universität Bochum, Deutschland

TYPICAL FRACTURES OF THE MAXILLOFACIAL REGION IN SOCCER-RELATED ACCIDENTS - DIAGNOSTIC AND THERAPEUTIC PROCEDURES

N. HARTMANN and G. NEHSE
Dept. for Oral, Maxillofacial and Plastic Surgery,
City Hospital, Münsterstr. 240, 4600 Dortmund 1, Germany

1 Introduction

Soccer is the most popular ball game in Germany. Played very often in leisure time by non-professionals there is a high incidence of fractu res seen in traumatology units. Because of the way the game is played most injuries happen to be at the lower extremities. In some cases however, the maxillofacial region is involved.

2 Aetiology and location of fractures

2.1 General considerations
A fracture in the maxillofacial region typically happens when players are crashing into each other fighting for the ball. Jumping into the air when the ball is played high to gain possession with the head players can easily have contact with each other's head. This contact may be insignificant, normal or severe; it might be at any site of the head or face, but preferably the most prominent anatomical parts of the face are disconcerted, i.e. the zygoma, the nose and the mandible.

Fig. 1.: Left zygoma fracture with displacement of the medial antral wall; the orbital floor is dislocated (Coronal CT)

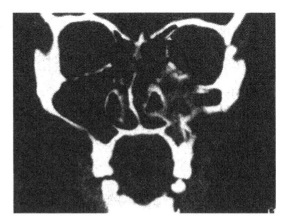

2.2 Zygoma fractures

The zygoma prominence is the point where the head of the opponent hits the face most often in fighting for the ball; other possibilities of hitting the zygoma include the fist of the goalkeeper on trying to punch away the ball, or when two players run side by side for the ball and the opponent's zygoma prominence is struck with the elbow. Rarely is a kick to the face a cause of fracture.
A fracture of the zygoma can be located ventrally or dorsally. Dependent on the intensity of the hit, in the ventral fracture one can see an impression of the malar complex with a periorbital haematoma, an infraorbital bony step, a disturbance of the infraorbital sensibility and a diplopia; if the fracture is located more dorsally at the lateral side of the face, an impression fracture of the zygomatic arch may impair the opening of the mouth.

2.2.1 Orbital blow out fractures

A fracture of the orbital floor and/or the medial orbital wall often isn't to be seen immediately. Either hitting the eyeball directly with a suddenly increased pressure in the orbit ("hydraulic force") with a consequence of a fracture at the weakest areas of this region, or striking the zygoma not strongly enough to fracture the thick bony structures at the orbital rim but still transmitted to the thin orbital floor with a consecutive fracture, are the causes of getting an isolated fracture of the orbital walls. Because of the hidden nature of this fracture type, showing clinical symptoms like diplopia sometimes as late as one week after the trauma, it is essential that the diagnostic procedures are done by a specialist (Hartmann and Haase, 1986).

2.3 Nasal fractures

The nose is a more prominent area in the face than is the zygoma. Therefore many fractures in soccer-related accidents are to be seen in this area. Fortunately the most prominent parts of the nose consist of soft tissue and cartilage which are pliable. Fractures take place at the small upper part of the nose regularly without any loss of function and only in few cases with aesthetic disturbances and the need fo therapeutic intervention.

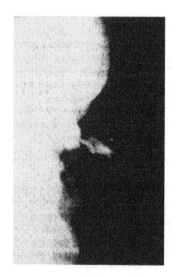

Fig. 2: Nasal fracture with dislocation (Lateral nasal x-ray)

Fig. 3: Fracture of the
right mandibular condyle,
nondisplaced (Lateral
part of an orthopantomo-
graphic x-ray)

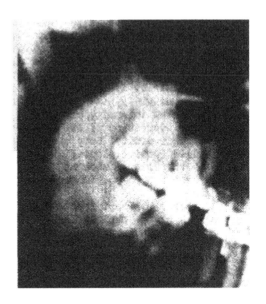

2.4 Mandibular fractures
The weakest area in the
normally configurated mandible is the condyle, i.e.
the region below the tem-
poro-mandibular joint. In
about 40 % of all mandi-
bular fractures the con-
dylar region is involved
(Hartmann, 1991). A frac-
ture of the condyle, spe-
cially when its a displa-
ced or even a dislocated
one shows the clinical
signs of pain, swelling,
haematoma and malocclu-
sion.

3 Material and Methods

296 patients with fractures were seen at our unit. Diagnostic procedures consisted of clinical examination, different x-rays (OPG,
Waters' view, Clementschitsch's view) and in special cases computerised tomography (CT); therapeutically we either did conservative treatment with the fracture in an idle position or, if necessary, an open reduction and internal fixation (ORIF) with
titanium miniplates.
All patients were followed up at least six months until the plates
for the internal fixation could be removed at the earliest.

4 Results

From 1/89 to 12/90 a total of 296 patients with fractures either
of the mandible (30 %), the midface (63 %) or combined fractures
(7 %) had to be treated in our department. Out of the total number of patients eleven (3.7 %) had fractures related to soccer
accidents. In five cases a fracture of the zygoma (Fig. 1) or the
zygomatic arch was found, while four patients had a nasal fracture
(Fig. 2). One condylar fracture (Fig. 3) and one isolated orbital floor fracture (Fig. 4) completed our series. In 6 patients
the fracture was the result of a head-to-head-crash, elbow-to-
head happened in 4 cases; 1 patient got a kick to his face.

Fig. 4: Isolated fracture
of the orbital floor; a
"hanging drop" is to be
seen at the roof of the
maxillary sinus (Hypo-
cycloidal tomography)

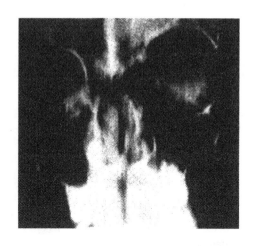

All 5 patients with the
malar fracture got an
ORIF; post operative
x-rays showed good re-
duction (Fig. 5), the
healing process was
uneventful. After 6-9
months the miniplates
were removed.

The nasal fractures were treated with a closed reduction. When the
typical post operative swelling was gone after 4-5 days the patients
could breathe through their noses without problems. Aesthetically
their noses showed almost the same configuration as before the
trauma.

The condylar fracture was openly reduced and fixed internally with
a miniplate by an intraoral approach, thereby restoring the vertical height of the mandible and giving the patient the possibility
of immediate funktion (Fig. 6). The plate is still in place but
will be removed soon; the mandibular function is undisturbed with
an opening of 41 mm without any deviation.

Concerning the isolated
orbital floor fracture we
brigded the fracture area
from a transconjunctival
approach with a polyglac-
tin plate (Höltje, 1983)
which will be resorbed
after about 6 months and
replaced by fibroblastic
scar tissue. At the last
control, 13 months after
operation, there was un-
disturbed motility, bin-
ocular view and no enoph-
thalmos.

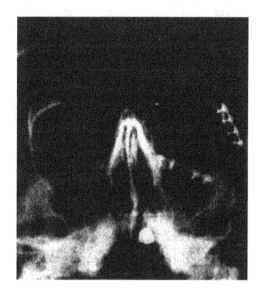

Fig. 5: Left zygoma frac-
ture after open reduction
and internal fixation; titanium miniplates at the
zygomatico-frontal suture
and the infraorbital rim
(Waters' view)

Fig. 6: Fracture of the
right mandibular condyle
after open reduction and
internal fixation; tita-
nium miniplate at the
fracture site (Lateral
part of an orthopantomo-
graphic x-ray)

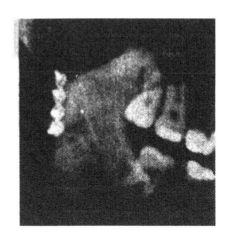

5 Discussion

In a study of 2901 acute maxillofacial fractures Schuchardt et al.
(1966) reported of 3.3 % sports-related fractures. Now, thirty years
later, in our series only the soccer-related maxillofacial fractures
had a higher incidence; together with 10 other sports-related fractures (squash, horse riding, hockey, wrestling) in our patients,
we had a total of 7.1 % of sports-related fractures. Interpreting
these numbers we see, as working time shortens, much more leisure
time with more possibilities to participate in sports than years ago.

Since diagnostic procedures like CT give us more opportunities to
detect fractures which were overlooked in earlier times and therapeutic procedures with extensive biocompatible materials allow us
to operate upon most situations there is a good chance for every
patient to get a restitutio ad integrum after a soccer/sports related fracture in the maxillofacial region.

6 References

Hartmann, N. (1991) Condylar and subcondylar fractures. Communication to First Maxillofacial Course for Rigid Fixation, Athens,
13-16 June 1991

Hartmann, N. and Haase, W. (1986) Isolated orbital floor fractures.
ORBIT, 5, 273 - 277

Höltje, W.-J. (1983) Wiederherstellung von Orbitabodendefekten mit
Polyglactin. Fortschr Kiefer-Gesichtschir, 28, 65-67

Schuchardt, K., Schwenzer, N., Rottke, B. and Lentrodt, J. (1966)
Ursachen, Häufigkeit und Lokalisation der Frakturen des Gesichts-
schädels. Fortschr Kiefer-Gesichtschir, 11, 1-6

LONG-TERM FOLLOW-UP OF INVERSION TRAUMA OF THE ANKLE

R.A.W. VERHAGEN and G. DE KEIZER
Maria Hospital, Department of Surgery, Tilburg, The Netherlands

1 Introduction

Lesions of the lateral ligaments of the ankle joint are one of the commonest diagnostic findings in accident surgery and are the most common injuries in sports. From the literature it is known that about 25 per cent of the patients who are treated at the emergency department of a central hospital for a sports-related injury have an acute sprain of the ankle. For The Netherlands this means that only 300,000 patients each year suffer a sprained ankle in sports. In soccer 30 per cent of all injuries of the lower extremities are in the ankle, and of these, 75 per cent involves the lateral ligaments. No wonder that there is a great amount of literature on this subject.

A review in the Journal of Bone and Joint Surgery of February this year refers to 77 publications in the English-language literature. The indications, treatment methods, and the results reported by different authors are not comparable because of the great variation in selection criteria and evaluation methods. Even the results of 12 prospective randomised trials, mentioned in this review (Kannus and Renström, 1991), are in some respects conflicting.

It seems logical that the prognosis following an inversion trauma depends on the grade of severity of the injury. In 1989 the results of our treatment policy after a 9 months follow-up were published (Schaap et al., 1989). At that time we could not demonstrate any difference between grade I, II and III lesions in 817 patients (Figure 1).

To examine the long-term follow-up results of inversion trauma of the ankle we conducted a retrospective study with the same group of patients after 5 years.

2 Materials and Methods

All patients with a sprained ankle were diagnosed and treated according to the protocol in our hospital. The diagnosis 'sprained ankle' was made on basis of the history and physical examination. Fractures were excluded by plain X-rays.

The sprained ankles were classified into the traditional three grades, depending on the extent of instability found on clinical examination. If necessary, the degree of instability was established under local infiltration anesthesia.

The classification was as follows: ankle sprain grade I - no demonstrable sign of instability; treatment consisted of compression with bandages; grade II - only mild or incomplete instability present; treatment consisted of partial immobilization by means of tape and physiotherapy; and sprain grade III - joint completely unstable; treatment of ankle sprain grade III consisted of primary surgical repair of the ruptured ligaments. After treatment consisted of 3 weeks in walking plaster followed by 3 weeks of partial immobilization in tape and physiotherapy.

As was done in the first study after 9 months, the data of the

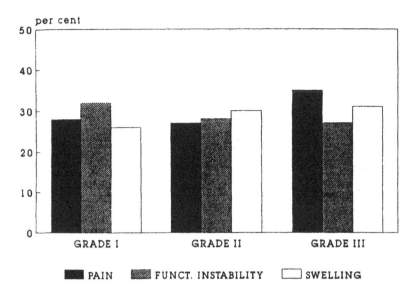

Fig. 1. Residual complaints 9 months post-injury.

residual complaints and degree of handicap were obtained via a ques
tionnaire. The questionnaire was filled in at home by the patients
themselves. For different reasons 67 patients were lost.

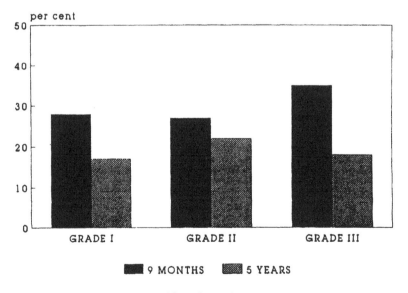

Fig. 2. Pain.

3 Results

Of the 750 questionnaires sent out, 577 were returned and appeared to be suitable for analysis. The overall respons rate was 77 per cent.

Return to work or physical activity is an important point because of economic reasons. In addition, athletes and other physically active people appreciate a quick return to training and competition. In our group 424 out of 577 responders participated in some way in sports. Because of residual complaints of the injured ankle 23 patients (5 per cent) had to change and 16 patients (4 per cent) had to stop their physical activities. So 9 per cent of the responders who participated in sports had residual complaints which interfered with their physical activities.

It appeared that after 5 years 15 per cent could only continue their original occupation with some handicap, for example with the help of an elastic bandage;six per cent was not able to maintain their occupational activities at all, due to residual complaints.

After 5 years pain diminished in each grade, as compared to after 9 months post-injury. The most pain was in the operated group grade III and the least in the grade II group (Figure 2).

In each group an increase in the number of patients with feelings of giving-way was seen. The highest progression was in the grade II group, increasing from 28 per cent after 9 months to 48 per cent after 5 years (Figure 3).

We also asked for recurrent re-injuries as an indication for actual instability. As was expected these numbers are lower than those for functional instability. The highest percentage of patients with recurrent re-injury was in the grade II group (Figure 4).

Ten patients appeared to be operated upon because of recurrent re-injuries. They were in the grade I and II group. None of the patients in the grade III group was re-operated at a later time.

The overall subjective judgement as given by the patients themselves, shifts from 85 per cent good after 9 months to a lower appreciation level after 5 years. The appreciation was lowest in the grade II group with only 62 per cent of the patients judging themselves 'good' (Figure 5).

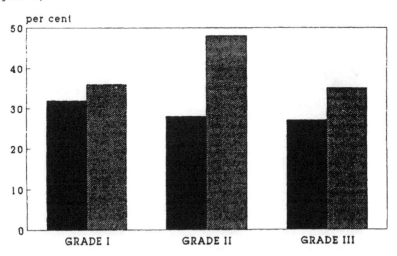

Fig. 3. Functional instability.

393

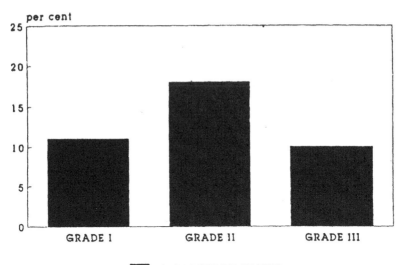

RECURRENT RE-INJURY

Fig. 4. Actual instability.

4 Discussion

The most striking result of our previously published study 9 months post-injury was the fact that no differences emerged between the three groups with regard to the frequency and nature of the residual complaints or the extent of the handicap. So it was concluded that the prognosis following a simple inversion injury without visible signs of instability was the same as that for a completely unstable ankle which

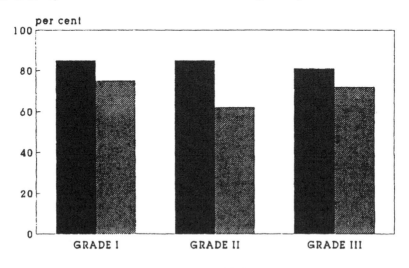

9 MONTHS   5 YEARS

Fig. 5. Judgement of treatment results 'good'.

had been treated by primary ligament suture.

In this study 5 years post-injury it became clear that some differences appeared. Although after 9 months the residual complaints of
pain and functional instability were the same in each grade, after 5
years, pain diminished in each grade, but the least in grade II.
Functional instability increased in each grade, but the most in the
grade II group. This was also the case for actual instability with
recurrent re-injury. The overall judgement of the results given by the
patients themselves shifted in time to a lower appreciation level,
irrespective of the grade.

Ankle ligament injuries are still considered as rather innocent
lesions and it is considered that patients can return to their pre-
injury level of activity without handicap. The results of this study
show that a sprained ankle, irrespective of the grade, interfered in 9
per cent of the patients with their physical activities and 6 per cent
could not regain their occupational activity level.

The aim of this study was not to compare the results of conservative
with operative treatment in a well defined group of patients. With our
study we tried to get insight in the long-term history of our patients,
diagnosed and treated according to our protocol. This history shows
that an operatively treated grade III lesion has about the same prognosis as a conservatively treated grade I lesion, in some respects even
slightly better, while after 5 years the results of the conservatively
treated grade II group show that this group has a less good prognosis.

5 References

Kannus, P. and Renström, P. (1991) Treatment for acute tears of the
   lateral ligaments of the ankle. J. Bone Joint Surg., 73A, 305-312.
Schaap, G.R. Keizer, G. de and Marti, R.K. (1989) Inversion trauma of
   the ankle. Arch. Orthop. Trauma Surg., 108, 273-275.

ANTERIOR ANKLE PAIN IN FOOTBALL
Aetiology and indications for arthroscopic treatment.

ROLAND BIEDERT
Sports Traumatology, Swiss Federal Sports School, Magg-lingen, Switzerland

1 Introduction

Persistent pain and swelling in the anterior part of the upper ankle are encountered very frequently in football. Because of an often long case history and especially because of their lack of response to various conservative treatments, these symptoms frequently represent a chronic problem and prove disconcerting both to the sportsmen themselves and to the therapists, in regard to the restoration of full sporting fitness and performance. Many different causes can be responsible for triggering and sustaining these complaints. Consequently, the case history and the previous therapies may also differ very considerably.

2 Aetiology and Pathology

Classically, in the patient with a long history of typical anterior ankle pain there is no instability. On the other hand, sudden pain occurs when the foot is put in a certain position, and also pain and discomfort after sporting activity. These are often combined with an effusion, swelling and a certain restriction of movement due to the pathology. Pinching effects, in the sense of an impingement, blocking, or the fear of a blocking, and a feeling of undsteadiness are frequently reported.

Various pathological changes can lead to the classical clinical symptoms:

a) **Adhesions, cicatrices**
   Practically all forms of trauma in the area of the upper ankle can lead to cicatrices and/or adhesions on the various structures within the joint. This hypertrophic synovial tissue is then responsible for the painful restrictions of walking and movement.

b) **Meniscoid-type lesions**
   This type of injury is manifested by cicatrices following damage to the lateral capsular ligament (Martin et al., 1989). The post-traumatic formation of such an adhesion between the lateral cheek of the talus and the fibular cartilage can lead to the painful symptoms.

c) **Osteophytes/exosotoses with synovitis**

   Also through a concomitant synovitis, repeated trauma of
   the anterior joint capsule can lead to symptoms in the
   anterior part of the joint. The typical pinching effects
   observed here are caused by the formation of bony ex-
   crescences or osteophytes. These develop on the one hand
   as a result of recurrent microtrauma to the joint capsule with maximum plantar flexion of the foot. The
   exostoses are formed, like the calcifications, by minute
   tears in the area of the anterior edge of the tibia and
   the neck of the talus. Through pinching effects in a
   compression trauma or a sprain, such osteophytes can
   cause injury to the synovia. With maximum loaded dorsal
   extension the same symptomatology is then manifested by
   an impingement of the altered soft-tissue structures by
   the exostoses, similarly to a nut-cracker effect.

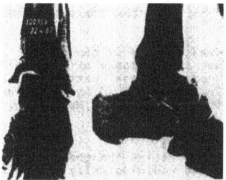

Fig. 1. Opposing osteophytes
causing capsule impingement.

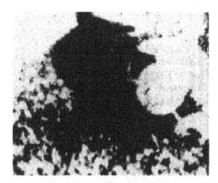

Fig.2. Extreme defor-
mation of the ball with
corresponding reaction
to the anterior joint
capsule.

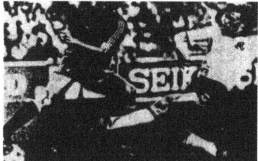

Fig. 3. Recurrent micro-
trauma of the anterior
joint capsule due to
exessive tensile strain
in maximal plantar flexion.

d) Folds, fibrotic subcutaneous fatty tissue

As a result of a direct contusion trauma of the anterior joint capsule, the subcutaneous fatty tissue lying on the neck of the talus can be injured and, trough fibrosis, can become painful.

e) Free arthrolits

In the case of a recent, undetected lesion, chondral or osteochondral fragments can spread through the joint and lead to pinching or blocking.

f) Osteochondral lesions of the talus

An injury is to be found in the case histories of more than 80 % of these patients (Biedert, 1989; Martin et al., 1989; Parisien, 1985). While chondral and osteochondral fractures belong to the recent acute lesions, with chronic symptoms, especially involving the talus, a posteromedial osteochondrosis dissecans is present in most cases.

g) Osteochondral lesions of the tibia

These occur, in the sense of a dorsal compression fracture with maximum dorsal extension, in the upper ankle, and are classified according to the usual classification for osteochondral lesions (Hempfling, 1987; Parisien, 1985).

h) Arthrotic changes

Advanced degenerative changes are easy to diagnose, clinically and radiologically. The symptomatology is mostly very advanced, with chronic pain and marked loss of function.

3   Differential Diagnosis

Various other clinical conditions can also result in symptoms involving the anterior part of the upper ankle. These have to be considered in the diagnosis of anterior ankle pain. Fatigue fractures, changes of the extensor retinacula and chronic tendinitis of the extensor tendons deserve particular mention.

4   Therapy

Typically, long-term conservative therapy has not provided a cure in the clinical syndrome described here. In view of the patient's wish to quickly regain his or her full sporting capability, surgical intervention becomes necessary. In place of the arthrotomy the indications in our patients for an arthroscopic intervention on the upper ankle was made with great caution. The difficulty certainly lies in correctly interpreting the arthroscopic findings and recognizing a definite connection between the symptoms and a 'pathological' arthroscopy finding.

4.1 Technical procedure

Arthroscopy of the upper ankle is performed with the patient in the dorsal position, with the lower leg placed horizontally. A tourniquet is applied to the thigh. After the 'land-marks' have been correctly drawn, the joint is first filled with about 20 ml of Ringer's solution. The arthroscope is then inserted from the antero-lateral portal. After filling of the upper ankle with liquid as filler medium, the anteromedial access can be used to insert all the necessary instruments (Johnson, 1981).

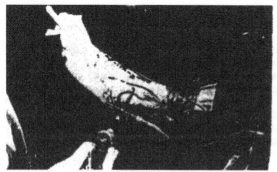 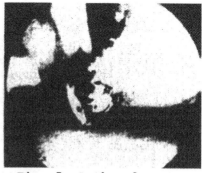

Fig. 4. Operation site with the arthroscope in the anterolateral access and landmarks.

Fig. 5. Arthroplasty drill inserted anteromedially for ablation of the osteophyte.

4.2 Indications

a) **Free arthroliths**
   The arthroscopic removal of a small fragment is technically relatively easy. Decisive for a good result, however, is an isolated lesion with no concomitant degenerative changes (Boe, 1986; Hempfling, 1987; Martin et al., 1989; Parisien, 1985).

b) **Cicatrices, adhesions, meniscoid lesions**
   These changes can be easily diagnosed by arthroscopy. The treatment is carried out using motorized instruments, with which the pathological tissues are removed.

c) **Chronic synovitis, osteophytes, exostoses, calcifications**
   These changes are mostly to be found in combination. From the therapeutic point of view it is important, with arthroscopy, to deal with both the primary causes (exostosis, osteophyte, calcification) and the sequelae (synovitis). Through alternate anterolateral and

anteromedial access, the whole anterior joint cavity can be examined and treated. The synovectomy can be performed with the shaver, while osteophytes can be completely removed with the arthroplasty drill.

d) Osteochondral lesions

Changes classified as Grades II or III are good indications for the arthroscopic treatment (Canale and Belding, 1980). Good results can be obtained in about 90 % of the cases (Martin et al., 1989). It has been shown (Parisien, 1985 a+b) that the long-term results are even rather better than the short-term results. The arthroscopic treatment consists of the removal of ostechondral fragments and curretage and debridement of the pathological parts.

5   Complications

If the arthroscopy is performed correctly, this operation is largely free from complications. Theoretically, the following lesions are possible: vasomotor-nerve and chondral lesions due to incorrect handling of the instruments, emphysaema due to gaseous filler medium, soft-tissue swelling with the use of liquid filler medium, compartment syndrome, infection and post-operative haemarthrosis due to inadequate Redon drainage.

6   Post-operative Follow-up Treatment

Arthroscopic interventions can be performed both in outpatient practice and with hospitalization. The patient is mobilized on the first post-operative day, with sole contact up to a load of 20 kg for 2 to 7 days. The crutches can be dispensed with after about one week, provided the joint is free from effusions and there is no longer any swelling. Physiotherapy starts from the first day after the operation. Strengthening and coordination exercises complete the follow-up therapy. Sporting activity (e.g swimming, cycling) can normally be resumed from the second week. More demanding sports (e.g. football) sometimes require a rehabilitation phase of up to 4-6 weeks.

7   Results

Arthroscopic interventions on the upper ankle were carried out in a total of 24 patients. In 81 % a synovectomy was performed and in 53 % osteophytes or exostoses were removed at the same time. Also in 53 % of the patients adhesions and cicatrices were removed. This shows the combined presence of different pathologies at the same time. The average age of the patients was 25.2 years. The follow-up time was between 12 and 42 months, with an average of 21 months.

Because of the small number of operated patients and the frequently multiple combined diagnoses these results can be considered only as trends. The best results were obtained in chronic synovitis with cicatrices or adhesions. Satisfactory results were observed with the removal of osteophytes and after the smoothing of Grade II osteochondral lesions. The results in the treatment of degenerative joint changes are not encouraging. Two thirds of all the patients showed a good to very good result, while in one third the results were unsatisfactory. These patients showed mainly degenerative changes. Our results are comparable to those reported in the literature (Andrews et al., 1985; Parisien, 1985 a+b).

8 Summary and Conclusion

In very carefully selected patients, therapeutic arthroscopy is a very helpful and elegant procedure. An exact diagnosis is essential, whereby the significance of a pathological change as the cause of symptoms can be problematical. The advantages of arthroscopic therapy are the low morbidity involved, the more rapid rehabilitation, the very good overview of the whole joint, the shorter hospitalization time, avoidance of an osteotomy and less pain.

9 References

Andrews, J.R., Previte, W.J. and Carson, W.G. (1985) Arthroscopy of the Ankle. Technique and Normal Anatomy. Foot and Ankle, 6, 29-33.

Biedert, R. (1989) Osteochondrale Läsionen des Talus. Unfallchirurg, 92, 199-205.

Boe, S. (1986) Arthroscopy of the Ankle Joint. Arch. Orthop. Trauma Surg., 105, 285-286.;

Canale, T.and Belding, R. (1980) Ostechondral Lesions of the Talus. J. Bone Joint Surg., 62-A, 97-102.

Hempfling, H. (1987) Farbatlas der Arthroskopie grosser Gelenke. Gustav Fischer Verlag, Stuttgart.

Johnson, L.L. (1981) The knee and other joints, in Diagnostic and Surgical Arthroscopy (eds). C.V. Mosby Company, St. Louis, Toronto, London, pp. 412-419.

Martin, DF., Baker, CL., Curl, WW., Andrews, J.R., Robie, DB. and Haas, A.F. (1989) Operative ankle arthroscopy; long-term follow-up. Am. J. Sports Med., 17, 16-23.

Parisien, J.S. (1985 a) Diagnostic and Operative Arthroscopy of the Ankle. Technique and Indications. Bull. Hos. Jt. Diseases Orthop. Inst., 45, 38-47

Parisien, J.S. (1985 b) Operative Arthroscopy of the Ankle. Three Years' Experience. Clin. Orthop. Rel. Res., 199, 46-53.

KINESIOLOGICAL ANALYSIS OF THE ANKLE'S ARTICULATION IN TRAINED AND UNTRAINED INDIVIDUALS, WITH OR WITHOUT HISTORY OF FORMER MUSCLE-LIGAMENT INJURY

A.D.P. BANKOFF, A.R. TOLEDO, J.L. COELHO and F.C. VIEIRA,
Laboratory of Electromyography and Posture of Biomechanics -
Physical Education, University of Campinas, Brazil.

1 Introduction

The ankle (talocrural) joint is formed by the articulation of the fibula and the tibia with the talus and is responsible for the dorsal and plantar flexion movements of the foot. The tibia and the fibula are intimately united by the inner bone membrane and by the inner bone ligaments, but also by the anterior and the posterior tibiofibular ligaments and by the transverse ligaments which also articulate with the talus. The weight of the body is transmitted by the trochlea of the talus.

The medial malleolus, a process of the tibia, articulates with the medial malleolar facet of the talus. The fibula supports little or no weight; the fibula goes downwards adjoining the lateral face of the talus forming the lateral malleolus, which articulates with the lateral malleolar facet of the talus. This way, the talus is encased in a sort of flanked cavity or notch, providing a considerable stability to the articulation.

Caillet (1978) considered the talus as the master key of the mechanics of the foot's apex, describing the articulation of the bi-malleolar pincers and affirming that inside the pincers, the talus would work like an articulation in ginglimo. Dorsiflexion and plantar flexion of the ankle occur around an axis that passes crosswise to the body of the talus. The lateral extremity of the ankle's axis passes by the fibula's apex and is centrally situated between the fixation of the external collateral ligaments, allowing them to remain tense during all the movements. At the medial extremity the transverse axis is placed eccentrically to the medial ligament's insertion point. In this position the anterior medial ligaments become tense at plantar flexion. The alteration of extension and relaxation restricts the ambit of the plantar and dorsal movements of the ankle.

Lindsjo et al. (1985) measured the dorsal and plantar flexions' degrees in three different ways - the individual in a supine position, sitting with no load and through a third and a new method where it was possible to evaluate the ankles under load. This method presented values closer to those obtained in osteo-ligamentary preparations from previous studies of several authors. Robinson et al. (1986) studied the stabilization of the ankle's articulation used as injury prevention, finding negative effects on the cases with insufficient or excessive control of the ankle's mobility. He concluded that a diminished arc of mobility in an

ankle's articulation can adversely affect the performance of an
individual in an agility procedure.

2 Methods

After a standardized warm-up of 3 min, the degrees of dorsiflexion
and plantar flexion (the articulation's movement in the sagittal
plane) were measured with load (body weight). In total there were 60
individuals (120 ankles) examined. They were divided into 2 groups:
a 1st trained group was formed by 30 individuals (60 ankles) with a
weekly load of physical exercise and training equal or superior to
20 hours and the 2nd group (untrained) was formed by individuals
that did not reach this level of weekly physical activity.

The method chosen to measure the dorsal and plantar flexions, in
degrees, of these ankles was described by Lindsjo et al. (1985).
The individual puts his foot on top of a bench, which is 30 cm high,
and leans forward as much as possible without lifting the heel from
the bench (dorsal flexion). The posterior muscles' relaxation
contributes to a higher dorsiflexion value, measured as being the
angle between the supporting line of the foot and the long axis of
the leg. For measurement of plantar flexion with load, the same
scheme is repeated, but the individual raises his heel as much as
possible without getting the ankle bone off the bench. The plantar
flexion degree is measured through the angle between the supporting
line of the foot and the long axis of the leg. To obtain the
measurements, a HEALTHFOCUS TM 0-180 degrees goniometer was used.

3 Results

The results that refer to the ankle's measurements are represented
in Tables 1, 2 and 3.

Table 1. Distribution of the number of individuals that didn't
present injury; that presented injuries in both ankles; that
presented injury in the right ankle and that presented injury in the
left ankle, trained and untrained, with the respective percentages

	ankle without injury	injury in both ankles	right ankle with injury	left ankle with injury
Trained	15(50%)	7(23%)	3(10%)	5(16.6%)
Untrained	9(30%)	7(23%)	11(36.7%)	3(10%)

Table 2. Distribution of the averages of the dorsal flexion angles (right and left) and plantar flexion (right and left) with the respective numbers of individuals: individuals without injury, individuals with injury in both ankles, individuals with injury only in the right ankle and individuals with injury only in the left ankle, trained and untrained.

Number of individuals	Average of dorsal flexion (degrees)		Average of plantar flexion (degrees)	
	right ankle	left ankle	right ankle	left ankle
TRAINED				
15 without injury	23.4	25.5	37.8	33.4
7 injury R/L	25.6	24.4	39.1	42.7
3 injury R	30.7	30.4	51.6	46.0
5 injury L	22.2	22.4	32.2	32.2
UNTRAINED				
9 without injury	32.6	27.7	43.6	43.4
7 injury R/L	27.6	28.4	43.7	42.1
11 injury R	27.5	25.8	46.2	44.3
3 injury L	30.0	30.0	48.3	47.6

Table 3. Distribution of the intensity of the injury for the cases of medial right ankle, lateral right ankle, medial left ankle and lateral left ankle, representing them as trained and untrained

		SERIOUS	MODERATE	LIGHT
TRAINED	medial right		1	
	lateral right		4	5
	medial left	1		
	lateral left		4	7
	Total	1	9	12
UNTRAINED	medial right	1		
	lateral right	2	3	12
	medial left			
	lateral left	3	2	5
	Total	6	5	17

According to the results presented in Table 1, we can observe that in the trained group 50% of the individuals did not present injury in the ankle, 23% presented injury in both ankles, 10% presented injury only in the right ankle and 16.6% presented injury only in the left ankle. In the untrained group 30% of the individuals did not present injury in the ankles, 23% presented injury in both ankles, 36.7% presented injury only in the right ankle and 10% presented injury only in the left ankle. The group of trained individuals showed a higher number of people without ankle sprains when compared to the untrained group.

The averages of plantar and dorsal flexion degrees for right and left ankles of trained and untrained groups indicated that the group of trained individuals obtained the following average values: right ankle dorsal flexion 24.4° and plantar flexion 38.6°; left ankle dorsal flexion 25.2° and plantar flexion 36.6°. The untrained group of individuals obtained the following averages: right ankle dorsal flexion 27.5° and plantar flexion 44.4°; left ankle dorsal flexion 27.4° and plantar flexion 43.9°. The untrained group had a bigger articular amplitude as reflected in the averages, in most instances, when compared to the trained group.

In Table 2, the opposite occurs with the articular amplitude in cases: i) average of the plantar flexion degree of the left ankle with injury in both ankes and ii) average of the dorsal flexion degree of the right ankle, average of the dorsal flexion degree of the left ankle, average of the plantar flexion degree of the right ankle and average of the plantar flexion degree of the left ankle with injury in the right ankle.

We observed (Table 3) that the group of trained individuals showed 10 cases with light injury, 9 cases with moderate injury and 1 case of serious injury. In the group of untrained individuals we noted 17 cases with light injury, 5 cases with moderate injury and 6 cases with serious injury.

Our results refer to the kinesiological analysis of the amplitude measurements, in degrees, of dorsal flexion and plantar flexion movements, in trained and untrained individuals, with and without a previous history of osteo-ligamentary injury. A list of our observations is as follows:-

i) The anterior osteo-ligamentary injuries in the ankles were more frequent in untrained individuals when compared to trained individuals.

ii) The incidence of anterior osteo-ligamentary injury in the right ankle was higher in the untrained individuals than in trained individuals.

iii) In the left ankle, the incidence of anterior osteo-ligamentary injury was higher in trained individuals than in untrained.

iv) The number of 'twisted ankles' was higher in the untrained group.

v) The measurements, in degrees, of the movements' amplitudes was significantly higher in the untrained individuals compared to the trained individuals in both movements and in both ankles.

vi) The average, in degrees, of the movements' amplitudes, when presented with the respective number of individuals with anterior osteo-ligamentary injury was higher in the trained group, specifically in those individuals who presented with injury in the right ankle.

vii) According to the information contained in our protocols, 52.3% of the untrained people who suffered some kind of ankle injury did not search for medical assistance for treatment. In other words, they searched for domestic treatment.

viii) According to the information contained in our protocols, the trained individuals (soccer players) that suffered some type of ankle injury were always assisted by specialized medical treatment.

ix) When classified, the injuries occurred in a higher number in untrained individuals, the only exception being in the moderate cases for trained individuals.

x) The anterior osteo-ligamentary injuries happened more frequently in inversion movements of the feet.

4 References

Caillet, R. (1978) Syndrome Dolorosas. Pe e Tornozelo. Editora Manole, Sao Paulo.

Lindsjo, U. Danckwardt-Lilliestrom, G. and Sahlstedt, B. (1985) Clin. Orthop. Rel. Res., 199, Oct.

Robinson, J.R., Frederick, E.C. and Cooper, L.B. (1986) Systematic ankle stabilization and the effect on performance. Med. Sci. Sports Exerc., 18, 625-628.

THE TREATMENT OF SPRAINED ANKLE, TAPE VERSUS MALLEOTRAIN. A COMPARATIVE, PROSPECTIVE STUDY OF THE TREATMENT RESULTS IN ONE HUNDRED PATIENTS WITH DISTORTION OF THE ANKLE

S.J.M. JONGEN, J.H. POT, P.B. DUNKI JACOBS
MCA, Dept. of Surgery, Alkmaar, The Netherlands

1 Introduction

Inversion injury of the ankle is one of the most commonly
occurring acute injuries in The Netherlands (Van der Ent,
1984). Injury of the lateral ligaments of the ankle joint
is for instance frequently seen in football players
reporting to the Emergency Ward of the MCA.
Treatment of ankle ligament injury is an issue still
subject to discussion. Although some still passionately
defend the surgical approach (Ahrend and Pollahne, 1989;
Bar and Tausch, 1988; Jaskulka et al., 1988), a number of
well implemented randomised prospective studies (Cramer
and Friedhoff, 1990; Klein et al., 1988; Sommer and Arza,
1989) have led to a current preference for early
functional treatment of acute distortion of the ankle.
This is linked with the fact that the results of this
treatment are as good as, if not better than, surgical
treatment, the lower health care costs and the
convenience for the patient (no hospital admission, a
more rapid recommencement of work and sports) being
additional factors in favour of conservative treatment.
The most frequently applied method in The Netherlands is
taping of the ankle, using Coumans' bandaging method
(Cramer and Friedhoff, 1990; Van Moppes and Van den
Hoogenband, 1982). This reliable and popular method does,
however, have some disadvantages; taping requires some
skill and is time-consuming, the tape has to remain in
position day and night and can cause irritation of the
skin. The application and changing of the tape is usually
performed as second-line medical care, which is rather
expensive.

Recently, a new method, that could possibly obviate some
of the disadvantages of tape, has been introduced. This
so-called Malleotrain is an elastic bandage for the ankle
joint with a grip seam on either side of the Achilles'
tendon (Fig. 1). In a prospective randomised study
treatment with tape was compared with treatment with
Malleotrain.

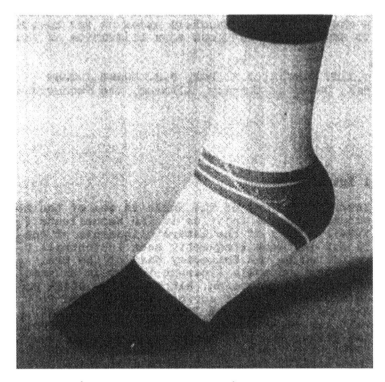

Fig. 1. The Malleotrain bandage.

2 Patients and Methods

One hundred patients were randomly allocated either to treatment with tape or to treatment with Malleotrain. The inclusion criteria were: recent inversion trauma, isolated injury, no ankle traumata in the medical history, and an age range of 18 to 50 years. The diagnosis distortion of the ankle was made on the basis of anamnesis and physical diagnosis. An x-ray was made to exclude fractures. Due to the limited value of ancillary diagnostic x-ray examination (e.g. stress radiograms or arthrography (Van Moppes and Van den Hoogenband, 1982), which is associated with poor reproducibility, lack of correlation between objective findings and complaints, and investigator-bound results, we refrained from this approach.
The primary treatment consisted of immobilisation of the joint for a week with a rear plaster splint. This was followed either by treatment with tape 3 times over 6 weeks, or Malleotrain treatment for 6 weeks.

The ankle function was assessed in the clinic after 3, 5, 7 and 15 weeks, respectively, and during these visits the patients also completed a questionnaire. The follow-up period covered a period of 15 weeks in total. After this the final result was determined and the patients voiced their opinions.
Results were recorded as: very good, good, moderate and poor. The parameters assessed in order to arrive at this conclusion were: pain, swelling, fear of spraining, recurrent sprain and resumption of work.
When all parameters were evaluated favourably, the result was considered very good. If only one parameter had given the evaluation inadequate, the result was good. Two parameters below the mark meant a moderate result and more than two inadequate parameters meant a poor result. If the patient recommenced sports, this was recorded, but not considered in the result. The opinion of the patients themselves, after 15 weeks, was expressed as very content, content, moderately content and discontent.

3 Results

Altogether 88 patients had evaluable results. Twelve patients (6 from each group) dropped out of the study, because of an incomplete follow-up or because they prematurely discontinued the therapy and decided for a different method of treatment.
The mean age was 28 years. Male/female ratio was 3:1. In the group using tape 34 patients (68%) were classified as very good and good. In the group using the Malleotrain method 35 patients (70%) were classified as such (see Fig. 2 and Table 1).

Table 1. Results by number of patients and percentages			Table 2. The patient's opinion, by number of patients and percentages		
RESULTS	TAPE n=50	MALLEOTRAIN n=50	PATIENT'S OPINION	TAPE n=50	MALLEOTRAIN n=50
very good	22(44%)	25 (50%)	very content	12(24%)	22 (44%)
good	12(24%)	10 (20%)	content	25(50%)	16 (32%)
moderate	7(14%)	4 (8%)	moderately content	6(12%)	3 (6%)
poor	3(6%)	5 (10%)	discontent	1 (2%)	3 (6%)
unknown	6(12%)	6 (12%)	unknown	6(12%)	6 (12%)

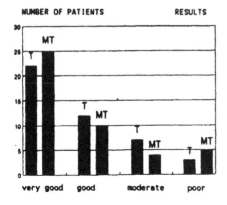

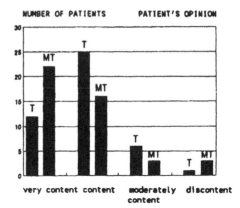

Fig. 2. Results by number of patients.

Fig. 3. The patient's opinion, by number of patients.

Regarding the patient's opinion, 37 patients (74%) in the group using tape were very content or content, versus 38 patients (76%) in the group using Malleotrain (see Fig. 3 and Table 2).

Work was resumed after 21 days on average (tape group 20 and Malleotrain group 22 days); this is in accordance with the time period stated in the literature (Van Moppes and Van den Hoogenband, 1982). After 15 weeks no difference could be found between the groups, both with regard to the recommencement of sports and to the use of preventive bandage during sports (see Figs. 4 and 5). Irritation of the skin under the tape was observed in 4 patients using tape bandage.

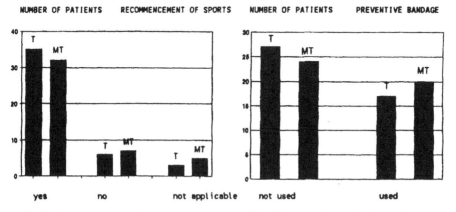

Fig. 4. Recommencement of sports by number of patients.

Fig. 5. Preventive bandage by number of patients.

4 Discussion

A condition for functional treatment of lateral ankle ligament injury is that adequate protection can be provided against inversion, by an external stabilisation method. Different methods have been developed to this end, varying from a simple foam rubber insole, a so-called "Pronationswurm" (Sandor et al., 1990), for example, to a specially made high leather shoe, the so-called "Adimed-Stabil-Z-Schuh" (Ludolph and Niezold, 1989).

As already mentioned, taping of the ankle is the most popular method of conservative treatment in the Netherlands. The study has shown that functional treatment of acute ligament injury with tape or Malleotrain gives good results in 68% and 70% of cases, respectively. The follow-up period lasts only 15 weeks. These early results contrast with the late results usually stated in the literature, varying from 6 months to 4 years (Cramer and Friedhoff, 1990; Klein et al., 1988; Sommer and Arza, 1989; Van Moppes and Van den Hoogenband, 1982).

In the literature, the criteria for diagnosing ankle ligament injury are not always unequivocal. Moreover, striking differences are encountered with regard to the method of classification of the results.

All these factors complicate the comparison of our percentages with those mentioned in other studies.

We conclude that early functional treatment of acute ankle ligament injury gives good results, a statement in accordance with current views. This study demonstrates that there is no significant difference, regarding objective and subjective results, between the two methods of functional treatment studied. Other factors will determine which method is eventually preferred. The disadvantages of taping, as mentioned above, can partially be overcome by the Malleotrain method. This bandage, being patient-friendly, easy to fit, and applicable in first-line medical care, and, furthermore, leading to lower costs, certainly deserves a place in the treatment of ankle distortion.

5 References

Ahrend, E. and Pollahne, W. (1989) Erfahrungen in Diagnostik, Therapie und Rehabilitation von frischen und alten fibularen Kapselbandverletzungen des oberen Sprunggelenkes. Sporttraumatologie, 83, 83-87.

Bar, B.W. and Tausch, W. (1988) Erste Erfahrungen mit
der ambulanten Bandnaht der frischen lateralen
Bandruptur am oberen Sprunggelenk in Lokalanaesthesie.
Zent. bl. Cir., 113, 1268-1272.
Cramer, E.A. and Friedhoff K. (1990) Eine sichere
Alternative in der frühfunktionellen Behandlung aller
Bandinstabilitäten am OSG? Unfallchir., 93, 275-283.
Jaskulka, R., Fischer G. and Schedl, R. (1988)
Injuries of the lateral ligament of the ankle joint.
Arch. Orth. Trauma Surg., 107, 217-221.
Klein, J., Schreckenberger, C., Roddecker K. (1988)
Operative oder konservative Behandlung der
frischen Aussenbandruptur am oberen Sprunggelenk.
Unfallchir., 91, 154-160.
Ludolph, E. and Niezold, D. (1989) Untersuchungen zur
Supinationsstabilität im Adimed-Stabil-2-Schuh bei
Kapsel-Bandinstabilität des oberen Sprunggelenkes.
Unfallchir. 92, 195-198.
Sandor, L., Suveges, G. and Nacsai, I. (1990)
Frühfunktionelle aktivkonservative Behandlung der
Aussenknochelbandrupturen mit dem "Pronationswurm".
Unfallchir., 93, 284-288.
Sommer, H.M. and Arza, D. (1989) Functional treatment
of recent ruptures of the fibular ligament of the
ankle. Inter. Orth., 13, 157-160.
Van der Ent, E.W.C. (1984) Lateral ankle ligament
injury. Thesis, Rotterdam, The Netherlands.
Van Moppes, F.I. and Van den Hoogenband, C.R. (1982)
Diagnostic and therapeutic aspects of inversion trauma
of the ankle joint. Thesis, Maastricht, The
Netherlands.

ANKLE INJURIES: PHYSICAL EXAMINATION AND ARTHROSCOPY

C.N. VAN DIJK
Academisch Medisch Centrum, Amsterdam, The Netherlands.
W. SMITH
Milwaukee, North America.

1 Introduction

The most frequently injured site in football is the ankle joint. Among
the ankle injuries the vast majority consist of supination traumas.
The physical examination after an acute supination trauma is usually
not reliable in discriminating between a distorsion or a rupture of
the lateral ankle ligaments. The first question that has to be
answered is if there is a fracture or not. If the patiënt can stand
and walk on the injured leg and there is no pressure pain on the
fibula then the chance of a significant fracture is less than 0.6
percent. If we can examine the patiënt on the "field" within a few
minutes after the trauma before swelling has occurred, then it is
usually possible to examine the ankle joint for instability. When
swelling has occurred and the pain is diffusely present, then
stability testing is not possible.

2 Physical examination

When we initialy treat the patiënt with ice, pressure bandage and
elevation and we examine the ankle 4 or 5 days after the trauma then
the physical examination appears to be very accurate.
   In a prospective study performed in the AMC, Amsterdam, 400
patiënts were tested and in this investigation the reliability of the
physical examination was even higher than that of the arthrogram. The
arthrogram was performed in all 400 patiënts within 48 hours after
trauma. The physical examination was then without knowledge of the
result of the arthrogram performed 5 days after trauma. Operation was
performed when either the arthrogram was positive or the physical
examination was positive (Beek, 1985).

3 Residual problems

Residual problems after lateral ligament rupture of the ankle occur
in a high precentage. In the literature 30 to 50% of the patiënts
complain of some pain, some swelling or some giving way. A minority
has real instability problems (van Dijk, 1991).
Most of the patiënts have pain and swelling, usually during or after

playing sports or performing demanding physical activity. Their complaints are observed despite the treatment modality. In the Amsterdam series of 400 patiënts (200 treated by operative means and 200 by elastic bandage) at 6 months follow-up, 26% still had complaints. The complaints were usually located over the medial side of the ankle. This pain on the medial side is present in most patiënts directly after a supination trauma.

In the Amsterdam series of 400 patiënts, in 60% there was pressure pain on the medial side 5 days after trauma. In a consecutive series of 30 patiënts who underwent operative repair of the lateral ankle ligament, arthroscopy was done to look at the medial structures. In these 30 patiënts there was one rupture of the deltoid ligament, 3 patients had synovitis, 2 had fibrous bands, while 19 patiënts had cartilage damage on the tip of the medial malleolus and the opposite medial talar facet.

Physical examination of the ankle joint in chronic ankle injuries is important in discriminating between the various types of pathology. Attention was drawn to the entrapment syndrome of the superficial peroneal nerve, peroneus tertius syndrome, plantar fasciitis, chronic achilles tendon problems and recurring dislocation of the peroneal tendons. The diagnosis of the above mentioned pathology relies usually on physical examination.

4 Arthroscopy

Arthroscopy of the ankle joint is gaining in popularity. With physical examination and examinations like infiltration, isotope scan, CT-scan or MRI almost any intra- and extra articular ankle pathology can be determined. In general there is no need for arthroscopy in the diagnostic strategy. Moreover viewing every corner of the ankle joint is demanding and is virtually impossible without using mechanical distraction. On the other hand there is hardly any intra-articular ankle pathology that can not be treated by arthroscopic surgery. Most of the intra-articular pathology is located in the anterior part of the ankle, like osteophytes, scar tissue, fibrous band and synovitis, osteochondral lesions , calcifications and so on. Osteochondral lesions of the talus can be located more to the posterior part of the joint and it is in those lesions that mechanical distraction has its place. In some cases a transmalleolar portal is then needed.

In a Dutch multicentre trial in which 256 patients were retrospectively reviewed with an average follow-up of 2 year in loose bodies, impingement lesion and osteochondral defects a good or excellent result was found in over 90% of the patients. In this study diagnostic arthroscopy had a poor outcome (van Dijk et al., 1992).

5 Conclusions

Physical examination appears to be very accurate in discriminating between a distorsion or a ligament rupture, when performed 4 or 5 days after an acute supinationtrauma. The frequency of residual problems after supinationtrauma is high. The main cause of these residual problems is not instability, but recurrent pain and swelling. An important cause for these residual problems is cartilage damage located on the medial side of the ankle joint.

Most chronic ankle problems can be managed by arthroscopic surgery. In treatment of impingement lesions osteochondral defect or loose bodies a good or excellent result can be expected in over 90% of patients. The role of diagnostic arthroscopy is very limited.

6 References

Beek v. J. (1985) Evaluation of ankle injuries using the Cybex II dynamometer. Acta Orthop. Scand., 56, 6, 516.

Dijk van C.N. (1991) Arthroscopie van het bovenste spronggewricht. Letsels van de enkel en voet, pp. 69-86. (eds. J.B. van Mourik en P. Patka).

Dijk van C.N., Fievez A.W.F.M., Heyboer M.P. et al. (1992) Arthroscopy of the ankle. NOV Jaarvergadering, Enschede 1992.

INJURIES TO THE FOOT IN SOCCER PLAYERS

R. SAGGINI, A. CALLIGARIS, G. MONTANARI, N. TJOUROUDIS and L.
VECCHIET
Postgraduate School of Sports Medicine, University of Chieti, Medical
Section of F.I.G.C., Coverciano (FI), Italy

1 Introduction

In soccer, the foot not only participates in the performance of a
motor action (understood here as an act of moving the whole body
structure in space), but most of all comprises the basic element in
many sporting movements. Thus it should be considered to have an
essential role especially in football.

   The foot, in relation to external stresses, proves to be most
adaptable and variable in interfacing with the ground which supports
it, so that the human is assured safe economical movement through
space. It is not a structure isolated from the general context of
the body but one which is completely integrated into the genesis of a
motor act. It can be affected by pathological processes deriving
from its manner of advancing over a surface such as grass, precarious
by definition, and by its manner of positioning itself for the act of
kicking a ball.

2 Materials and Methods

We have analysed, over 24 months, 200 players belonging to Italian
professional teams who have chronic pathological events on structures
of the foot.

   The method consists of both a clinical and x-ray evaluation and a
dynamic assessment by means of a podobarographic platform with 1024
piezoelectronic sensors. With this method it is possible to describe
the pressure and the forces during the stance phase of the foot. In
this representation it is possible to recognize the heel contact and
the support phase and after the propulsive phase (Saggini and Reale,
1983).

   Therapeutic approaches should always include an objective
examination of behaviour and integuments. After this the structure
can be analysed with diagnostic images, radiography, ultrasonography,
computed tomography or nuclear magnetic resonance, to highlight any
pathological processes also involving the osteo-musculo-tendinous
structure.

3 Results

From a statistical point of view the hallux rigidus represents the

most frequent pathology because in 34% of the subjects a hallux
rigidus of the first degree appeared. In 6% there was a third degree
hallux rigidus, heel pain appeared in 15%, the syndrome of sinus
tarsi in 10%, plantar fasciitis in 6%, sesamoiditis in 8%, hallux
valgus in 4%, metatarsalgia in 7%, metatarsalgia of Morton in 2%,
chondral injuries of trochlea tali in 2%. A more frequent pathology
but intercurrent with the others already mentioned has been a
subungual haematoma in 60% of subjects, hyperkeratosis in 35% and
unguis incarnatus in 6%.

Hallux rigidus

The hallux rigidus is a pathological process which has a high
incidence in soccer players. Three stages of hallux rigidus can be
distinguished clinically and radiographically. In 34% a hallux
rigidus of the first degree appears and in 6% it is of third degree.

Clinically the pain is around the joint especially in the forward
propulsion phase of the foot during the stance phase on the ground.
In severe cases, chronic inflammation of the long extensor tendon of
the hallux is evident and the sheath of the tendon becomes thickened
at the point where it meets the typical dorsal exostosis.

Radiographically, there is degenerative alteration with reduction
of the rima and subchondral osteosclerosis and also increase of the
tranverse diameter of the articular head with the presence of the
osteophytes in the border.

The phenomenon of localised osteochondral fracture from direct
trauma rarely occurs in soccer players. If it does occur, it will
rapidly give rise to third degree hallux rigidus.

Heel pain

Heel pain is a very common phenomenon, caused by direct trauma or
microtrauma. The tendinitis of the Achilles tendon is the first
cause of pain but often there are microtraumatic forms of heel pain
with neuretic involvement which develop in relation to particular
neural and regional anatomy.

Clinically pain appears on the medial border of the heel. It is
noticeable proximally along the course of the Achilles tendon.

The causes of the form of pain are to be found in an alteration in
the 3-D movement of the hindfoot, especially the sub-talar joint.
This is combined with the stretch of the neural structures described
above in contact with the fascial border and the calcaneal crest.

For talalgia in a posterior location, two distinct pathological
phenomena can be distinguished. These are insertional pathology and
pathology caused by appearance of bursitis because of the retro-
calcaneal spurs.

Sinus tarsi syndrome

Clinically referred elective pain is evident on palpation on forced
inversion of the foot. Always clinical and case history reveal a
history of sprain in inversion or a predisposing anatomical status
such a valgus of heel or valgus flat-foot or varum cavum (Valenti,
1977).

The gait analysis shows a reduction of internal rotation during
the contact phase. These data are correlated with the pathological
process.

Plantar fasciitis

Inflammation of the plantar fascia from overload with pain in the plantar aponeurosis and the insertion at the heel is present very often. This is an insertional syndrome caused by repeated microtraumas on the plantar fascia and its insertions at the calcaneus and the metatarsal eminences. It may be monolateral or bilateral.

The x-ray can often show calcification situated on the fascial insertion in line with the calcaneal tuberosity. Scintigraphic examination in an acute phase reveals an increase in the flow of the microcirculatory system in the soft tissues. The presence of calcaneal spurs, scintigraphically passive in this case, only demonstrates continuous traction taking place at the insertion of the plantar fascia. The traction causes osseous metaplasia at the insertion.

Sesamoiditis

The sesamoid bone is situated in the body of the tendinous structure. The sesamoids are situated in the middle of the flexor tendon of the hallux. Usually, two sesamoids are present, one medial and one lateral.

A state of acute inflammation is often present, accompanied by pain and, at times, swelling of the plantar aspect of the first metatarsus. In this case, there will be a pathological process of the sesamoids, the medial in particular (just here, in fact, a foot stud is situated). When a sesamoid shows bipartite on a radiogram and clinically presents pain when pressure is applied locally (exactly on the bipartite point in particular), it would be correct to assume the presence of a microfracture from direct stress. In this case, radiograms with special projections, use of computed tomography and scintigraphy may highlight an irregular separation with unequal but well separated fragments. A state of inflammation is often present (6%), accompanied by pain and, at times, swelling of the plantar aspect of the first metatarsus.

Hallux Valgus

This is a pathological process which is rare in soccer players, but if it does appear, can limit performance, mostly because of the counteraction between the osseous structure and the foot. By "soccer players' hallux valgus" is understood a deviation, usually quite small, at the beginning of the hallux and mostly associated with a varus state of the first metatarsus. This is the anatomical condition in soccer players which is most predisposing to bring out the pathological phenomenon. Following continual microtrauma to the foot from violent blows of the ball, when articular instability (anatomically described above) is present, axial disarrangement of the first ray may result.

Metatarsalgia

This is a syndrome from overload of the forefoot which, in the soccer player, arises either because of a predisposing anatomical functional situation or is related to the practice of the game on hard ground with the contributory presence of studs which are positioned on a metatarsal eminence. It should be remembered that the soccer player tends to execute vigorous spurts and abrupt stops which act mainly on the forefoot. The analysis of ground reaction clearly shows that, during the thrust forward of sprinting, the subject develops not only vertical forces far in excess of those which the osteoarticular fore-foot can absorb but also very high shear forces during the abrupt stops. Thus, along with irritation of the bone at metatarsal eminences, there is also metatarsophalangeal instability and, thereafter, besides friction of the integuments, there is hypermobility of the osteoarticular structures, greatly facilitating the metatarsus in assuming a position of plantar flexion.

Morton's metatarsalgia

This is a pathological process which has its cause in extrinsic and intrinsic factors (Bossley and Cairney, 1980). Among these are:- (i) playing footwear; (ii) the violent twisting movements which the player performs during a winding run at maximum acceleration: in this case the torque moment of ground force greatly increases, thus creating a situation of high friction correlated to a very high peak force. Intrinsic factors include:- (i) the presence of a marked external rotation on the horizontal plane of the lower limb; (ii) progress of the foot-ground reaction characterised by an involvement of only the fourth and fifth rays during the thrust phase and by a time period which is increased by 25% compared with normal duration time during the intermediate phase (Saggini et al., 1988).

The factors cited above can be concurrent in the production of neural phenomena in the interdigital parts of the fourth and fifth spaces and, in the final analysis, of the formation of a "neuroma" which will have to be ablated.

Chondral lesions

Chondral lesions are found in 2% of cases. These lesions are caused by movements of the talus in eversion or eversion. The locations were anterior-lateral in one case and posterior-medial in three cases. The degree of lesion was classifiable: (i) one case with cartilaginous cleavage; (ii) two cases with osteochondral fracture without displacement of the fragment; (iii) one case with osteo-chondral detachment with displacement of the fragment.

4 Conclusions

The pathological processes that can develop in the foot of a soccer player during a game are caused by either simple acute trauma from contact or microtrauma from repeated stress to the foot, which develop when the player is running (with or without the ball), stop-ping, suddenly changing direction or speed, or in the act of kicking itself.

5 References

Baxter, D.E. (1982) Nerve entrapment as cause of heel pain. Communication to the Orthopaedic Foot Club, New Orleans, May.
Bossley, C.Y. and Cairney, P.C. (1980) The itemetatarso-phalangeal bursa: its significance in Morton's metatarsalgia. J. Bone Jt. Surg., 62, 184-187.
Saggini, R. and Reale, S. (1983) L'analisi della deambulazione nel

piede cavo e piatto come ausilio nello sviluppo e valutazione di procedure terapeutiche. **Rasegna di Bioingegneria**, 8, 1-3.

Saggini, R., Migliorini, M., Vecchione, P. and Cardini, M. (1988) Sindrome metatarsalgica di T.C. Morton: valutazione biomeccanico-clinica e correlazioni eziopatogenetiche. **Chir. Piede**, 12, 255-259.

Valenti, V. (1977) La rappresentazione nervosa nella istologia del legamento a siepe. **Chir. Piede**, 1, 1-4.

CLINICAL AND INSTRUMENTAL ASSESSMENT IN YOUNG SOCCER PLAYERS

V. GUZZANTI, F.M. PEZZOLI and *A. BAGARONE
Ospedale Bambino Gesu' Div. Ortop. and Traumat. Rome-Italy
* CONI - Istituto Scienza dello Sport Rome - Italy

1 Introduction

Orthopedic assessment of growing soccer players was perfomed in order to detect paramorphia and\or dysmorphosis of the spine. Assessment was based on a thorough orthopedic examination and a series of instrumental examinations. Clinical judgement was based on the detection of paramorphia and\or dysmorphosis of the spine. Athletes underwent telethermographic screening and, in some cases, x-ray examination.

The choice of telethermographic examination was dictated by the need to use a valid, non-invasive method. The telethermographic method made it possible to analyze the results and print them on photographic film.

2 Materials and Methods

The sample population consisted of 90 junior soccer players, aged between 10 and 12 years. The athletes had no record of previous trauma and had played soccer at a competitive level for about three years.

The training schedule was three two-hour sessions a week. The first part was dedicated to the potentiation and elasticity of the muscles of the trunk and the upper and lower limbs. The second part included lessons for the improvement of individual technique.

Assessment consisted of two essential steps: clinical examination and instrumental evaluation. Clinical examination was based on case history, objective examination of the spine and study of the morphological and functional characteristics of the upper limbs with particular attention to the work load in competitive soccer.

In all 90 subjects dynamic instrumental thermography of the spine was effected using a Digital Philips machine capable of revealing the temperature differences for values lower than 0.15 C. Thermography was chosen because it involves no risks and can be repeated. The validity of this examination in the study of paramorphia and dysmorphosis of the spine has been recognized by various authors. In particular, Woodrought (1976) reported the peculiarity of thermography in evidencing the different muscular activities between one side and the other of the spine, sometimes anticipating the clinical manifestation of dysmorphosis. This examination is based on the detection of the normal thermographic map. Negative thermographic images (Th-) are characterized by a uniform and symmetrical distribution of the thermal gradients on both sides of the spinal column. In positive thermographic images (corresponding to scoliosis, muscular hypertrophy and scoliotic posture), the result is asymmetrical.

In positive thermographic images (Th+) there are different thermal gradients characterized by hypo- and hyperthermic areas with an asymmetrical distribution on the left and right sides of the posterior surface of the thorax and the lumbo-sacral region. The greater or lesser significance of this asymmetry is determined by the extent of the calorimetric difference, that is range, between one side and the other of the paravertebral muscles, using the reference scale in the photographic image obtained.

3 Results

Clinical and instrumental examination of the 90 junior soccer players showed:

a) twenty-three had clinical asymmetry of the paravertebral muscles (consisting of muscular hypertrophy corresponding to the posterior region of the scapular girdle and the dorsal muscles). Twenty of these had a positive thermographic response;

b) there were three cases of scoliosis confirmed by X-ray and thermography;

c) four had a scoliotic posture (consequent to slight length inequality of the lower limbs) and positive thermography;

d) three had positive thermography and negative clinical assessment (Th+, clinical examination-).

In scoliosis the thermographic response showed more evident hyperthermic areas than the images obtained in the cases of simple muscular hypertrophy and a distribution of the hyperthermic area corresponding to the hump, a sign of the different activity of the paravertebral muscles.

In the four cases of scoliotic posture with positive thermography, slight hyperthermic areas were observed with thermal gradients lower than those obtained in scoliosis and muscular hypertrophy.

Table 1. Results of Clinical Examination (CE+)

	Pathology	No. of cases (%)	
A	Muscular hypertrophy	23	(20.7%)
B	Scoliotic posture	4	(3.6%)
C	Scoliosis	3	(2.7%)
	Total CE+	30	(27%)

The incidence of structural deviations of the spine in the soccer players examined was not different from that obtained by other authors for preadolescents and adolescents not involved in competitive sports.

From an analysis of the results, we feel that subjects with muscular hypertrophy and positive thermographic findings (CE+, Th+) represent a group "at risk" to be followed up because they could in the future develop spinal dysmorphosis. We feel that also young soccer players with a negative clinical examination and positive thermography (CE-, Th+) should be followed with particular attention, in that the latter could be a warning sign of future development of spinal dysmorphosis. In this situation thermographic examination could offer a contribution to clinical assessment.

4 Conclusions

Clinical and instrumental examination of 90 adolescent soccer players made it possible to show that the sport practised did not cause significant alterations in the development of the spine. Telethermography of the locomotory apparatus in young soccer players was of valid support to the clinical examination in recording and documenting calorimetric asymmetry consequent to hypertrophy of the dorsal paravertebral muscles and the scapular girdle.

Table 2. Results of Thermography Examination (Th+)

	Pathology	No. of cases (%)	
A	Muscular hypertrophy	20	(18%)
B	Scoliotic posture	4	(3.6%)
C	Scoliosis	3	(2.7%)
D	Ce- with Th+	3	(2.7%)
	Total Th+	30	(27%)

It must be mentioned that telethermographic examination in subjects with scoliosis sometimes does not show up a different distribution of thermal areas. The presence of Th- in scoliosis is most likely due to already structured deformities which have reached an equilibrium between paravertebral tensions. For this reason we consider telethermography as useful for confirming clinical findings but not able, by itself, to permit typing of the curves by way of evaluation of calorimetric asymmetries corresponding to the concavities and convexities of the curves.

In the final assessment we consider "at risk" with a high possibility of developing in the future towards spinal dysmorphosis, not only those subjects who besides clinically observed muscular hypertrophy have a positive thermographic examination (CE+, Th+), but also those three cases with a positive thermography and a negative clinical examination (CE-, Th+). For a correct interpretation of the results, also those subjects with muscular hypertrophy and negative thermography (CE+, Th-) must be subjected to long-term follow-up.

Whereas these results still need further analysis and follow-up, they do permit us to evaluate the type of athletic and technical preparation undergone by this sample of adolescent soccer players. The thermographic findings obtained cannot be univocally evaluated, but merely compared with the objective clinical observations.

5 References

Chandler, J. Kibler, W.B. Uhl, T.L. Wooten, B. Kiser, A. Stone, E. (1990) Flexibility comparisons of junior elite tennis players to other athletes.Am. J.Sport Med., 18, 2, 134-136.

Daenens, L. (1981) Thermography in a rheumatological private practise. Medicamundi, 26, 2, 107-111.

Woodrought, R.E. (1978) Telethermography of the back. Acta Th., 3, 76, 1-2.

ARTHROSCOPIC RECONSTRUCTION OF THE ANTERIOR CRUCIATE LIGAMENT IN PROFESSIONAL SOCCER PLAYERS USING THE LEEDS-KEIO LIGAMENT

P.A.M. Vierhout, Tramatologist, Medisch Spectrum Twentre, Enschede, The Netherlands.

1 Introduction

Rupture of the anterior cruciate ligament (ACL) can often lead to mechanical instability of the knee and progressive degenerate changes. These have been demonstrated in both experimental animal models and clinical studies (Noyes and Grood, 1976).

In a prospective study of 1,154 arthroscopic operations of the knee, 178 cases of ACL injury were found. Of these patients, 85% also had meniscal damage. All patients exhibiting arthroscopic evidence of ACL injury had positive Lachman and Pivot shift scores ranging from 1+ to 3+. The majority of the injuries were the result of sporting activities, primarily soccer. Of the patients with ACL injuries, 60% did not complain of any pain or instability preventing them from continuing their usual sporting activities; some even continued playing professional soccer at international level. Of the 40% who experienced problems associated with their ACL deficiency, half consciously accepted reductions in their sporting activities and eventually returned to sport at a lower level, while half required an ACL reconstruction because of continued function instability.

In the case of a professional soccer player who exhibits functional instability preventing him from returning to professional soccer, a fast and reliable rehabilitation is required following ACL reconstruction. Surgical techniques available for treatment of the deficient ACL include the use of autografts, allografts, intra-ligamentous repairs and synthetic materials.

The autograft, usually the middle third of the patellar tendon, is one of the most common repair materials. The success rates of patellar tendon reconstruction of the ACL have varied greatly (Feagin and Curl, 1976; Johnson et al., 1984) and require long periods of immobilisation and rehabilitation. As a consequence the patient is often prevented from returning to normal sports activities for at least one year until the graft has been incorporated and the tissue had time to mature into aligned collagen. This length of time is unacceptable for the professional soccer player.

Despite several reports of good results obtained from conservative treatment of acute ACL injuries, at least a third of patients end up undergoing a reconstruction of the ACL. One method for providing immediate post-operative stability involves replacement of the ACL with the Leeds-Keio Ligament. The Leeds-Keio Ligament is both a strong permanent implant and a scaffold type device. It is made from polyester in an open weave mesh-like structure and is anchored to the

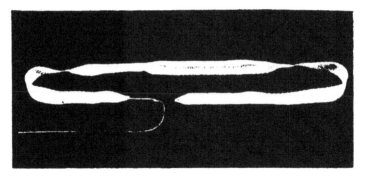

Fig.1.   The Leeds-Keio Ligament.

femur and tibia with bone plugs.

These plugs unite with the host bone through the mesh of the
ligament, providing a biological fixation for the ligament. Tissue
ingrowth also occurs along the intra-articular and extra-articular
section of the ligament. The ligament is tubular in cross-section
with an outside diameter of 11 mm. One end has a pouch for inserting
one of the bone plugs, whilst the other is simply split open (Fig.1).
The implant is completely flexible and has a maximum tensile strength
of approximately 2,220 N, which is well above the average tensile
strength (1,730 N) of the normal ACL of young adults (Noyes and
Grood, 1976).

The stiffness of the Leeds-Keio Ligament measured in soft grips
(thus simulating the manner in which it is held in the bone) is close
to that of the natural ligament (Seedhom, 1988). This is regarded as
a vital feature of the design since its comparable stiffness with the
natural ACL ensures that ingrown tissue around the ligament will be
subjected to appropriate levels of tensile strain during normal
activities. These tensile strains cause this tissue to mature into
aligned collagen parallel with the axis of the implant. More
importantly, these tensile strains are only generated if the attachments of the artificial ligament are correctly situated at the
original sites of attachment of the natural ACL, that is to say the
ligament is placed isometrically.

The use of arthroscopic techniques in the reconstruction of the
ACL has changed the diagnostic and therapeutic possibilities in knee
surgery. Arthroscopic ACL reconstruction minimises the post-
operative morbidity of the knee joint whilst at the same time
provides the surgeon with the opportunity to directly identify the
attachment sites for the prosthetic ligament.

2 Operative Technique

Prior to reconstructing the ACL, a careful inspection of the articular cartilage, retro-patellar space, menisci and synovial capsule is
made. Any associated pathology should be diagnosed and treated.

The intra-condylar area is then inspected, often remnants of the
ACL can be found. When distal remnants of the ACL have attached themselves to the PCL, these should be disected away, as this attachment
does not provide stability to the knee.

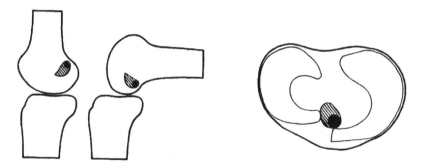

Fig.2. The isometric attachment site for the reconstruction.

The posterior plica between the PCL and lateral condyle is identified, and the most posterior part of the condyle located using an
arthroscopic probe. By moving 3 to 4 mm from this position in a
cranial direction, the isometric attachment site for the artificial
ligament is located. The guide arm of the universal clamp is then
inserted into the joint through the anterior portal and the pin
inserted into the lateral condyle at the chosen attachment site. As
much of the surrounding ligamentous and synovial tissue as possible
is preserved.

The universal clamp system is then used to remove a small bone
plug and create a stepped tunnel through to the isometrical
attachment site on the lateral condyle. Once complete, a similar bone
tunnel is prepared in the tibia. The isometric attachment site on the
tibia is located as far anteriorly and medially within the area of
attachment of the ACL, but without damaging the anterior attachment
of medial meniscus (Fig.2).

The sheathed ligament is then threaded through the two tunnels and
the sheath removed. Both bone plugs are placed inside the ligament
and pushed into the bone tunnels. The ligament is therefore anchored
in the annulus around the bone plugs, between two freshly cut bony
surfaces. The open mesh structure of the ligament allows bone and
connective tissue to unite through the ligament, hence creating a
biological anchorage. The ligament is then fixed extra-articularly
with a Fastlok fixation device at each end. The Fastlok is for
primary fixation to ensure that the ligament will not slip around the
bone plugs and hence loosen, in the early post-operative stages prior
to biological anchorage.

Once fixed, the intra-articular section of the ligament is
examined using arthroscopic flexion and extension. Only if the
ligament remains in tension throughout the full range of motion will
the ligament become successfully ingrown with new tissue. This
usually takes approximately 6 months and is essential to the success
of the reconstruction.

3 Rehabilitation

If arthroscopically, the function of the ligament looks normal and
the patient has full range of motion, the patient is encouraged to

move the joint through a full range of motion at one day post-operatively. Otherwise, a Continuous Passive Motion Device (CPM) is used to passively move the joint. On the second day post-operatively the patient is allowed to walk with the aid of crutches.

Two weeks post-operatively patients are encouraged to walk without the use of crutches, with the knee protected using a knee brace. After 6 weeks the ingrowth around the bone plugs is assessed radiographically. Three months post-operatively sportsmen are encouraged to start jogging, until 4 months post-operatively when a professional soccer player should be back in training with his team. After 6 months the player should be back to playing competitive league matches.

The use of arthroscopic reconstruction in conjunction with this rehailitation programme, minimises muscle wastage on the injured leg. Where patients are actively reaching complete range of motion, muscles around the knee should regain their strength within 4 weeks of the operation.

4 Results

So far, more than 150 patients have received an ACL arthroscopic reconstruction, using the Leeds-Keio Ligament. At one year post-operatively, 90% of patients experience little or no problem in performing routine activities of daily living. The post-operative incidence of pain and giving way was less than 10%, and in these cases were occasional and usually associated with strenuous activities. All patients showed a marked improvement in the clinical laxity of the knee post-operatively. Most of the patients examined one year post-operatively are very promising, 87% being excellent.

Our experiences with the Leeds-Keio Ligament show that recovery from ACL injury can be successful and quick. Professional international soccer players have returned to play for their league teams in five months following their reconstruction.

5 References

Noyes, F.R. and Grood, E.S. (1976) The strength of the anterior cruciate ligament in humans and rhesus monkeys: age related and species related changes. J. Bone Jt. Surg. (Am), 58A, 1074-82.

Feagin, J.A. and Curl, W.W. (1976) Isolated tear of the ACL: 5 year follow-up study. Am. J. Sports Med., 4, 95.

Johnson, R.J., Eriksson, E., Haggmark, T. and Pope, M.H. (1984) Five to ten-year follow-up evaluation after reconstruction of the anterior cruciate ligament. Clin. Orthop., 183, 122.

Seedhom, B.B. (1988) The Leeds-Keio Ligament: biomechanics, in Prosthetic Ligament Reconstruction of the Knee (eds M.J. Friedman and R.D. Ferkel), W.B. Saunders Company, Philadelphia.

THE ATTACHMENTS AND LENGTH PATTERNS OF THE ANTERIOR (ACL) CRUCIATE LIGAMENT IN MAN - an anatomical basis for ligament replacement.

L.POLIACU PROSÉ, H.R.KRIEK, C.A.M.SCHURINK and A.H.M.LOHMAN
Dept. of Anatomy, Free University, Amsterdam, The Netherlands

1 Introduction

Knowledge of the role of the ligaments in movement and stability of the knee joint is crucial for the diagnosis of ligament damage and for orthopaedic interventions such as ligament repair and replacement. From studies of the geometry of the articular surfaces and of the anterior (ACL) and posterior (PCL) cruciate ligaments in models of crossed four-bar mechanisms it has been suggested that the ligaments are important for the control of fine-tuned motion of the knee (Müller, 1983) such as occurs in football and soccer. Essential in this concept is that the links of the mechanism behave isometrically during movement.

The ACL functions further as the primary restraint that limits anterior tibial displacements and, it is known that in almost all cases of ACL-insufficiency an instability of the knee joint develops (Müller, 1983). Hirshman et al. (1990) reported that football and soccer account for 25 % of all knee instabilities (grade II and III) caused by sport activities in which the ACL was injured.

The goal of knee ligament surgery is to restore the normal knee motion and the limits of the motion (Müller, 1983). In the actual concept of ACL reconstruction, Odensten and Gillquist (1985), Seedhom and Fujikawa (1987) and Daniel (1990) indicated that the ligament substitute must be fastened in such a manner that it behaves isometrically during knee movement. Unfortunately, conflict persists concerning both the anatomical and functional aspects of the ACL (Amis and Dawkins, 1991; Fuss, 1989; Odensten and Gillquist, 1985; Sapega et al., 1990).

The aim of this study was to quantify the attachment sites and to calculate the lengths (distances between centres) of the whole ACL and PCL and of the different bundles (distances between the outermost attachments) of the ACL in 10 embalmed knees.

2 Material and Methods

At 10 knee joint angles, ranging from 0° to 140° of flexion, the position of the femur against the fastened tibia was recorded three-dimensionally (3-D) in 10 knees by means of a "Sony LM12S-31T Magnescale Computer Digital System" measuring frame (measurement error 0.01 mm). The 3-D coördinates of the oval-shaped tibial and femoral attachment sites of the ACL (and PCL) were recorded after disarticulation of the knees. The magnitude of the attachment sites, the centre (geometric midpoint) of the attachments and the length of the ACL were calculated from the 3-D coordinates. In addition, the cross-section of the ACL was calculated (IBAS system) and the course of the ACL was studied in sagittal sections through the ligament of 4 knees positioned at 0° or 120° of flexion.

3 Results

The surface of the cross-section area of the ACL is 40.4 mm^2 (SD 10.7).

The tibial and femoral attachment sites of the ACL are approximatelly equal in magnitude (ratio:0.9). The calculated parameters are given in Table 1.

Table 1. Magnitude (mean value and SD) of the attachments sites of the ACL.

Parameters	Tibial		Femoral	
	mean	SD	mean	SD
Surface (mm^2)	153.8	43.2	157.3	34.7
Antero-posterior diameter (mm)	21.2	2.0	21.5	2.1
Medio-lateral diameter (mm)	13.3	2.1	15.7	2.7

All distances calculated between the attachments of different bundles of the ACL during flexion and extension of the knee are non-isometric. The length of the central bundle of the ACL (distance between centres) is maximal (Lo= 33.7 mm;SD 3.9) at 0° of flexion. During flexion the central bundle of the ACL decreases in length, being minimal (about 90% of Lo) at angles from 105° to 140° (Fig.1). This is similar to the length-pattern of the central bundle of the ACL recently reported by Sapega et al. (1990). The length of the central bundle of the PCL (distance between centres) is maximal (Lo = 37.7mm; SD 3.9) at 120° of flexion. The length decreases between 120° and 0° of flexion and is minimal (about 80% of Lo) at 0° of flexion (Fig.1).

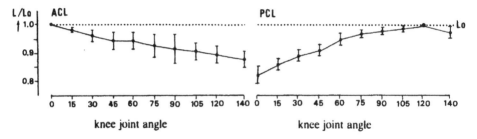

Fig.1. Graph representing the relative lengths (L/Lo) of the central bundles (distance between centres) of the ACL and the PCL at different knee joint angles.

The lengths of the antero-posterior and of the postero-lateral bundles of the ACL are maximal (Lo= 47.6mm; Lo=26.0mm) at 0° of flexion. Both bundles are shorter in flexed positions of the knee. In contrast, the length of the antero-medial bundle of the ACL is maximal (Lo=43.5mm) at 105° of flexion and minimal at 0° of flexion. This pattern is similar to that of the central bundle of the PCL.

The role of the intercondylar eminence (IE) of the tibia in the tension of the cruciate ligaments during knee movement appears to be more important than hitherto has been recognized: the PCL is bent around the IE during extension, whereas the same holds for the ACL during flexion (Fig.2). This bending may influence the course and perhaps also the tension of the ligaments during knee joint movement.

4 Conclusions

The present results show that the positions of the centres of attachment of the ACL and PCL are different from those indicated in studies of ligament reconstructions (Seedhom and Fujikawa,1987;

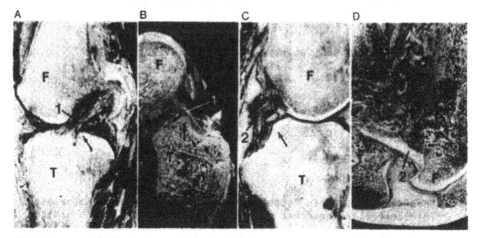

Fig.2. Photographs of sagittal sections showing the femur (F), the tibia (T) and the intercondylar eminence (arrow) and

    A. the straight course of the central bundle of the ACL (1) at 0° of flexion;

    B. the bent appearance of the central bundle of the ACL (1) in a flexed knee;

    C. the bent appearance of the central bundle of the PCL (2) at 0° of flexion;

    D. the straight course of the central bundle of the PCL (2) in a flexed knee.

Daniel, 1990) and in models of crossed four-bar mechanisms (Müller, 1983). Furthermore, the different bundles of the ACL do not behave isometrically during knee joint movement.

From an anatomical point of view we conclude that an artificial ligament should be placed so that it connects the centres of the attachment sites. This is in accordance with the notion of Odensten and Gillquist (1985). Ideally, the length-pattern of the artificial ligament should reproduce that of the central bundle of the initial ligament during knee joint motion.

5 References

Amis, A.A. and Dawkins, G.P.C. (1991) Functional anatomy of the anterior cruciate ligament. J.Bone Jt.Surg., 73-B, 260-267.

Daniel, D.M. (1990) Knee Ligaments - Structure, Function, Injury and Repair. Raven Press, New York.

Fuss, F.K. (1989): Anatomy of the cruciate ligaments and their function in extension and flexion of the human knee joint. Anat.Rec., 184, 165-176.

Hirshman, H.P. Daniel, D.M. and Miyasaka, K. (1990) The fate of unoperated knee ligament injuries, in Knee Ligaments (ed D.Daniel), Raven press, New York, pp.481-504.

Müller, W. (1983) The Knee - Form, Function and Ligament Reconstruction. Springer, Berlin.

Odensten, M. and Gillquist, J. (1985) Functional anatomy of the anterior cruciate ligament. J.Bone Jt.Surg., 67-A, 2, 257-262.

Sapega, A.A. Moyer, R.A. Schneck, C. and Komalahiranya, N. (1990) Testing for isometry during reconstruction of the anterior cruciate ligament. J.Bone Jt.Surg., 72-A, 2, 259-267.

Seedhom B.B. and Fujikawa K. (1987): The Leeds-Keio Anterior Cruciate Ligament Replacement, Howmedica, Kiel.

SHOULDER INJURIES: PHYSICAL DIAGNOSIS AND ARTHROSCOPY

C.N. VAN DIJK
Academisch Medisch Centrum, Amsterdam, The Netherlands.
G. DECLERQUE
Antwerpen, Belgium.

1 Introduction

Shoulder injuries in football are not as frequent as lower extremity
injuries. Like in other contact sports the chance of a direct injury
to the shoulder joint is still present. Dislocation of the shoulder
joint or AC-joint results usually from a fall or a forced abduction-
exorotation injury of the arm.
  The shoulder joint lies deep in the body and is therefore not
easily accessible for palpation. Evaluation of a patient with a
shoulder problem by physical examination has always been considered
to be difficult. Many tests are available and it is difficult to
interpret the validity and value of all these tests. Shoulder
pathology can be subdivided under 5 headings: cuffpathology,
instability, arthritis, frozen shoulder and other "pathology"
(neurological problem, cervical problems and acromio-clavicular (AC)
joint problems). To discriminate between the different groups a
simple strategy of physical examination can be used.

2 Examination

Any examination starts with the patient's history; this usually gives
us a working hypothesis. The physical examination consists of:-
1. Inspection: we look at both shoulders from behind whereby we look
especially at the contour of supraspinatus and infraspinatus muscles
(atrophy?). 2. Active abduction: the patient is asked to abduct the
shoulder actively up to 180°. If he can do so without complaints we
go on to palpation. If the active abduction is restricted we test
for passive abduction. 3. Palpation: the shoulder joint is hidden
deep in the body and is therefore not readily accessible for
palpation. Usually the whole C5 dermatoma is painful on palpation.
  Another factor is the subacromial bursa which overlies the cuff.
Any irritation somewhere in the cuff will cause irritation of the
bursa and thereby pain on palpation around the whole shoulder joint.
The AC-joint and the biceps tendon are accessible to palpation due to
the fact that they lie superficially. 4. Resistance test: supraspinatus, infraspinatus and biceps muscles. 5. Other tests: appre-
hension test and stability test.
  When, by performing these tests, we have gathered conflicting
information, or we feel we have not yet confirmed our working hypothesis, we can extend our physical examination by performing other

tests like range of motion in other directions, other resistance tests and so on. In all patients we need to look for neck function, neurological and vascular status.

With this simple strategy of physical examination we are usually capable of diagnosing the problem without missing essential pathology. In some patients there is a need of further investigation like X-ray, Isotope scan, CT scan, echography or magnetic resonance imaging (MRI).

3 Arthroscopy

An increasing number of pathological conditions of the shoulder joint nowadays can be managed by arthroscopic surgery. Arthroscopy gives us the opportunity to visualise the joint from inside.

One of the important structures in the shoulder is the glenoid rim. Pathology of the anterior labrum finds its origin usually in a hyper-abduction exorotation trauma of the shoulder. When the distal anterior part of the labrum is detached, the middle and distal glenohumeral ligaments are detached with it and therefore the shoulder is anteriorly unstable. In selected cases arthroscopic or open reattachment offers a good solution. Injury of the posterior part of the labrum is usually caused by a fall on the outstretched arm. Most of the time the posterior superior part of the labrum gets injured. Another possible injury mechanism is impingement between infraspinatus posterosuperior part of the labrum and humeral head, as happens in volleyball players when the arm is brought backwards to perform a smash. Injury of the superior part of the labrum is called a SLAP-lesion.

4 Conclusions

Using a simple strategy of physical examination we are usually capable of diagnosing the problem without missing essential pathology. In a selected number of patients there is need for further investigation like X-ray, isotope scan, CT-scan, echography or MRI. Arthroscopy in general does not play a role in the diagnostic strategy.

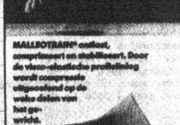

PART ELEVEN

Managing a:
Coaching

RELATIONSHIP BETWEEN PSYCHOLOGICAL ASPECTS OF SOCCER TRAINERS AND
PLAYERS

R. VANFRAECHEM-RAWAY
Université Libre de Bruxelles, ISEPK, Psychologie Appliquée à l'Education Physique - Laboratoire de l'Effort, Brussels, Belgium

1 Introduction

Our purpose is to analyse the personality characteristics of players
and trainers in higher and lower level soccer teams by means of the
Thill's athlete personality questionnaire and to analyse trainers'
evaluations of the athletes' personality with a scale based upon Thill
test (1984).
   It is thought that sport situations have an influence on the
athletes' behaviour. The athletes' behaviour is adapted, thus, in a
team as well as in teams of personality profile (Grassarth-Maticek
et al., 1990 ; Kosbowscky and Maoz, 1988).
   In the same way, the role could reach a great importance in
players' behaviour. For a trainer, a real knowledge of the athlete
could have an influence on the trainer-athlete relation and therefore
upon the team efficiency (Horne and Carron, 1985 ; Strach, 1979 ;
Weiss, 1986).

2 Methods

We used Thill's QPS (1984) in five fields prevalent for athletes
personality analysis : motivation, control, activity, relation and
sincerity. Each field contains items with two opposite behaviour
polarities. A scale with a maximal value of 10 points expresses the
trait's intensity. This test shows high validity and is well adapted
to sport situations. We used it with 13 trainers of higher level teams,
age : $\bar{X} = 49.2 \pm 1.92$, 17 trainers of lower level teams, age : $\bar{X} =$
42.5 ± 2.99 and 100 players, half of whom were higher players, age :
$\bar{X} = 23 \pm 2.35$.

3 Results and Discussion

3.1 Trainers' personality profiles
The statistical analysis comparing trainers of higher and lower levels
shows many differences (Table 1). The lower level trainers are
situated in the test standard mean score. The top level trainers have
the highest stress resistance capacity. They have a good emotional
control even against an important stress. They are deeply motivated
and present a good self-esteem. Dominant in their relation, they
prefer safety and show a good control of their activity. Their specific
motivation is high. We believe that for trainers the team efficiency
appears like a valorization process. This could justify their

particular status in the club. Moreover, the attitude of the media amplifies these elements. They are dominant and have a poor level of sociability in contrast with lower level trainers. Those results are significant and correspond to literature, except for sociability of the higher level trainers (Ogilvie and Tutko, 1976 ; Rush and Ayllon, 1984 ; Strach, 1979 ; Weiss, 1986).

Table 1   Comparison between higher and lower level trainers

| | Higher level trainers | | Lower level trainers | | |
	$\bar{X}$	SD	$\bar{Y}$	SD	t
Motivation	7.4	0.55	4.5	0.85	7.6***
Selfesteem	6.6	0.41	5.0	0.73	5.5***
Psychol. endurance	7.0	0.56	5.3	0.75	5.6***
Impulsivity	2.4	0.23	5.0	0.99	7.2***
Risk taking	3.2	0.56	5.0	1.8	4.5**
Emotional control	6.2	0.65	5.3	0.8	2.8*
Resist. against stress	6.4	0.43	3.9	0.75	9.7***
Extraversion	3.8	0.55	5.4	0.6	5.5***
Dominance	6.9	0.24	4.9	0.7	7.9***
Sociability	2.8	0.55	5.4	0.83	8.3***

   * significant at $P \leqslant 0.05$
  ** significant at $P \leqslant 0.01$
*** significant at $P \leqslant 0.001$

Nevertheless, the group of higher level trainers reached a high level of homogeneity.

3.2 Players' profile analysis
Lower level players are in the test standard mean (Table 2). In contrast, some personality characteristics of top level players are:- a high degree of motivation, good psychological endurance and great vivacity . This appears with a high homogeneity in the test results. Top players are more aggressive and they are less likely to take risks but these characteristics present a high level of heterogeneity.

Table 2. Comparison between higher and lower level players

| | Higher level players | | Lower level players | | |
	X	SD	Y	SD	t
Motivation	6.9	2.6	4.2	1.0	10.9***
Psychol. endurance	6.3	1.5	4.8	0.77	6.9***
Vivacity	6.9	1.9	4.8	2.6	6.9***
Impulsivity	4.9	1.7	5.0	2.5	0.34
Risk taking	2.7	1.8	4.6	3.0	6.07***
Emotional control	4.3	1.7	4.4	2.8	0.75
Dominance	4.5	3.0	4.8	1.6	0.97
Aggressivity	6.7	4.9	5.6	2.4	5.33***
Cooperation	2.6	2.4	3.1	1.9	1.94

*** significant at $P \leqslant 0.001$

Although the present measurements are in concordance with the
literature on professional players, there are some discrepancies in
the "relation" field and in the "control" field (Grassarth-Maticek et
al., 1990 ; Kosbowscky and Moaz, 1988 ; Vecchiereni et al., 1977).
These discrepancies can be explained by the different positions on
the green (Figure 1).

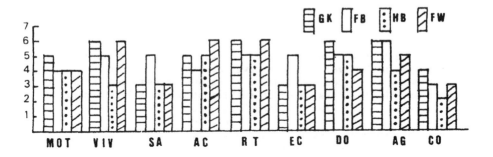

Fig. 1. Comparison between positional roles

    The profile of the goalkeeper is quite different from offensive
players (forward and half-back). The goalkeepers have a greater basic
motivation (MOT), they are more dominant (Do), more aggressive (AG).
They have more vivacity (VIV) and they take more risks (RT) than
full-backs and half-backs. The full-backs have more emotional
stability (ES), but they have a greater self affirmation (SA). The
forwards have a greater vivacity (VIV) but they are also impulsive
and improvident (AC). The half-backs have less vivacity and less

aggressivity (AG) but less cooperation (CO) too.

These results show an adaptation to the team requirements.
The personality differences according to the positional role show
remarkable differences in the highest divisions. Complementarity
between players is more important in top level soccer.

3.3 Players' evaluation by the trainers

Mood is known to be·important for motivation (Pritchard and Karasick,
1973 ; Tutko and Ogilvie, 1967). In the same way, the knowledge of the
players' personality seems important with regard to team efficiency.
This reflects the "Pygmalion effect" (Rosenthal and Jacobson, 1968).

For higher level trainers, we measured more or less seven
equivalences between trainers' evaluation of players' personality and
actual players' responses. For the defenders, those personality
characteristics are emotional stability, aggression as well as limited
risk taking, psychological endurance, sociability and domination. They
are proper to the defenders.

Concerning the forwards, the trainers recognize vivacity, risk
taking, motivation and extraversion. Although 57 % of the equivalences
are present in the defenders and 42 % in the forwards. With lower
level trainers, only 28 % was noted for the defenders and 21 % for
the forwards.

The results, in comparison with the literature about team sport
demonstrate that the trainers in this study have a bad perception of
the soccer player's personality (Horne and Carron, 1985 ; Kosbowscky
and Maoz, 1988 ; Nicaise, 1990 ; Weiss, 1986).

4 Conclusions

Players' personality characteristics show a good adaptation to their
function and thus to the game situation especially for high level
players. The high level trainers have personality characteristics
corresponding to a good emotional control and stress management.

However, the trainers have not sufficient human understanding ;
moreover the results are confirmed by the poor level of their
perception of players. Such results are especially remarkable for the
lower level trainers. The results are limited to the population
studied but emphasize the poor care given to the psychological aspect
in our country during soccer trainers' education.

5 References

Grassarth-Maticek, R., Egrenek, H.J., Rieder, H. and Raskic, L. (1990)
    Psychological factors as determinants of success in football and
    boxing. Int. J. Sport Psychol., 21, 237-255.
Horne, T. and Carron, V.A. (1985) Compatibility in coach athlete
    relationships. J. Sport Psychol., 7, 137-144.
Kosbowscky, M. and Maoz, O. (1988) Commitment and personality
    variables as discrimination among sports referees. J. Sport Exerc.
    Psychol., 10, 262-269.

Nicaise, M. (1989-1990) Etude approfondie d'équipes de volleyball. Mémoire de licence en Education Physique, U.L.B., non publié.

Ogilvie, B. and Tutko, T.A. (1976) Problem's Athletes and How to Handle Them. Pebham, London.

Pritchard, R.D. and Karasick, B.W. (1973) The effects of organizational climate on managerial job performance and job satisfaction. Org. Behaviour Hum. Perform., 2, 126-146

Rosenthal, R. and Jacobson, C. (1968)Pygmalion in the Classroom. Halt Renckart and Winston, New York.

Rush, D.B. and Ayllon, T. (1984) Peer behavioral coaching : Soccer J. Sport Psychol., 6, 325-334.

Strach, C. (1979) Player's perceptions of leadership qualities for coaches. Res. Quart., 60, 679-686.

Thill, E. (1984) Questionnaire de personnalité pour sportifs. Edit. Psychol. Appliquée, Paris.

Tutko, T.A. and Ogilvie, B.C. (1967) The Role of the Coach in the Motivation of Athletes in Play, Games and Sport. Thomas, Springfield.

Vecchiereni, Bleneau, M.F. and Ginet, J. (1977) Comparaison des données psychologiques de 32 jeunes sportifs aspirant à devenir professionnels. Génériologie, 66, 47-57.

Weiss, M.R. (1986) The influence of leader behaviors coach attributes and institutional variables on performances of college basketball team. J. Sport Psychol.. 8, 332-346.

SELF-HYPNOSIS FOR ELITE FOOTBALLERS

Colin P. Davey
Deakin University, Rusden Campus, Victoria, Australia

1 Introduction

Collingwood Football Club in the Australian Football League has been without a premiership for 32 years, despite playing in 10 grand finals and over 20 semi-finals. All have been lost. So consistent has failure been, that the sporting writers coined the name "Colliwobbles" to indicate that the team wobbled when the pressure mounted in the final series.

Teams striving for a premiership need three things:

(a) Skill or talent
(b) Fitness and
(c) The correct psychological or mental approach.

Collingwood's record over 30 years indicated it had the necessary skills and fitness, but had been suspect in the psychological approach. Hence it was decided to rectify this.

At the first World Congress in Science and Football held at Liverpool, Davey (1988), has outlined many alternative approaches to psychological training including, visual motor behaviour rehearsal (Suinn 1980), and sports psyching (Tutko 1976). Since each of these procedures uses some form of relaxation, and imagery, the preferred term to be used when these procedures are used immediately before a game is self-hypnosis.

According to Morgan (1980), although the results of experiments in hypnosis have been equivocal, nevertheless some experiments have demonstrated its potential use in sport. This paper describes one such successful use.

Hypnosis has been defined (Orne, 1980) as an altered state of consciousness in which the mind is susceptible to suggestion. This state is a natural one similar to sleep and day-dreaming. It allows the subject to narrow his attention, and dissociate from distracting cues, whilst the brain switches from the left side (cognitive analytical thinking) to the right side, which processes sensory information used in imagery. Football players were encouraged to use internal or proprioceptive imagery, rather than external or visual imagery, especially before a game.

2 Methods

Before using imagery 25 players on the first teams training list were encouraged to use a relaxation response, such as sitting or lying comfortably, closing eyes, breathing easily, relaxing all muscles, and maintaining a passive attitude. This should lead to a decreased heart rate, blood pressure, breathing rate and a decreased body metabolism. Although this state is usually necessary before imagery can be commenced, especially in the early stages, it is the complete opposite of what is required for the fight or flight response, ie., increased heart rate, blood pressure, breathing rate, and an increase in blood flow to the muscles. Hence, exertion arousal should be used with a 10 to 15 minute vigorous, strenuous activity which will optimise arousal levels before play (Davey, 1989).

In general, relaxation lowers arousal to prepare for imagery, whilst physical exertion raises arousal level prior to performance. The procedure before play is, relaxation, imagery (self-hypnosis) followed by exertion arousal. Such a procedure may be termed "instant pre-play", the opposite of the more commonly used term, "instant re-play".

In addition to self-hypnosis, other procedures were also used throughout the year. Lectures were given to players on goal setting, anxiety, arousal, attention, concentration, relaxation, imagery, and self-coping statements, together with individual counselling interviews. The education of the players in each of the psychological concepts that affect performance is considered essential.

3 Results

Such procedures allowed Collingwood Football Club to win the 1990 Australian Football Championship for the first time in 32 years. In addition to the skill and fitness aspects which they had had many times before, they at last used the correct psychological preparation to produce a premiership team.

4 Discussion

Because of the confidential nature of the procedure and the possibility of identification of individuals in the team as named, examples of footballers who have successfully used the above procedures will be taken from two other Australian football teams in the same competition.

(i)   One footballer who had always played as a centreman lost favour with the coach and was played in another position. He lost confidence and was relegated to the seconds, when the author took him through the self-hypnosis procedure. After several weeks using the procedure his replacement in the centre was injured and he was returned to his original position. His general play began to improve immediately as his confidence was restored, and at the end of the season he led the Australian Football League in the number of possessions gained, and won the medal for the best and fairest player.

(ii)   Another footballer whose goal kicking inaccuracy led to his being replaced as a full forward, the position from which most goals are scored. Using the same procedure he was instructed to image himself, kicking goals from various positions on the football field. After kicking 8 goals one week, and 11 goals the next in the reserves team (a large number even for Australian football), he was returned to the firsts and eventually made the State team.

(iii)   Another example was a footballer who played in the full back position, where it is his duty to negate the play of his forward opponent, and stop him kicking goals. So aggressive was this player that his rugged play often broke the rules of the game, and his opponent was awarded a free kick, which many times resulted in a goal. Using the self-hypnosis procedure he was instructed to visualise himself playing against many different aggressive opponents, and to use acceptable methods to counter his play. Again, after many weeks of training his play became acceptible, and he too, made the State team as a full back.

These are a few examples of individuals who have successfully used self-hypnosis to their own advantage. In the team that recently won the premiership, the Sports Psychological Skills Questionnaire (Nelson, 1990) showed that 21 out of 25 or 84% of the players had consistently used the self-hypnosis procedure.

Finally research over ten years (Davey, 1985) in eight of the twelve leading teams in the Australian Football League, showed that the answer to the question, "What makes a good footballer psychologically"? is

(i)   His personality is slightly extraverted, slightly anxious.
(ii)   His motivation is high in desire to win, confidence, coachability, conscientiousness and determination.
(iii)   He has an incentive to achieve excellence and success, he likes stressful situations, is aggressive and affiliative.
(iv)   His mood profile is less tense, depressed, angry, fatigued and confused, and he shows more mental vigour.
(v)   He can process information, is not overloaded, and has high self esteem; and
(vi)   Finally, he sets goals, practices relaxation, imagery, and self-hypnosis, before a game.

5 REFERENCES

Davey, C.P., (1985) What makes a good footballer psychologically? **Australian and New Zealand Association for the Advancement of Science,** Melbourne.

Davey, C.P., (1988) Psychological assistance for footballers, in **Science and Football,** (eds T. Reilly, A. Lees, K. Davies and W. Murphy), E. and F.N. Spon, London, pp. 519-530.

Davey, C.P., (1989) Self-hypnosis and exertion arousal, **Seventh World Contress in Sport Psychology,** Singapore.

Morgan, W.P. (1980) Hypnosis and sports medicine, in G.D. Burrows, and L. Dennerstein, **Handbook of Hypnosis and Psychosomatic Medicine,** Elsevier, Oxford, pp. 359 - 375.

Nelson, D., 1990 Sports psychological skills questionnaire, **World Congress on Sport For All,** Tampere Finland.

Orne, M.T. (1980) On the construct of hypnosis, in G.D. Burrows, and L. Dennerstein, **Handbook of Hypnosis and Psychosomatic Medicine,** Elsevier, Oxford, pp 29.-51.

Suinn, R.M., (1980) **Psychology in Sports,** Burgess, Minnesota.

Tutko, T., (1976) **Sports Psyching,** Tracker, Los Angeles.

ANALYSIS OF STRESS IN SOCCER COACHES

D. Teipel, Deutsche Sporthochschule Köln, Germany

1 Introduction

According to Nitsch (1981) stress can be perceived from a
biological, psychological and sociological perspective. In
general, various stressors from a specific environment and
particular tasks may result in a destabilisation of a
person. The consequences of long-lasting and severe
psychophysiological, psychological and sociological
stressors can either be overload in terms of fatigue or
cognitive/emotional stress or underload in terms of
monotony and satiation. The degree and duration of stress
basically depend on the subjective evaluation of specific
demands. In this respect soccer coaches especially at a
professional level are almost permanently confronted with
winning or losing and also with the manifold expectations
and demands from club officials, players, referees,
spectators and journalists. These aspects of stress were
rarely systematically investigated up to now. There are
only few studies which dealt with aspects of psychophysiological and psychological stress of soccer coaches.

The psychophysiological stress of soccer coaches before,
during and after games is apparently high. According to the
study of Trzeciak et al. (1981) the heart rates of soccer
coaches changed in relation to individual factors and
specific game situations. The heart rates of 14 out of 18
professional coaches showed an average of 104 beats/min
half an hour before the start of the observed games. During
the games the heart rates varied between 108 and 156
beats/min. Comparing the heart rates of two age groups it
was found that the younger, less experienced group
manifested slightly, but not significantly higher heart
rates than the older, more experienced group of coaches. In
this study the specific actions of the coaches during the
games were not related to their heart rates.

Selected aspects of psychological stress were
investigated by Biener (1986). He analysed specific stress
factors and coping strategies in 227 soccer coaches by
means of a questionnaire. Altogether, 83% of the coaches
defined stress as psychological load, 7% as physiological
load and 10% as the feeling of pressure from all sides,
continuous criticism, fear of losses and necessity of
success. Of the coaches 79% evaluated the feeling of stress
during the game as medium to high, whereas only 21%
experienced only a low degree of stress. Concerning coping
strategies, the coaches frequently mentioned conversations
with their partners or family members, physical activity,

walking, relaxation procedures, watching television and sleeping for long periods.

The psychophysiological study did not take the specific actions of the coaches before, during and after games into account. The study concerning psychological stress focused only on general, but not soccer-related evaluations and coping strategies. In this study following problems of psychophysiological stress of soccer coaches were analysed:

1. psychophysiological stress in terms of heart rates before, during and after games in dependence of coaches' actions and game events;

2. psychological stress in terms of evaluations of specific environment- and success/failure-related aspects.

2 Method

For the analysis of psychophysiological stress two professional coaches of opposing teams were investigated in respect of heart rates and specific behaviour before, during and after a specific game. The heart rates were measured by means of short-range radio telemetry (Sport Tester PE 3000, Polar Electro, Kempele, Finland). This equipment allowed the measurement and storage of the heart rates of coaches in 15-second intervals over a period of 4 hours. In order to relate these actions of the coaches to the specific game events, two observers wrote a protocol of the game. The two observers cooperated in watching the game and making notations of game events such as goals, dribblings, passes, free kicks, penalties, injuries of the players, and so on. This procedure was conducted in order to associate important game events with the coaches' actions. Thus, the game was videotaped and reanalysed. In particular, the behaviour of the home and away team coach was videotaped before, during and after the game and categorised in respect of positions and movements such as sitting, standing, walking slowly, walking fast, giving instructions to the players, talking with the assistant coach or the linesman and in respect of emotions especially in response to goals, good or bad actions of the players such as joy, fear, anger and disappointment. As the timers of the telemetry equipment and the video camera were started at the same time, the actions of the two coaches could be directly related to their heart rates in specific game situations.

For the analysis of aspects of psychological stress a specific questionnaire concerning environmental and game- and season-related stress factors was applied. Forty five stress factors were evaluated on a 7-point-scale from

'1=not stressful' to '7=very stressful'. Twenty eight
soccer coaches from professional and high amateur levels
answered this specific questionnaire.

3 Results

3.1 Psychophysiological stress

For the analysis of psychophysiological stress the heart
rates and the behaviour of two coaches were analysed. Both
coaches of opposing teams of the second professional league
participated in this case study. The home team needed a win
to take part in a promotion game for the first league,
whereas the visiting team held a mid-table position.

The measurement of the heart rates of both coaches and
their behaviour observation started about 33 minutes before
the game and lasted more than 150 minutes for both coaches.
The behavior of both coaches was videotaped during the
whole game, apart from the half-time period. The home team
scored in 22nd minute, but after a close game and many
chances the opposing team scored in the 87th minute to draw
level.

The heart rates of the home team coach varied between
110-160 beats/min with an average of 126 beats/min over the
whole period of 170 min. The heart rates of the opponent's
coach also varied between 110-160 beats/min with an average
of 124 beats/min over the period of 150 min.

From the beginning of the heart rate analysis until the
start of the game, the heart rates of both coaches
oscillated between 110-120 beats/min. The joyful movements
of the home team coach after the goal for his team in the
22nd minute resulted in a significant increase of his heart
rate from 130 to 147 beats/min. In contrast, the heart rate
of the opponent's coach remained fairly constant on the
level of about 130 beats/min, due to his rather motionless
behaviour. Even 2 min after the goal the heart rate of the
home team coach was about 20 beats/min higher than that of
the opponent's coach.

During half-time both coaches went to the dressing
rooms, held their team talks and came back to the benches.
During this period the heart rate of the home team coach
decreased from about 140 to 120 beats/min, whereas the
heart rate of the opponent's coach varied around 120
beats/min.

In the second half the heart rates of both coaches
fluctuated between 110 to 140 beats/min. After the goal for
the visiting team in the 87th minute the heart rate of its
coach increased rapidly from about 130 to about 160
beats/min, due to his short actions of enjoyment. Also, the
specific behaviour of the home team coach, who stood still,
put his hand over his eyes and shook his head, thus
indicating severe disappointment and frustration, resulted

in an increase in his heart rate from 135 to about 150
beats/min. As both teams had good chances to score in the
last minutes of the game, both coaches showed comparatively
high heart rates of about 150 beats/min. After the game the
heart rate of the home team coach decreased from about 150
to 120 beats/min during his slow walk to the cabin and his
participation in the press conference over a period of
about 30 minutes.

These findings of the two coaches of opposing teams on
the second league professional level prove that the
psychophysiological stress measured by heart rates
approaches almost maximal level with comparatively little
motor activity in some game situations. Apparently a close
correlation between important game situations, more or less
motion- and emotion-related actions of the coaches and
their individual heart rates can be detected.

3.2 Psychological stress

The specific questionnaire consisted of 22 environmental
stress factors concerning the relationship between coaches
and club officials, spectators, referees, journalists and
opponents and 23 game- and season-related conditions which
were evaluated on a 7-point-scale from '1=not stressful' to
'7=very stressful'. Coaches (n=28) from professional and
high amateur levels answered the questionnaire.

All in all, the coaches assessed the specific
environmental stress factors as low to medium stressful.
The highest comparative evaluations of stress were found in
the relation of coaches with referees in home games, short-
term reserve players and newspaper journalists. The coaches
evaluated low degrees of stress in their relation with the
assistant coaches, sponsors, opponent coaches, opponent
players and home spectators.

The evaluations of stress in respect of environmental
factors were in most cases by far lower than in respect of
the game- and season-related aspects. The coaches assessed
the following five conditions as 'rather' to 'very'
stressful: necessity of relegation avoidance only by a win
in the last game, relegation rank at the third last game,
relegation rank at mid-season, high loss and possibility of
promotion only by a win in the last game. In contrast, a
high lead before the end of the game, a win, top rank after
five games, top rank at mid-season and a draw in an away
game were regarded as 'low' stressful.

4 Summary

In this study specific aspects of psychophysiological
and psychological stress in soccer coaches were analysed.
In respect of psychophysiological stress the heart rates of
two opposing coaches on the second professional level were

investigated before, during and after a specific game. The heart rates of the two coaches varied between 110-160 beats/min with peaks in situations of goals for their own or the opposing team. There seems to be a close relation between essential events on the field, emotional reactions (e.g. joy, anger, frustration) and/or motion reactions (e.g. sitting, standing, walking, jumping) and their heart rates.

Concerning psychological stress the evaluations of specific environmental and game- and season-related conditions by of group of 28 soccer coaches on professional and high amateur levels were investigated. The relations with assistant coaches, sponsors, opponent coaches and opposing players were assessed as low stressful. But the interaction with reserve players and referees in away and home games was evaluated as medium stressful. The highest evaluations of stress were found in situations of severe threats of relegation in the last game, three games before the end of the season, at mid-season and in case of a big loss. The possibility of promotion only by a win in the last game was regarded as highly stressful.

The findings of this study prove that the psychophysiological stress of soccer coaches before, during and after games can reach a high level and that fear of losing, bad results at the beginning, at the middle and before the end of the season can mean high psychological stress. Thus soccer coaches must learn to perceive, evaluate, appraise, attribute stressors adequately and act in specific game situations effectively. In this way various stressors can be prevented from resulting in actual or long-lasting overload or destabilisation of soccer coaches' behaviour.

5 References

Biener, K. (1986) Stress bei Fussballtrainern. Deutsche Zeitschrift für Sportmedizin, 5, 107-110.
Nitsch, J.R. (1981) Stress. Theorien, Untersuchungen, Massnahmen. Huber, Bern.
Trzeciak, S., Heck, H., Satomi, H. and Hollmann, W. (1981) Über das Herzfrequenzverhalten bei Fussballtrainern während eines Punktspiels. Deutsche Zeitschrift für Sportmedizin, 5, 127-140.

THE POSITION OF A PROFESSIONAL SOCCER-COACH IN THE NETHERLANDS: A CLOSER LOOK

W. MOES & D.W. MAANDAG
Dept. of Educational Sciences, University of Groningen, Groningen, the Netherlands

1 Introduction

The aim of this research study was to investigate the position of professional soccer- coaches in the Netherlands. The motivation behind this work was the lack of research in this field. As there seems to be a continuous discrepancy between the individual interest and the interest of the branch as a whole, the results provide suggestions relating to normalization of labour-facilities specifically concerning soccer-coaches.

2 Methods

A questionnaire, composed mainly of closed answering-categories, was distributed in June of 1990. Only coaches who were working for a professional soccer-organization at the moment of the investigation were included in the analysis. The questionnaire was constructed with the help of an independent group of experts. This group was composed by the Foundation for Labour Matters in Professional Soccer (Stichting Arbeidszaken Betaald Voetbal, SABV) in which organization the Coaches' Union (Vereniging Van Voetbaloefenmeesters Nederland, VVON), the Players' Union (Vereniging Van Contractspelers, VVCS) and the Federation of Professional Soccer-organizations (Federatie Betaald Voetbalorganisaties, FBO) are united. It consisted of (former) coaches, club managers and representatives (on personal title) from the above mentioned organizations with the exception of the Players' Union. Some of the representatives had more than one function.

In general the task of this group was to check and interpret results, to clarify problems and otherwise to provide information which could be of use. After the first results were available, they were discussed in the expert-group. According to the expert-group some of the observations in a more objective matter of speaking did not correspond with the actual situation. To check this we interviewed three, at that time, unemployed soccer-coaches. These results were included in the conclusion.

3 Results and discussion

Of the 155 questionnaires that were sent, 83 were returned, constituting a response of 53.5%. So as to receive an optimal number of completed questionnaires the coaches were allowed to respond anonymously. In the meantime, the expert-group indicated the salary- scales for different levels of coaches. After analyzing the respondents' annual income, it was found that the ratio of the different types of coaches included in the analysis was the same as the ratio of the different types of professional soccer-coaches in general.

However, there was one exception: the so called 'top level coaches' (3 to 5 persons) were less represented in the analysis than should have been. With respect to the outcome of previous research (namely personality profiles of top level trainers), the response problem can be regarded as a result. "The top level trainers have the highest resistance capacity. They have a good emotional control even against an important stress. They are deeply motivated and present a good self-esteem. Dominant in their relation, they prefer safety and show a good control of their activity. Their specific motivation is high." (Vanfraechem-Raway, 1991). Furthermore it is hypothesized that top-level coaches are in a less vulnerable position than other soccer-coaches. This might explain the reason why top-level coaches were under-represented: they have already reached the top and the actual system is therefore benefitial to them.

Two thirds of the coaches had played professional soccer. Another 24% had performed at amateur and/or youth-team level. One could assume therefore, that coaches are mainly recruited from this branch and by this branch of sport. The professional soccer-branch is hardly influenced by other branches.

Of all the coaches, 45% stated they were interested in (more) schooling. Most areas of interest were not directly soccer-related, for example, areas such as sport psychology, coping with media and coping with conflicts. Approximately 20% of the coaches who in the previous two years had taken part in a course were involved in an area that was directly soccer-related. The reason for this most likely had to do with the content of the courses being offered.

We have come to the conclusion that the profession of a soccer-coach is a very individualistic one. Moreover,

it is not a very organization-specific profession, rather more branch- specific. This means that a coach can be replaced rather easily. The facts that support this are:
I) a coach only works as a coach; if he has ever been unemployed as a coach he has not had another job - in other words, in a coach's career there is only horizontal mobility within the branch;
II) whenever a coach decides to educate himself, he must do so at his own expense. Clubs argue that it is not in their direct interest, strategically speaking, to invest in what could possibly become a future rival. This situation is comparable to a characteristic of the soccer-branch as a whole: there is a constant rivalry between players, coaches and clubs;
III) the role of the coaches' Union (the Vereniging van Voetbaloefenmeesters Nederland, VVON) consists mainly of solving problems, instead of career-planning and professionalization of the occupation;
IV) and (Figure 1) whenever a coach obtains another job he is usually approached personally by a club: other ways or even strategies of getting a job or a new job seem to be of secondary importance.

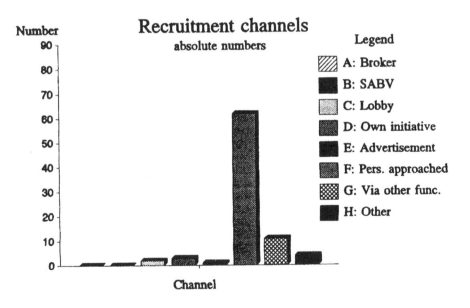

Figure 1. Different means of how professional soccer-coaches are recruited.

We have come to the conclusion that the role of the Dutch
Soccer Association (Koninklijke Nederlandse Voetbal Bond,
KNVB) is strongly regulatory. It could be formulated that
the Association determines the career of a coach. Facts
are that:
    I) the KNVB formulates the necessary preconditions
    for participating in coaches- training courses;
    II) the KNVB is in charge of the execution of these
    courses;
    III) the KNVB is in charge of the issuing of
    necessary licenses, and once acquired by a coach the
    license is valid for five years. It is therefore up
    to a coach if he wishes to professionalize and/or to
    acquire knowledge by educating himself.

Since their job, as we have already seen, is very much an
individualistic one, coaches must know their way and have
and maintain contacts with many people. Moreover, they
find a lot of satisfaction in their work, partly due to
the fact that they consider the influence of the media,
sponsors and the audience in their work as minimal. Apart
from this they very much like the freedom of their job,
the soccer-game, the variation in their work, the
excitement and so on. The only negative aspect is the
insecurity of their position (Figure 2). These outcomes
indicate some characteristics of a soccer-coach in
general. The persons who become soccer-coaches seem to be
people with very specific individual qualities, such as:
maintaining-strategies, coping with stress, leadership-
abilities and leadership-styles.
1In relation to this there is evidence (Hameleers, 1989)
that coaches of top-sport teams view themselves primarily
as quiet, self-assured people who keep cool at critical
moments.
    In cooperation with the expert-group some 'core-tasks'
were formulated. These concerned: determining game-
tactics, deciding on work-out exercises, composing the
broad players- selection, determining the weekly line-up,
formulating long-term technical policy, organization
training of youth-players, decisions concerning new
players, scouting of players, contracting (new) players,
negotiating with players about contracts and determining
of premiums. The most important people carrying out
certain job-functions in a professional soccer-
organization (in the Netherlands) were also determined.
These were the coach, the rest of the technical staff,
the scouts, the players, the medical staff, the technical
director, the general manager, the daily committees, the
general committees, the commercial manager and the
sponsor(s). Next, the coaches had to indicate from their
perspectives which person (including themselves) had
which level of influence (1=no influence/ no arrow,

2=advising role/ no arrow, 3=co-deciding role/ thin arrow, 4=autonomous deciding role/ thick arrow) (Figure 3).

Appreciation of coaches' jobs

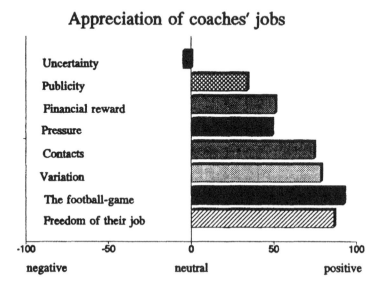

Figure 2. *Factors in the appreciation of soccer-coaches' professions.*

It can be noted that a coach has autonomy as far as technical core-activities immediately related to optimizing the product of the game are concerned (Figure 3). Although a coach perceives himself as highly influential in regard to soccer-technical aspects concerning his team, it has been argued that his actual position is more subtle than he perceives it. What is meant by this is that, also as a result of increasing professionalization of committees - the ones who formulate the club-policy and contract players - the coach sometimes has to produce good results which obviously can not be realised if there is a lack of good players on his team. Moreover, there is an increasing influence, mostly indirect, and dependence of sponsor(s) and their money. This often leads to a shift in responsiblities. For a coach the consequence is that his position becomes more dependent and therefore vulnerable

FUNCTION   CORE-TASK

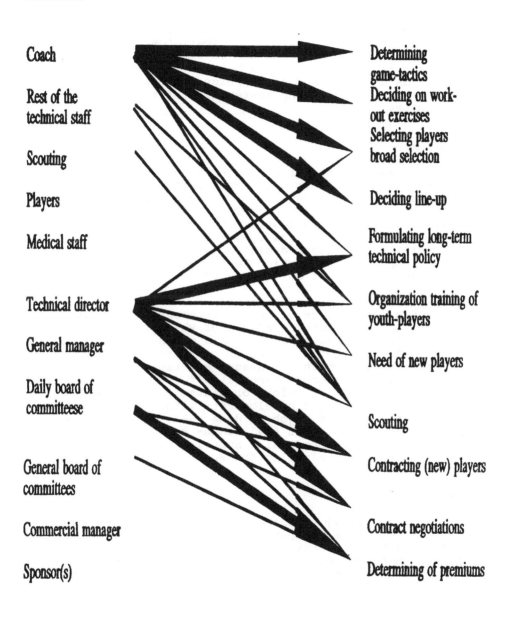

Coach	Determining game-tactics
Rest of the technical staff	Deciding on work-out exercises
	Selecting players broad selection
Scouting	
Players	Deciding line-up
Medical staff	Formulating long-term technical policy
Technical director	Organization training of youth-players
General manager	Need of new players
Daily board of committeese	
	Scouting
General board of committees	Contracting (new) players
Commercial manager	Contract negotiations
Sponsor(s)	Determining of premiums

Figure 3.   Organigram of a soccer-club from soccer-coaches' perspectives. No arrow: no influence/ advisory role; thin arrow: moderate influential role; thick arrow: autonomous deciding role.

455

Finally it is mentioned that the number of Dutch coaches working outside the Netherlands is much larger than the number of foreign coaches working in the Netherlands. Of all the coaches working in the Netherlands, 96% have Dutch nationality. Only 11% have experience outside the Netherlands. It appears that due to what can be referred to as external pressure of the branch, the Netherlands function as a nurse-pond for foreign professional soccer, resulting in an increasing instability of the branch in this country.

4 Conclusion

This study makes a number of suggestions. It seems that the time has come for the different parties involved (the employers, the employees and the soccer-association), to create a climate of constructive thinking and co-operation. This is a necessary precondition for arriving at a well pre-conceived policy-making instead of permanently making adhoc decisions. In general, this is the most important suggestion that can be taken into account as a result of our study.

More specific suggestions concern:
I) the formulation of common interests and goals (by the above mentioned parties) of which the professional soccer-branch as a whole can benefit;
II) the institutionalization of a professional organization which is managed and financed by the professional soccer-branch itself (separate from the amateur section), which formulates policies and monitors different developments within the branch;
III) to judge if a job is done well, that is more than just looking at the league- table, a system should be developed which supplies more objective criteria for evaluating the work of a coach/manager.

5 References

Hameleers, T. (1989) Leiderschapsopvattingen bij coaches vantopsportteams. (Unpublished research study) (pp. 14). Maastricht, Rijksuniversiteit Limburg.
Vanfraechem-Raway, R. (1991) Relationship between psychological aspects of soccer trainers and players (pp. 1-2). Communication to the 2nd World Congress on Science and Football. Brussels, Universite Libre de Bruxelles.

FINANCING SAFETY AND STADIA REFURBISHMENT: TOWARDS A NEW BALL GAME

JOHN SUTHERLAND, GERRY STEWART AND WOLFGANG KEINHORST
Leeds Business School, Leeds Polytechnic,Leeds LS2 8BW,
United Kingdom.

1 Introduction

An intense level of activity is reported among soccer
clubs in the English Football League, with almost half of
the 92 clubs already having made planning applications
for the redevelopment or relocation of their stadia.
Unlike most investment decisions, however, where the
relevant costs and benefits of a project are assessed
prior to a decision on whether or not to proceed,
football clubs have little choice but to comply with the
recommendations of the Taylor Report(1990) that all
stadia covered by the 1975 Safety of Sports Grounds Act
be all-seated by August 1999.

This paper identifies three methods of investment
appraisal, successively based upon financial, economic
and social criteria and applies these to an examination
of the potential viability of stadia refurbishment
projects. Pessimistically concluding that none of these
methods would rationalise the expenditure necessary to
finance the projects, the authors advocate an alternative
relationship between club and community mediated by Local
Authorities and modelled on systems operating in a number
of European countries, most especially what was West
Germany.

2 Lord Justice Taylor's Report

The Taylor(1990) Report on crowd safety and control at
football grounds was the ninth such report in the history
of professional soccer in the United Kingdom. Justice
Taylor cited six features which were claimed to
"disfigure football to-day" (para.58). Two of these were
soccer grounds - described as "elderly" (para.27) - and
their facilities - described as "lamentable" (para.29).
Seeking a better future for soccer, Justice Taylor argued
that although there was no panacea for achieving crowd
safety and curing problems of crowd behaviour, he was
"satisfied that seating does more to achieve those
objectives than any other single measure." (para.61)

Identifying an increasing proportion of seated
accommodation as a trend already apparent in England and
Wales and throughout Europe (and stipulated as a FIFA

requirement for preliminary competition in the 1994 World Cup), Justice Taylor recommended that stadia of all clubs in the First and Second Divisions of the Football League (and national stadia) should be all-seated by the start of the 1994-5 season, and that all other clubs designated under the 1975 Safety of Sports Grounds Act progressively move towards this objective by August 1999. It was conceded that the construction/reconstruction programme associated with such proposals would "require heavy expenditure." (para.99) The Report quoted Football League estimates of £30 million to provide all-seated stadia, and an extra £100 million to provide cover for the same. These estimates have proved to be somewhat conservative given the desire of many clubs to combine refurbishment with commercial development and the difficulties of this in unsuitable inner city areas (Shepley, 1990).

Having acknowledged the funding from such authorities as the Football Trust (currently £7.73 million to support projects totalling £27 million), and having suggested that further consideration might be given to potential sources of finance such as levies on transfer fees, Justice Taylor concluded that "in the end the bulk of finances for ground improvement must be raised by the clubs themselves." (para.116) In this respect club management was exhorted to be "enterprising" and "resourceful" (para.117) and to seek additional sources of revenue income such as might come from advertising and sponsorship and the sale of television rights: to seek to diversify the activities of the club (eg. into the marketing of sportswear and similar merchandise): and to seek access to long-term finance via debentures or equity.

For most clubs even with additional finance from advertising and sponsorship, current annual expenditures exceed current income. Such operating deficits mean that, on the one hand clubs cannot finance stadia refurbishment/relocation by internally generated surpluses and on the other hand access to external finance is restricted. The latter is made even more difficult by the very nature of the projects under consideration and the problems in establishing acceptable criteria for assessing their viability.

3 Methods of Investment Appraisal

Refurbishing stadia in accordance with Justice Taylor's proposals will entail costs; simultaneously, it will create benefits. What costs and benefits are to be identified, and how they are to be valued, and who are perceived to pay the costs and reap the benefits will differ according to the method of investment appraisal used. Similarly, the decision whether or not the project is deemed to be viable may change according to the method chosen. This section discusses three distinct methods of investment appraisal which may be used to evaluate such projects, namely financial appraisal, economic appraisal and social appraisal.

3.1   Financial Appraisal

Central to modern methods of private investment appraisal is discounting. This reduces, or "discounts" the nominal value of future sums of money to the present, giving decision makers a means of assessing a project's current net worth.

In single project exercises, the decision rule is to accept all projects with a net present value greater than zero. A variant of this method is to calculate the yield or "internal rate of return" associated with the project. With this method, the decision-making rule is that all projects with an internal rate of return above a pre-determined "target" rate are deemed viable. Both approaches may be extended to problems involving a selection between competing projects, each, for example, creating different streams of revenue and costs to the organisation at different points through time. Additionally, and of importance in the current context, both may be used to evaluate the relative merits of refurbishment or relocation projects.

From the perspective of the professional soccer club, the primary source of project associated revenue to be set against costs is gate money. An assessment would have to be made of the effect that higher prices associated with seated accommodation would have on consumer demand and total revenue. The little empirical evidence which exists is not too discouraging, Bird(1982) having estimated a price elasticity of - 0.2 for the Football League as a whole. Nevertheless, these market constraints, in addition to the latent threat of poor playing performance and perhaps relegation to a lower Division, both of which would adversely affect gate revenues, have necessitated diverse strategies by clubs to attempt to modify the cost and revenue streams. These strategies include :- a, the search for sponsors to share construction and operating costs; b, the selection of projects which aim to add to and diversify revenue streams, either from leisure related (eg. sports club facilities) or non-leisure related (eg. shops and offices) activities; c, the search for co-operating private developers to share construction costs, if maintaining independence with respect to associated revenues (Shepley, 1990).

3.2   Economic Appraisal

Since it allows for an evaluation of the relative merits
of projects exclusively from the perspective of the
organisation, financial appraisal is most commonly
adopted by private, commercial organisations. Yet, all
project expenditures have economic impacts beyond the
organisation which ought to be taken into account.

In principle, these impacts are three-fold :- 1,
direct effects - measured in terms either of the number
of jobs created, or the income received by the employees;
2, indirect effects - measured in terms of either the
employment or income created in the local economy as a
result of the expenditure patterns both of the
organisation and its employees; 3, induced effects -
often described as "multiplier" effects - measured in
terms of the additional employment or income generated as
a result of expenditure on locally produced goods and
services by income recipients which would not have
occurred in the absence of the project.

The direct effects of professional soccer clubs on the
local economy are, in principle, observable from clubs'
annual accounts and reports. They are seen to be of more
consequence in income than in employment terms. What has
not been undertaken are assessments of indirect and
induced effects. For example, how much of what clubs buy
in as services, such as catering, publishing of club
related literature, club memorabilia an so on is locally
produced? How many of its employees live within the local
economy and spend there? Given the results of empirical
work which attempted to value local multiplier effects
with respect to considerably larger projects, such as
institutions of Higher Education (Lewis, 1988), little
can be expected from refurbishment investment though more
would be expected from a relocation decision,
particularly during the construction phase.

Consequently, even when adopting an approach capable
of calculating the wider economic impact, it is unlikely
that the results would appear to justify the expenditures
envisaged.

3.3   Social Appraisal

Social cost benefit analysis entails the enumeration and
evaluation of all costs and benefits, including those
experienced by individuals and groups, producers or
consumers, who are not directly involved in the activity.
While most often used to measure the economic and social
impact on communities of economic contraction, this
method is capable of being applied to new projects
undertaken to expand economic activity. It offers,
therefore, the most comprehensive perspective possible
and is of particular relevance when examining projects
undertaken by what have been described as "community"

clubs (Sutherland and Stewart, 1987).

Whether as a result of their own independent initiatives or under the auspices of the Professional Footballers Association's "Football in the Community Scheme", one laudable feature of the recent history of many clubs is their recognition of the positive role they can play in their community. For example, in their nomination for the Football Trust's Award Scheme in 1989-90 Preston North End cited weekly functions and special facilities for the elderly and disabled, creches, children's film shows, school holiday programmes, sports coaching at local schools, hospital visits by players and organised soccer competitions for the unemployed amongst a host of activities undertaken by the club. (Sutherland and Stewart, 1987).

These and similar activities currently undertaken by the majority of Football League Clubs are not without costs although these are often lessened by the willingness of other local business organisations to co-operate in producing the host of tangible and intangible benefits associated with the schemes. From this perspective all such activities are capable of identification, valuation and incorporation into the calculus. To the extent that these social activities are counted, this will modify the cost-revenue profile and perhaps affect the potential viability of the project. Most probably, however, and notwithstanding the long stream of benefits which may accrue to a host of individuals and groups within the community, these are unlikely to outweigh the discounted costs of project construction.

Irrespective of the method of investment appraisal adopted then, it would appear that few refurbishment/relocation projects would be deemed "viable" and certainly not so for all clubs in the Football League. This conclusion is likely to exacerbate the problems of Football League clubs in their quest for finance.

4 Financing Refurbishment

Business organisations have, in general, two sources of external finance. Firstly, they can seek "equity" finance by selling shares in the company's assets, offering buyers the right to receive a portion of the company's profits and an opportunity to participate in the decision making of the company. From the company's perspective, this is an ideal method of acquiring long-term finance. It has two principal disadvantages. Firstly, it carries the risk of diluting the degree of control exercised by the original owners of the company, possibly to the point of takeover. Secondly, it requires the company to be profitable in order to attract investors, unless these investors are more interested in psychic than pecuniary returns.

Until recently these considerations have made this source unpopular. Soccer is an industry with a tradition of low dividends making it financially unattractive to outside investors advancing risk capital. The recent experiences of Tottenham Hotspurs provide a salutary lesson in this respect. In addition, most clubs in England and Wales are, by deliberate choice, private limited companies where restrictions are imposed on the transfer of ownership.

The second principal source of investment finance is "debt". This may be bank borrowing, whereby a bank or similar financial institution charges an annual rate of interest and requires the capital to be repaid at a specified date in the future. No loss of control is implied in this method of financing, though failure to repay interest or capital could result in foreclosure. Debt financing is most suitable for short-term projects, although professional soccer clubs have been known to resort to such sources for longterm capital projects with almost calamitous results as interest rate cost rises coincided with reduced capacity to repay as attendances fell.

Debenture issue is another method of debt financing, where the same considerations apply. Whereas lending by financial institutions is mostly based on the value of assets as collateral, debentures can be more flexible. Rather than rely upon single, or a few, large creditors who would have a fixed charge on assets, soccer clubs could issue debentures "in series". For example, with Glasgow Rangers and more recently Arsenal, these are bonds which guarantee the purchaser a seat with privileges for all home matches. As these examples illustrate, this option is exercisable only by the largest, already wealthy clubs.

For the majority of soccer clubs, therefore, not only are there difficulties in justifying the required expenditures, there are problems in raising the necessary finance. The increasing role of the Football Trust in co-financing many of the current and proposed developments must, therefore, be seen as a result of the market's failure to fund these.

5 Towards a New Approach

Ironically, in exhorting clubs to be "enterprising" and "resourceful", Justice Taylor was neither. For a number of years, Football League clubs have responded to the periodic crises affecting soccer in exactly the manner suggested. Thus, rather than take the opportunity provided by the enquiry to initiate fundamental change, the report advocated the status quo as far as the supply of professional soccer in England and Wales is concerned. In essence the recommendations were based on a variant of the dominant economic paradigm which proffers "market" solutions to "market" problems. Clubs merely have to adopt a suitable "marketing mix" (advertising, sponsorship etc.) and, in conjunction with the appropriate diversification strategies, ways of financing improvements will be found. Where such cannot be found, clubs will go out of business and the market thus ensures that supply changes to meet demand

Even within the limitations of this "simple-minded economic analysis" (Taylor, 1984), the accuracy of this perspective is open to question. A major component of this paradigm is the idea of firms in a market producing a purely private good. An alternative, though still orthodox approach suggests that professional soccer exhibits classic symptoms of "market failure". The product of the industry may be seen to possess the characteristics of "merit" goods whereby many, not party to the production/consumption of the good, nevertheless derive satisfaction from it. Any analysis based solely on the private costs and benefits of professional soccer therefore is deficient because "there is a social demand for international and local success far greater than the private demand revealed by the paying spectators at the turnstiles." (Grattan and Lisewski, 1981).

There are several policy options to resolve this problem of potential under supply. Abroad, it is possible to see the extent to which governments have favoured the option of selective subsidy, especially for large scale capital projects, the stadia for "Italia '90" and the concept of "stadia communale" being excellent examples of central and local government involvement in stadia refurbishment. In this respect, the public sector was following the precedent of France in the 1984 European Championship and West Germany in the 1974 World Cup and 1988 European Championship.

The relationship which exists between many Bundesliga clubs and central and local government in Germany is especially instructive. The former recognise Bundesliga clubs as sporting clubs and they are treated in law as "verein". They are neither private nor public limited liability companies. Rather, they are bound constitutionally to produce a variety of sports facilities for the general public. They are recognised as charitable and non-profit making institutions and as a result receive numerous concessions in important areas of taxation. This is almost the opposite from the situation in the UK where, as Justice Taylor (1990) pointed out, "football clubs have a strong fiscal inducement to spend on players rather than ground improvements. Payments for players are allowable revenue expenditure. Improvements to the ground are not" (para.115).

Local governments participate also in the financing, if not operations, of soccer clubs. Given the extent to which the "verein" makes possible facilities of a sporting nature, the stadium is seen as a community asset to be exploited. The soccer club as well as the stadium and its immediate environment are viewed by the local authorities as important symbolic manifestations of civic pride.

In the UK, with limited exceptions such as Halifax Town, Preston North End, Leeds United, local authorities play no role in organising the supply of professional soccer. Lord Justice Taylor envisaged no change in the future, other than local authorities continuing to carry out their statutory duties with respect to safety certificates etc. Paradoxically, in putting the case for all seated stadia he used the examples of Utrecht and Nimes, both owned by the municipality, and providing communal facilities for a variety of sports. While Taylor may be justified in asserting that "in the current financial climate and with our different approach to communal funding, local authorities are unlikely to provide subsidies for such stadia" (para.124), there is little doubt that many local authorities would be willing to assist their local soccer clubs (Shepley, 1990) and more would be were the economic and political environment to change.

The nature of the policy recommendations made in the Taylor Report is one of "retrenchment" designed to preserve the existing form of the club rather than to "reconstruct its internal and external social relations."(Taylor, 1984) These recommendations compare with those advocated and implemented by the "unpaid but monied members of the local commercial bourgeoisie " who both own clubs and administer the game at a national level and who regularly obstruct attempts to democratise clubs by opening them up to the local community.

What is required is an alternative political economy of soccer which focuses upon club ownership and control and the material and ideological forces which prevent each being exercised in a manner which recognises clubs' social responsibilities. Inter alia, this approach would necessitate the incorporation of supporters and players, both of whom have long argued for such in several positive action plans.

6 References

Bird, P.J.W.N.(1982) The demand for league football.
Appl. Econ.,14, 637-647.
Gratten, C. and Liewski, B. (1981) The economics of sport
in Britain, a case of market failure. Brit. Rev. Econ.
Issues,3, 63-75.
Lewis, J.A.(1988) Assessing the effects of the
polytechnic: Wolverhampton and the local community. Urban
Studies,25, 53-61.
Shepley, C.(1990) Planning and Football League grounds.
The Planner, September.
Sutherland, R.J.and Stewart, G. (1987) Community
football. Leisure Management, July, 46-48.
Taylor, I.(1984) Professional sport and the recession.
Int. Rev. Sociol. Sport,19, 7-30
Taylor, Lord Justice (1990) The Hillsborough Disaster.
Final Report. HMSO, London.

ALAN CLARKE AND LAWRIE MADDEN
Centre for Leisure and Tourism Studies, The Polytechnic of North
London, United Kingdom.

1 Introduction

In the Summer of 1990 thoughts in the English Football League turned
to stadia. On the positive side there were the glowing reports of
the billions of lira which had gone into constructing and reconstructing the Italian grounds for the World Cup. Images of these
architectural wonders were beamed back to audiences of millions
throughout the tournament and more importantly witnessed by the
large numbers of supporters and officials who attended the tournament. On the other hand, arguably more positive but stemming from a
more depressing source were the findings of Lord Justice Taylor, who
had been commissioned to look into all aspects of safety following
the tragedy at Hillsborough football ground during the F.A. Cup
Semi-final between Liverpool and Nottingham Forest where 95
spectators died.

The Taylor Inquiry delivered a final Report which made many
important recommendations about the development of football grounds
in the 1990s. This Report was: "directed to making final and long
term recommendations about crowd control and safety at sports
grounds. Indeed to consider in depth information, opinions and
arguments from a wide range of sources and contributors both here
and abroad."

These recommendations into safety standards at sports grounds
have caused many clubs to take a hard look at their grounds and
recognise the limitations of their traditional homes. Lord Justice
Taylor was clear in his views that Hillsborough should not be
regarded as some sort of freak incident and condemned the general
level of facilities at football grounds. "Apart from the discomfort
of standing on a terrace exposed to the elements, the ordinary
provisions to be expected at a place of entertainment are sometimes
not merely basic but squalid. At some grounds the lavatories are
primitive in design, poorly maintained and inadequate in number.
This not only denies the spectator an essential facility he is
entitled to expect. It directly lowers the standards of conduct.
The practice of urinating against walls or even on terraces has
become endemic and is followed by men who would not behave that way
elsewhere. The police, who would charge a man for urinating in the
street, either tolerate it in football grounds or do no more than
give a verbal rebuke. Thus crowd conduct becomes degraded and other
misbehaviour seems less out of place." (p.36)

Lord Justice Taylor made a total of 76 recommendations including the provision of all-seater stadia; monitoring and amending safety certificates; the duties of the football clubs; police planning; communications; co-ordination of emergency services; first aid; medical facilities; ambulances; offences and penalties; and policing planning and implementation. The two which have continued to be debated are the ones which concerned the dismantling of the Government's plans for the national membership scheme and the ones concerning the licencing and development of all-seater stadia.

Much serious thought has gone into how the recommendations will affect the clubs and what the cost of implementing the changes will be. The estimates vary greatly but most are set above the £20 million mark for a First Division club and the total of over £500 million estimated for the whole of the Football League in the Chartered Surveyor Weekly (31.5.90) with the schedules for implementing the proposals designed to see all First Division grounds with all-seater stadia by 1993. Although the costs of the changes pose serious questions for the clubs and there has already been speculation that the reduction in player transfer activity witnessed during the last months of the 1990-91 season will be followed by large numbers of redundancies amongst professional footballers during the close season, there are other considerations which have to be taken into account because of the changes.

2 Into the future

There are three clear options for clubs, and many combinations of the elements which these three demonstrate. They are:
   i)   stay in the ground and rebuild within the fabric of the old stadium;
   ii) relocate to new or green field sites;
   iii) consider ground sharing proposals.

2.1 Rebuilding
The prospect of major rebuilding to accommodate the legislative necessity of all-seater stadia has been favoured by many clubs who have alrady invested heavily in the state of their grounds over recent years. There are also some geographic arguments about finding suitable new spaces which some clubs have used to rule out moving from their traditonal homes. Arsenal F.C., for instance, will have to battle with Islington Council for the right to redevelop the existing ground and are under no illusions that a new ground would be made available to them if they choose to move from Highbury.

Where there has been little investment or the value of the land makes relocation a financially viable possibility, there has been a move to consider a formal relocation. This has prompted some clubs to consider the option of relocation either through engineering a ground sharing option with another club or through the move to a green field site, where there is adequate space to develop a model of 1990s design. These plans have been discussed up and down the country, although some of the new sites being discussed may not qualify as perfect examples of 'green fields. Millwall F.C. is moving less than two miles (3.2 km) to a new stadium, even within one of the central areas of London.

2.2 Green fields and blue skies

There are several problems involved with relocation proposals and two are worth considering in some detail. The first concerns the question of planning agreements and whether the construction of football grounds will be an acceptable use of large areas of 'green belt' land around England's major conurbations seems questionable. A survey undertaken by the Royal Town Planning Institute revealed that 42 clubs, of the 92 in the league, expressed an interest to their local planning body in moving to a new site (Shepley, 1990 p.16). Taylor called for a "presumption in favour of requests for planning permission involving football clubs" and the Football League has gone further in asking for a separate body, modelled on the Urban Development Corporations, to adjudicate on footballing matters. Taylor's request only restated the general presumption that proposals will be allowed to go ahead unless there is demonstrable harm to interests of acknowledged importance. The call for an extra body which would give special consideration to football clubs seems likely to be counter-productive, especially as there is little evidence to suggest that the existing bodies are unduly obstructive at the moment. A more realistic response from the Football League would be to offer some guidance to its clubs on how to prepare and present applications in the way most likely to achieve acceptance and planning approval.

Identifying sites which are suitable has proved more difficult than some 'greenfield visionaries' had imagined. Yet the criteria for such a location are daunting: easily accessible, readily available, relatively inexpensive (compared to the value of the old ground and the land that occupies), not committed to other uses and yet capable of being developed commercially alongside the footballing proposals. This shortlist is then complicated by issues of public concern about the effects of a stadium on the site - traffic, noise, hooliganism (Bale, 1991) - and the loss of the public amenity and existing green belt/countryside policies. Even the offer of 'planning gain', where the local authority receives an asssociated benefit from the developments, does not allow a development to take place which would otherwise not be allowed to proceed. The recent discussions have nearly all focussed on the creation of 'community facilities' in or around the football stadia and yet these cannot be allowed to mask the real purpose of the proposals, which in most cases is to build a new soccer stadium.

Alongside these official difficulties are the unofficial considerations of what relocation would mean to the supporters themselves. Very little concern has been shown for the feelings of the 'customers' in these discussions, despite several instances where the fans have raised serious objections to the clubs' proposals. Even if we look just at the London area, we have seen more of Fulham's supporters attending a meeting to campaign for the preservation of Craven Cottage than attended the club's home games and Charlton Athletic's supporters gaining nearly 15,000 votes in the local elections when the Council threatened the club's return to its home ground. Such emotive and irrational pressures (Shepley, 1990) cannot be ignored when dealing with a subject as embedded in tradition and popular feeling as football. We do not live in a society where the buying and selling of franchises as seen in the American Football league would be readily accepted. There is more work to be done with supporters on their attachment to the home gound before we fully understand the relationship but the feeling is a genuine and a powerful force when it is mobilised.

2.3 Ground sharing
The Sports Council has advocated the use of ground sharing to help solve the problems of cost and this has been backed by the Football Trust in the schedule of payments for the improvements. For some the idea seems such an obvious solution. They cite the examples of Milan, Genoa and Rome so why not Liverpool, Manchester, North London and Sheffield. The arguments are based on sound economics, two clubs maximising usage of the same facilities and sharing the costs of improvements. This arrangement makes a number of assumptions which have not been properly explored. It presupposes an equal interest in the maintenance and development of the site which comes from a sharing of equals. However, where one club owns the ground and the other becomes a tenant, there is clearly an inequality of benefit. If we examine Charlton's experience of ground sharing with Crystal Palace, we see a team which has contributed to the stadium through paying rent but has seen its attendances fall and is on the brink of returning to its own stadium for the start of the 1991-92 season without any lasting benefit.

The obvious differences between the examples cited from the main-land of Europe and those mooted on the British island seem to be twofold. The first is that many clubs do own their own ground and the land surrounding it and have become used to being responsible for its upkeep. There is little sense of tradition of public involvement in the maintenance of soccer facilities. In even the hardiest bastions of soccer local councils have facilities which would have benefitted the club and the community and also served to modernise the oldest parts of the stadia. It is interesting that Hillsborough involved two of the councils at the centre of these allegations. Liverpool City councillors suddenly found themselves supporting the Stadia Mersey proposed to move Liverpool and Everton to a greenfield ground share, and Sheffield City Council spent £8 millions to build a sports complex less than a mile away from where councillors refused a partnership with Sheffield Wednesday some years before.

Without some form of restructuring of the ownership of the grounds, sharing is always going to be undertaken on unequal terms. Where the stadium is separately owned and/or operated, the terms of the sharing may be equal between two clubs and a third party, there would appear to be a greater opportunity for successful partnership. It also seems that a third party which is concerned solely with the development of the stadium may be in a position to guarantee those developments even before they become statutory requirements. There is a role here for local authorities to take a much greater respons-ibility for the provision of facilities in their area, which can then be operated through a management contract with a management company. This was the proposal for the redevelopment at Arnhem, where the city stood to gain a major venue from the redevelopment of the Vitesse stadium with Leisure Management International of Houston amongst the interested bidders for the rights to stage concerts and exhibitions at the ground.

One other aspect of ground sharing which has been resolved on the mainland is what the supporters feel about their own territory being a shared space. At Milan the home end alters between the two clubs except for the local derbies where a pattern of sharing is now established, but the negotiations between the Liverpool and Everton faithful for who gets the Kop at Stadia Mersey would be interesting. As most ground shares will not take place in a vacuum of tradition, there will be two sets of established patterns of support which are disrupted by the changes. These may be of minor consideration if the two clubs are never likely to meet in competition and the two ends can be preserved intact, which has been the experience at Bath with Bristol Rovers. Even the extra travelling and the loss of sense of locality can prove a barrier to supporters. We have already referred to the loss of support for Charlton F.C. when the club moved first to Crystal Palace and then to West Ham United but it will be interesting to monitor the pattern of support when the 1992-93 season begins and the supporters can go 'home' again.

3 Redeveloping the old, bringing in the new

This offers the most likely solution for most clubs, as it requires the least additional resources and involves the least disruption to the existing position. However, the problems involved with redevelopment are almost as complex as those involved in moving grounds. The argument for staying at the traditional ground cannot be used as an excuse for failing to meet the most exacting standards of the new grounds. Patching up the old ground has been a process long beloved of many of the English clubs and most pre-seasons have seen the painters try to cover the rust and create the impression of ground improvements. Very few clubs have gone through the fundamental reappraisal of their grounds which the creation of a new ground allows. There are likely to be many missed oportunities with old grounds being made good, rather than striving for perfection. Safety considerations and lines of sight have to be as important in old stadia, and indeed possibly more so, than in new ones. It is to be hoped that the new Football Licencing Authority will have an evangelical role as well as its statutory enforcement one in promoting the highest possible standards.

The Sports Council (1991) published its propsoal for a six stage redevelopment of football grounds which allows a club to undertake the redevelopments in several stages and to greater or lesser degrees as finances allow. In 'A Stadium for the Nineties' it is stated that the "viewing angles, viewing distances and circulation areas satisfy not only current UK good practice and standards but also draw on the team's considerable international experience." As with all Sports Council guides, this offers a blueprint which can be adapted to individual circumstances and provides the starting point for discussions within clubs, although where clubs do take it as the final word they will find themselves with a well designed 20,000 all-seater stadium. We feel that redevelopment is best illustrated by a real rather than an idealised case and would urge people to consider the Ibrox project as a good example of what can be achieved. This 50-year old stadium was transformed with a capacity of 40,000 and three new all-seater stands over a three phase operation costing just under £10 million in 1981.

470

A major concern for clubs involved in redevelopment will be the financing of the project. Many of the green field proposals recognise the value of the old ground as being a major asset which, when realised, would finance the new stadium. However, the gaining of benefit from the old ground whilst retaining it as a football ground is a more problematic option. Many councils have demonstrated their reluctance to mixing commercial interests with football by blocking proposals over the years which would have allowed office complexes, hotels, retail and leisure developments to finance the ground improvements. Shepley (1990) cited twelve which are currently being considered but many of these are reapplications and little seems to have changed from previous submissions to make their acceptance more likely. Diversification in the ground complex and the surrounding areas makes very good commercial sense, given the right combination of location and circumstances, but the local planners are bound to look very closely at the increased exploitation of land already deemed to be problematic because of the 'nuisance' of football matches. Retail developments with their large attraction of Saturday shoppers have been most heavily criticised for combining two heavy uses of the space on the same days.

Arsenal F.C. was the first club in England to go public on the idea of raising the funding for an all-seater stadium through offering an Arsenal Bond. This registers the subscriber's name on the back of the seat and gives him the opportunity to purchase a season ticket to sit in the same seat. By creating new money, the club hope to avoid the crippling impact of interest repayments by having over half the money for its developments in the bank before any building work commences. However, club officers are also aware that this may change the nature of their support. With a smaller capacity, the cost of watching Arsenal is likely to increase and the sort of person able to pay the price may change. The implications of this are unknown but are the subject of research being undertaken at the Polytechnic of North London. We can make some guesses that all-seater stadia will change the nature of support for clubs and how those changes will work through. We do not know whether the changes will be significant either for the clubs or for their supporters.

4 Patterns of support

That patterns of support will change is largely an assumption but clearly one which can be supported by several examples. One from Germany where Hamburg SV was attracting lower crowds, to the tune of 5,000 spectators less per game in 1990, to its games in the out of town stadium than its less fashionable neighbours St. Pauli, who play in the inner city, demonstrates that it is not just a problem facing the U.K. Certainly increasing travelling distances to stadia where there is ample car parking conjures a view of soccer very different to the one seen today, where local grounds are well supported by public transport routes.

The behaviour of supporters so condemned in the Taylor Report is not so widespread that we can inhibit changes because the supporters are so uncivilised that they would not appreciate them. In most stadia the cages have been taken down and the animals have not

471

bitten the hands that fed them. There is hope that better facilities will be greeted in the same way. They are what loyal supporters deserve anyway and the stadia which fail to provide them will become more anomalous as the decade progresses. All-seater stadia will not stop the singing but they have to be introduced with all the other benefits to make it appear that the supporters are worth the investment, rather than clubs bowing to the force of the law. This is a good opportunity to build closer links with their supporters.

5 Damascus Entertainments Inc.

The lessons which need to be heeded before the boom in stadia redesign takes off is that the major concerns have to be taken as an integral whole with the safety of the spectator and the well-being of the spectator held in harmony. No one would claim that soccer supporters have always demonstrated a commitment to progress and they have protested vigorously at changes which have been forced on to them and their game in the past. The opposition to new stadia comes not from the multi-functional designs which are being put forward but to the secondary role that soccer seems to occupy in these grand schemes. The economics of the game are now well enough known that diversification is recognised as a potential life saver for many clubs, although Tottenham Hotspurs' supporters may take a less relaxed view of the process given the losses accumulated by the club off the playing field which gave such sharpness to the Midland Bank's demand on the club in 1991.

A stadium designed for the playing of soccer and other sports, with community facilities and the possibility of hosting major 'events' such as pop concerts and exhibitions, does not threaten the sense of ownership that fans have with their own 'home' grounds. But a concert hall turned into a football stadium once a fortnight might be viewed very differently by many supporters.

6 References

Bale, J. (1991) Space, Location and Power: a Geography of Football. E. and F.N. Spon, London.
Shepley, C. (1990) Planning and Football League Grounds. The Planner, 28.9.90.
Sports Council (1991) A Stadium for the Nineties. Sports Council, London.

'ALL THINGS TO ALL PEOPLE': FOOTBALL IN THE COMMUNITY

ALAN CLARKE AND LAWRIE MADDEN
Centre for Leisure and Tourism Studies, The Polytechnic of North
London, United Kingdom.

1 Introduction

The argument in this paper is based on our impressions of schemes we
have visited rather than on empirical research. Rather than
presenting a definitive account of the schemes, we would like to
highlight some of the features which we think are important within
community programmes and to encourage responses about how these
themes fit in with initiatives in other countries. The themes
considered are:
· links to the clubs through involvement of players and other staff
· use of facilities
· development and outreach work
· range of activities undertaken
· justification and performance criteria
   Both authors have a long involvement with community schemes,
having been involved in such schemes, in one way or another, since
the early 1980s. We have witnessed the growth of the schemes with
great interest and their diversity with approval. The narrow
regimes proposed in some original attempts to link the club with the
community were almost a recipe for disaster. However, the schemes
have blossomed and now offer a wide range of alternative approaches
to the original task of building links between clubs and their
communities. We do not adhere to any strict notion of community in
dealing with this topic, using it more as an encompassing term for
all those people defined as a community by the clubs - so we include
young and old, men and women, supporters and non-supporters, and
participants and non-participants. Much of the club's attention is
directed locally, but a neighbourhood definition is difficult to
adopt when catchment areas between clubs may be very narrow and far
larger in rural areas, say around Norwich and Ipswich in Suffolk.
Area based work will be an important dimension to clubs' activities
but so will work at away grounds when the community of travelling
supporters may become an equally legitimate focus for activities.
To maintain their importance the schemes must find a concept of
community which they can operate with and follow it through in their
programming, otherwise the conceptual creation will present the full
flowering of the scheme.

2 Links to the clubs through involvement of players and other staff

What support for the schemes comes from the club itself? Some are
left to run largely independently of the club which gives the scheme
its name, whilst others are visited regularly by the people who work
for the organisation. We would ask whether the commitment to the
schemes is present throughout the club - do the Directors share in
the work of the scheme? Do the manager and coaching staff join in
events or do they delegate the responsibility to the players?
Furthermore, it could make a difference which players get involved.
Are they the youngsters keen to make a good impression with their
new managers or are they the established stars, already well known
to the public and established in their careers?
The types of involvement also vary from club to club. Are the
players there to make an appearance or are they there to become a
part of what is happening? In our report on the "Sportacular"
scheme, we emphasised the role of the players being actively
involved with the disabled and handicapped children on that scheme
as a crucial element in its success (Clarke and Madden, 1987). We
see no reason to suspect that one reason people, of all ages, like
to come to events at the football clubs is the chance to meet the
people who to them constitute the club. The greater the activity of
the staff, in all sorts of capacities, the richer the schemes for
those taking part.

3 Use of facilities

The needs of the club must obviously come before those of the
schemes, but unnecessary disruptions to the schemes can be avoided
with a little foresight. The idea of regular evening meetings on
the same night as the mid-week games causes a problem unless the
game becomes a focus for the evening; it may put some people off
attending on those nights or even coming along at all.
What is made available for the schemes seems to vary considerably
from club to club. Sports halls are almost universal but the state
of the hall and the equipment provided within it can be worlds
apart. There is a gap in many clubs' sponsorship packages, as some
do not solicit items for the schemes. Again it is argued that the
schemes and the scheme coordinators can generate their own ideas,
thus creating a greater sense of involvement for those participating
in the fund·raising. There is some merit in this but given the
amount of effort put into raising funds by the clubs it seems a
little disingenuous to leave it to the spirit of self-help.
Another key resource in terms of facilities is transport. This
is sometimes determined by the club's own lack of transport but some
clubs are more generous than others. The ability to take groups
out, away from the base of the scheme, can provide a massive boost
to the scheme and allow a greater sense of adventure to be built
into the programmes. Do the schemes have access to the main stadium
or are they kept at arm's length from the real work of the club?

4 Development and outreach work

There are two concerns about development and outreach work which we
would want to register. The first is that many of the schemes have
inscribed within their terms of reference a demand that they work
with disadvantaged, ethnic and minority groups. This raises serious
questions about the nature of those groups and their relation to
football. Are the groups listed, the ones that football clubs are
best suited to serve? Put another way, are the actions of football
clubs the 'natural' location for these groups to consider as working
in their interest? Admittedly much can be done to challenge such
'natural' perceptions but then these lists of target groups mirror
the target groups which other leisure providers have also drawn up.
If we accept that these groups are the correct targets for the
schemes and the schemes cannot but do so, how are they to set about
recruiting the support of these groups? What forms of contact are
available for them to begin to explore issues of programming with
these groups?

Secondly, there must also be questions asked about whether the
football clubs have the best people to be undertaking such work.
The pattern of recruitment to the schemes is still a largely unknown
area, but many have succumbed to ex-players. The attraction of
ex-players working within the community is hard to deny. Whether
these ex-players have the skills to develop effective outreach
strategies is another matter altogether. Some have and others have
not. We would argue for selection criteria which reflected the
ability to do the job and not just attract publicity headlines.

5 Range of activities undertaken

One of the most welcome indications from the first round of prize
awards for community schemes in 1990 was the sheer diversity of
activities being undertaken in the name of developing links between
the football clubs and their communities. It will be interesting to
see if this diversity is continued and how it can be moved forward
to offer developmental programmes for the groups involved. Where
diversity is an accidental product rather than a planned consequence
of the programming, there may be costs rather than benefits to the
diversity.

The diversity should be meaningful. For instance, the list of
sports which are offered should reflect a blend of activities rather
than a collection of comparable substitutes. They should also offer
individuals with a range of abilities the chance to participate in
the programme, without putting barriers in the way of extending the
range of the programme. The use of expert sports development
officers and teams of coaches can provide a valuable opportunity to
develop centres of excellence which cater for all ages and all
abilities. This has been taken one stage further at Arsenal F.C.,
for example, where the teams also take part in the outreach work of
the scheme. These aspects of programming can be worked through to
produce a well rounded programme.

Sports are not the sole component of diverse programmes. To
maintain an attraction for all the community, the blend has to find
elements which appeal to all ages, both sexes and a range of ethnic

communities. It is here that the challenges facing scheme
programmers is at its most difficult because for many of the
communities being targeted the sports hall focus of the schemes can
be a very unfamiliar location. This underlines a feeling that some
ethnic communities have little connection with the traditions which
value the position of the football club. If the schemes work
closely with their community and develop programmes with those
communities, these problems can be overcome.

6 Justification and performance criteria

Fundamental questions about the schemes may now be raised. If we
are to follow current practice in all forms of leisure provision, we
should be looking towards developing performance criteria for the
community schemes. When the schemes were conceived there was a
range of objectives set for them by the different authorities
involved. There are some parts of these grand plans which can be
monitored and others which are difficult, if not impossible, to
assess. For instance, the hope that the community schemes would
help to covercome the problems of hooliganism was very well
publicised at the creation of the schemes. Yet the impact of the
schemes on the hooligan problem is almost impossible to estimate,
alongside the other initiatives which have been introduced to help
to curb the 'problem'. In this area the investment in time and
effort, not to mention the financial resources put into the schemes,
is very difficult to justify. However, there are difficulties in
expecting performance to be seen mirrored in the reduction of the
crime figures, let alone the equally unmeasurable standards of
behaviour which the schemes were also expected to address.

Other aspects of the objectives were capable of being monitored
but the emphasis put on such monitoring will depend upon the working
practices of the scheme. How many organisers could honestly claim
to maintain the sorts of detailed records which are required if user
profiles are to be analysed for age, sex and ethnicity? Furthermore, the phrase 'extending the presence of minorities' was included
in some schemes and this presupposes two sets of figures, neither
one of which is immediately obvious from the operation of several of
the schemes in existence.

The actual performance of the schemes has been rightly welcomed
as a major advance for football clubs, although some have questioned
whether the initiative has come from the right quarter and how far
the clubs themselves are committed to the schemes. Where the clubs
have been prepared to resource the schemes properly with the help of
the Football Trust and the Professional Footballers Association,
there have been some significant developments. The challenge will
be to demonstrate the continued value which the schemes contribute
to the communities and we are beginning to work on performance
indicators which will demonstrate the impact of the schemes on the
communities, rather than on the clubs. The schemes will fail if
they are assessed only on the narrow contribution that they make to
the club in any financial or numerical sense. There are important
aspects of the schemes' work in presenting the clubs in a positive
light to people who might otherwise only see the negative side of
football disrupting their peace and tranquility.

It is important for clubs to be seen to be involved in their communities. This is partly because they are major community institutions and Bristol Rovers' intention to formalise this by using part of its new ground as a community centre/village hall is a significant point in realising this relationship. Furthermore, the clubs are going to require the support of the local communities as they attempt to update their grounds and an active community profile, for all age groups, both sexes and all races may help to smooth their path with the local councils and local councillors. The relationship will truly be one of 'give and take' rather than a one sided one, where the private institutions are seen to benefit from the local community without putting anything back.

7 Reference

Clarke, A. and Madden, L. (1987) Sportacular: the making of a partnership. **Leisure Management** (May).

INDEX

Leeds Keio ligament 425
Ligament injury 369,402,425
Ligament replacement 345,425,429

Malleotrain 407
Mandible injury 386
Match analysis 3,73,151,160,167,
   174,180,186,194,203,206,215,221,
   232
Match play 121,124,129,140
Medical check-up 383
Mental fatigue 261
Metabolism 86,107,281
Metatarsalgia 407
Middle-aged 53
Morton's foot 407
Motivation 307,442
Motor skills 313,319
Movement symmetry 194
Muscle strength 53,62,92,95,98,295,
                327,362
Muscular hypertrophy 421

Nose injuries 386
Notation 3,151

Orbit 386
Oxygen pulse 37,295
Oxygen uptake 121

Passing 221
Penalty taking 239,250
Personality 437
Physical fitness 3,21,27,31,37,40,
                47,59,62,146,292,
                295,304,319
Plantar fasciitis 407
Plantar flexion 402
Plyometrics 104
Podobarography 341
Positional role 3,27,40,62,135,190
Power output 47
Prevention 327,369,375,383
Proprioceptive training 383
Protection 369

Re-injury 391
Rugby League 3,104
Rugby Union 3,15,21,27,62
Rule changes 186
Running 341
Running speed 21,31,124

Safety 457
Scoliosis 421
Scouting 160
Seasonal variation 21,98
Self-hypnosis 442
Serum iron 135
Sesamoiditis 407
Sexual maturity 298
Shoes 335
Shooting 194,254
Shoulder injuries 432
Sinus tarsi 407
Skills tests 313,319
Small-sided games 140
Soccer boot 335
Soccer simulation 47,107,261,281
Soccer trainers 437
Somatotype 27,59,292
Specificity 277
Spine 421
Stacking 190
Stadia 457,466,473
Strength training 92,95,98
Stress 327,445
Synovitis 396

Tackling 327
Tactics 151,160,167,180,206,215,
                221,232
Taping 383,407
Task analysis 186
Taylor Report 457,466
Technique 194,313,319,327
Test construction 313
Therapy 396
Thermography 421
Throw-in 327
Training 3,73,86,104,114,135,232
                277,298
Translation 345
Treatment 407

Ventilatory threshold 43
Video 73,174,239
Video analysis 73,174

Women's rugby 27
Women's soccer 114,140
Work-rate 3,121,124,335

Zygoma injury 386

Printed and bound by CPI Group (UK) Ltd, Croydon, CR0 4YY

01/11/2024

01782626-0018